Lifestyle and Cancer

The facts

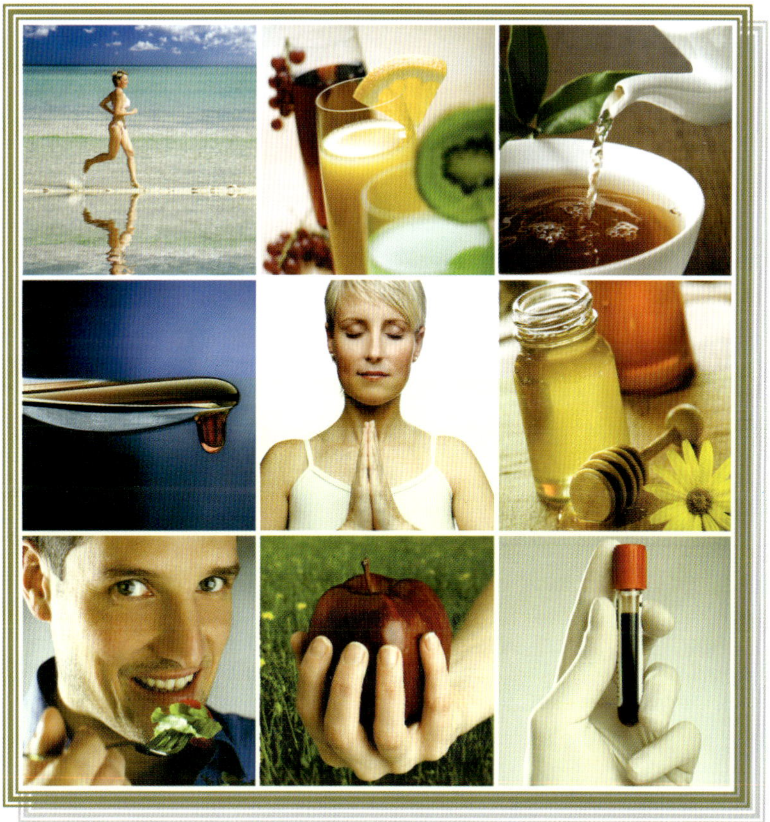

New revised second edition

Foreword by Paula Radcliffe
World champion marathon runner

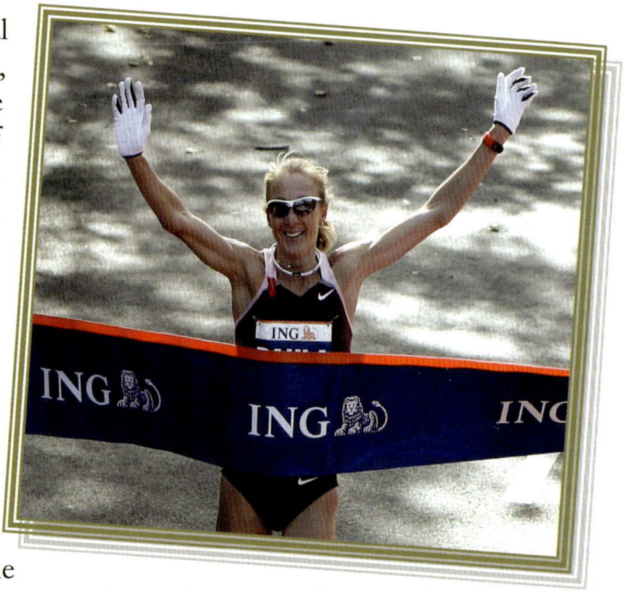

My mum, although exceptional in many ways, is, I'm sure, similar to thousands of people who have had the trauma of cancer thrust upon them. As well as wanting to make sure she had the best possible medical care and fully understand her treatment options, she had a strong desire to know the best ways to help herself. Day to day questions which seem straight forward before cancer now had an added complexity especially after the side effects of surgery, radiotherapy, chemotherapy and herceptin started creeping in. For example; What to eat, what not to eat, should I exercise less or more, if so how and where to exercise, would a supplement help, are they safe?

The problem is where to look for these answers? Medicine is similar to sport science in this regard, despite the great benefits of the *information age*; it is still difficult to sort the wheat from the chaff, to know which advice is based on myth and hearsay and which is based on fact and proof. Just as there are hundreds of books explaining how to run faster for longer, there are countless books telling you how to you how to live better for longer. On top of this there are literally thousands of websites, usually trying to sell you something, which claim to have the answer to fighting cancer, ranging from coffee enemas to magnets.

As a cancer expert who has worked closely with patients for many years, Professor Thomas is very aware of the concerns which many patients have, not only with conventional treatments, but with dietary, exercise and lifestyle issues after cancer. I know, from my mum's contact with him during her treatment, that he is sensitive to fact that patients like her need to feel in control and have a strong positive desire to help themselves. As a scientist and a doctor, he has an exceptional knowledge of the important topics around lifestyle and cancer, not only from his own research, but from regular scrutiny of the world literature. This book, therefore, provides just what people need to empower themselves - a reliable tool based only on best available evidence, containing relevant practical guidance sensitive to the psychological, cultural and physical needs of people after cancer.

We, as a family, have already striven to win, most obviously in sport and careers, but now with this recent turn of events in fighting cancer. To do this, as well as determination, effort and dedication, we needed, and continue to need, accurate advice and help. Certainly for my mum, this book has been fundamental in providing this well needed support and arming her with the tools to win her own personal marathon. I know she cannot thank Professor Thomas enough for his dedication, professional expertise and commitment.

Paula Radcliffe

This book will have a wide appeal but will be of particular interest to:

- Those who want to life a healthy lifestyle to avoid cancer
- Those who want to empower themselves after a diagnosis of cancer
- Those who want to reduce their risk of their cancer relapsing after treatment
- Those who want to improve their overall chance of long term cure
- Men who want to slow the growth of their indolent prostate cancer
- Families and friends of those affected by cancer
- Professionals interested in the evidence for lifestyle and cancer

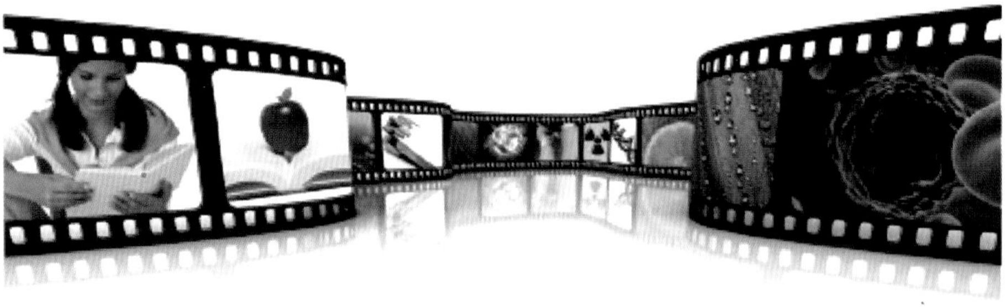

Published by Health Education Publications
Email: health-education@clara.co.uk
Web: www.cancernet.co.uk

ISBN 978-0-9558212-4-0

Papers used by Health Education Publications are natural, recyclable products made from wood grown in sustainable forests.

Graphics by Erika Silling
Photographs by the author or supplied by Unreal Ltd, London.
Proof reading: Great thanks to Mr Michael Vogel and Mrs Cecilia Nicholson

For more information, to review this book or order more books please refer to our website:

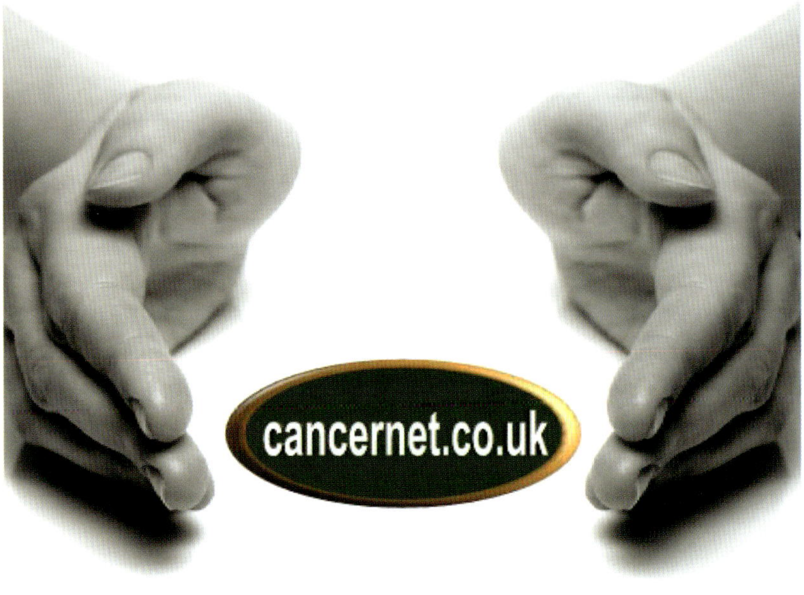

Contents

PART 3 Lifestyle to influence relapse rates and improve cure

"What to do more of / less of"

PART 4 Everyday lifestyle tips – specific guidance

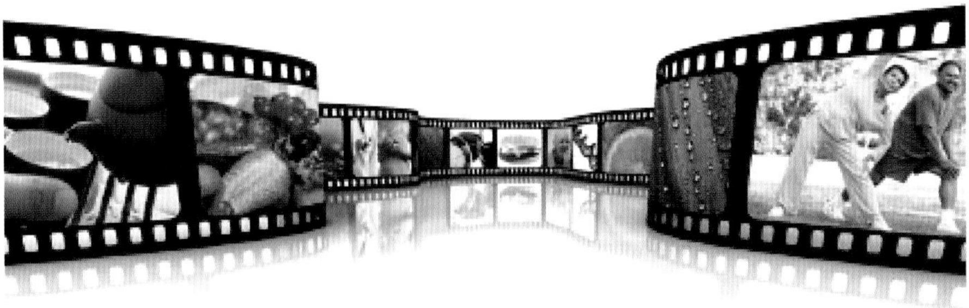

PART 1

Cancer & lifestyle

Introduction & background

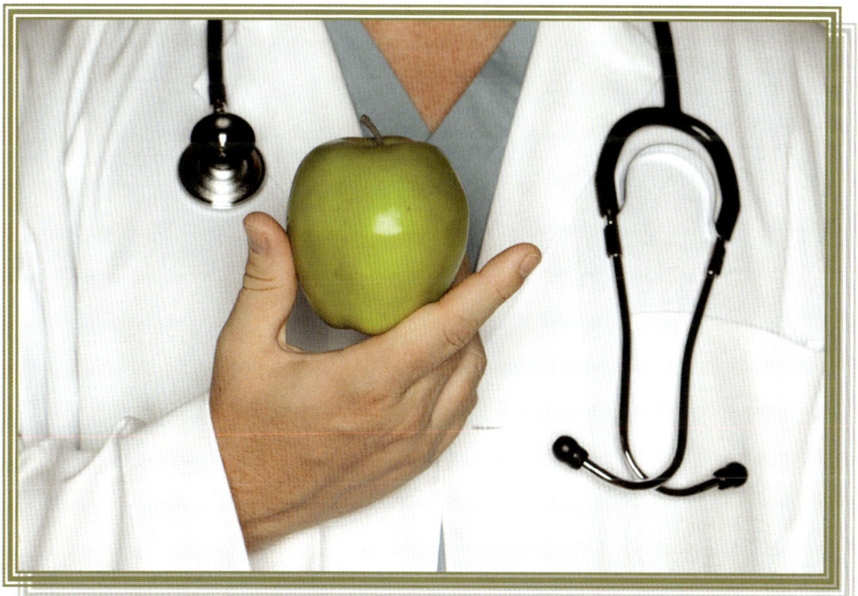

Chapter One

Introduction
About this second edition

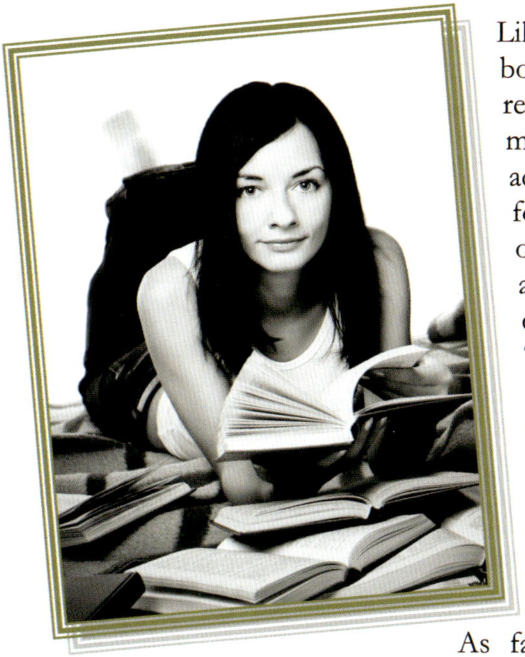

Like the successful first edition, this book aims to empower individuals with reliable information to ensure they can make the right lifestyle choices. The advice in the next twenty chapters, if followed, will ensure the best possible outcome after the trauma of cancer and its treatments - maximising the chances of living better and longer. This edition has been expanded to include information and advice on cancer prevention so, as well as being an ideal resource for those with a survivorship agenda it is now also highly relevant to anyone concerned about cancer in general.

As far as possible, the information and advice is based only on the facts or, in medical terms, reliable, high quality published research evidence from around the world. For this reason it dispels hearsay and urban myths but instead provides the reassurance and confidence that the efforts required to change an established and often comfortable lifestyle are worthwhile and likely to reap major benefits.

Since the first edition many more studies have been published in international medical journals as the importance of lifestyle is now beginning to be realised by health professionals and academic institutions. These have been included into this edition making it more up-to-date, topical and relevant to the stresses of modern day life. New chapters have been added on quality of life, psychological well-being, complementary therapies and nutritional testing making it bigger, better and more focused on issues which affect people in all aspects of their daily lives, not just those which affect hospital treatments..

Many readers, including patients who have survived cancer, their friends and relatives, have also written with valuable feedback and useful tips. This feedback from individuals from a wide range of cultural backgrounds ranges from the best ways to exercise, how to communicate with relatives and friends, practical tips such as how to grind linseeds and what happens if you eat too many goji berries! This feedback has also been incorporated into this edition making it even more readable and applicable to individuals from all walks of life. Likewise, if you have any comments of what should be included, expanded or omitted from the next edition please feel free to contact us (health-education@clara.co.uk)

The structure of the book has been simplified to make it more enjoyable and easier to read. It is now split into three main parts:

Part one: The book begins by describing the background to cancer, what causes it, how it is inherited and how environmental and lifestyle factors aid or interfere with our body's ability to fight it and stop it spreading.

Part two: Breaks down the most important specific factors in our lifestyle which influence how we cope with the effects of the disease and treatments and how they influence its progression or relapse. The information within each section has been divided into three categories:

1. **The evidence.** For those of you who don't need to lift up the car bonnet to see how it works, you may wish to move on as this section is rather technical. It summarises the published literature from across the world, describing studies proving the benefits or risks of this or that particular element of lifestyle.

2. **The underlying mechanism**. Again rather technical but describes how the chemical and physical elements of the individual lifestyle interact with cancer, or our bodily processes, to confer a benefit or cause harm.

3. **The everyday lifestyle advice.** This is the real meat on the bones, providing easy to follow practical tips describing the activities of daily living we ***should do more of*** and what we ***should do less of*** to stop cancer progressing or relapsing and to improve the overall chance of cure.

Part three: Refers to the symptoms and effects commonly experienced after cancer either caused by the disease itself or the subsequent treatments. For ease of explanation it breaks down these symptoms into specific topics and describes practical tips to relieve them or minimise their effects on the body.

Rationale for this book?

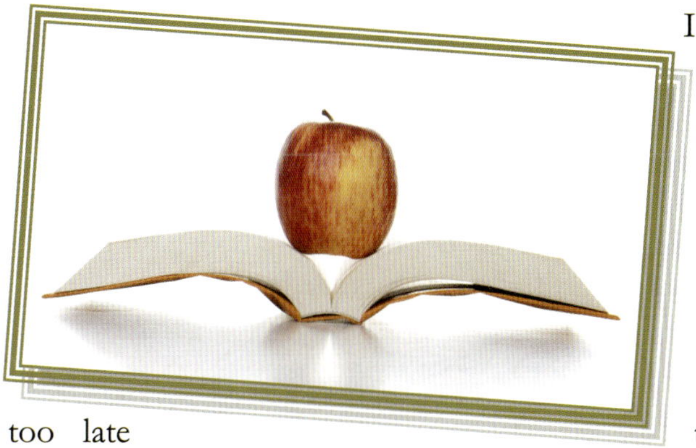

It is universally accepted that what we do or don't do to our bodies significantly contributes to the risk of developing cancer. What has been less well accepted are the benefits of a good lifestyle **after** a diagnosis of cancer. In fact, it is still heard said that once cancer has developed it is too late to change your lifestyle. This unhelpful myth implying *"there is no point closing the stable door now the horse has bolted"* could not be further from the truth. What this book sets out to demonstrate is the enormous importance of a healthy lifestyle after a diagnosis of cancer.

Changing the way you choose to live your life, however, is by no means an easy task at the best of times, but especially after the shock of cancer and during disruption caused by its complex treatments. So if you are to embark on a programme of unaccustomed exercise, ignore your cravings and eat food you previously thought only fit for a hamster you must be totally convinced that your efforts are all worthwhile. For these reason, this book emphasises the background and underlying mechanisms as well as the proof of benefit so readers really understand the reasons why these measures are needed and have the reassurance that they are worthwhile. This emphasise on facts hopefully will also help to resolve the ever increasing conflicting information from newspapers, magazines, the internet or simply over the garden fence which often bamboozle an individual when facing daily lifestyle choices.

Although the importance of lifestyle is now beginning to be recognised by health professionals, there remains a shortfall between what patients want and need and what they are formally given in UK oncology units. This data was confirmed in one of the lifestyle studies conducted at our cancer treatment centre which looked at the information needs and desires among patients and their relatives after their diagnosis. This study used a series of questionnaires designed with professionals at Cranfield, Hull and Cambridge Universities and involved patients over a one-year period with a range of cancers and therapies. In terms of the level of information, over 80 percent indicated that they wanted as much information as possible. When information was broken up into separate subcategories most were fairly satisfied with general information on cancer and its treatment – whereas less than 30 percent were satisfied with the lifestyle advice they were given. Over and above the benefits of lifestyle that will be described in this book, this unpleasant feeling of being inadequately informed has been shown to be linked with more ominous psychological and physical consequences. It is associated with an inability to make a proper decision, thus preventing patients exercising their full autonomy, leading to frustration, anger, confusion and poor adjustment to illness. On the other hand, patients satisfied with their level of information have been shown in clinical studies to have a greater involvement in their own treatment and lifestyle decisions. Furthermore, this exerted a protective effect on their well-being, including lower levels of anxiety and depression, better adjustment to work, and more positive attitudes towards the future.

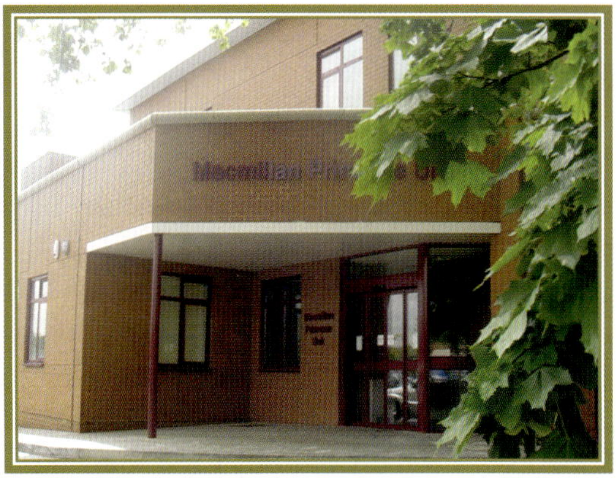

For the majority of patients with such a shortfall between what they want and what they are given, it is no wonder they and their carers and relatives turn to unsolicited sources of information from the myriad of Internet or lay published materials. Despite the great advances in the 'information age', the majority of patients still report difficulties sorting out the wheat from the chaff. Most patients were confused by the conflicting advice they had read but, more importantly, were frustrated with the material's lack of credibility and lack of an adequate explanation of any background evidence as to why a particular strategy may be helpful. With little justification as to why and how interventions work, their advice all too often fails to instil enough confidence in the reader to persuade them to significantly change their daily activities. In our experience there has to be a powerful motivation to put on a leotard after six months chemotherapy and walk into a local aerobics class. Even if patients have jumped this first hurdle, they have to be even more convinced when the novelty wears off and the aches and pains set in!

Other pitfalls confronting patients, especially from the Internet, are the numerous reports of wonder cures and miraculous recoveries that are commonplace in lay literature. Some of these are written in good faith but are frankly misleading, even lacking a solid diagnosis of cancer in the first place, or failing to mention the contribution of simultaneous conventional or alternative therapies. Others are of a more sinister nature, preying on the insecurities of patients and their relatives, persuading them to spend their hard earned money on *cure-alls* that are unproven, are unlikely to work or, more alarmingly, could even cause harm. This book clearly cannot compete with the enormous scope and range of the Internet, but what it loses in diversity it makes up for in accuracy and credibility.

Who would benefit from this book?

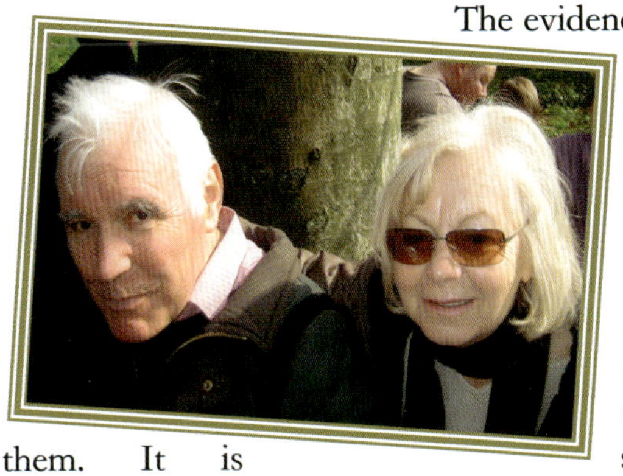

The evidence and advice in this book is relevant at every stage in the cancer journey and involves a wide variety of anticancer treatments, ranging from surgery, chemotherapy radiotherapy, hormone therapies, biological therapies or even those on active surveillance. Its advice not only benefits the patients themselves but their friends, relatives and the health professionals helping them. It is suitable for the young, old, sporty, previously sedentary, male or female from all walks of life, racial and cultural backgrounds. On a cautionary note for readers who have bought this book for someone with cancer, it must be remembered that the patient's themselves must be willing participants in the concept of a lifestyle change, and not everyone is keen. In the study mentioned above, up to 20 percent of patients wanted no extra information about their disease and preferred to let the doctor make decisions for them – without any outside interventions of their own. In this group, levels of anxiety were found to be almost as low as the fully informed group. The old saying 'ignorance is bliss' therefore stands for this group, and should be respected. This attitude can be found amoung individuals from any educational level, religious or cultural group. For example, Franz Ingelfinger, former editor of the New England Journal of Medicine, who himself had carcinoma of the oesophagus, sensed 'immediate and immense relief' when he abrogated responsibility to his doctor. It is therefore unwise to force advice and information on this small but significant group of patients, as they may be quite happy as they are and, more importantly, unless they want to, are unlikely to change their lifestyle anyway.

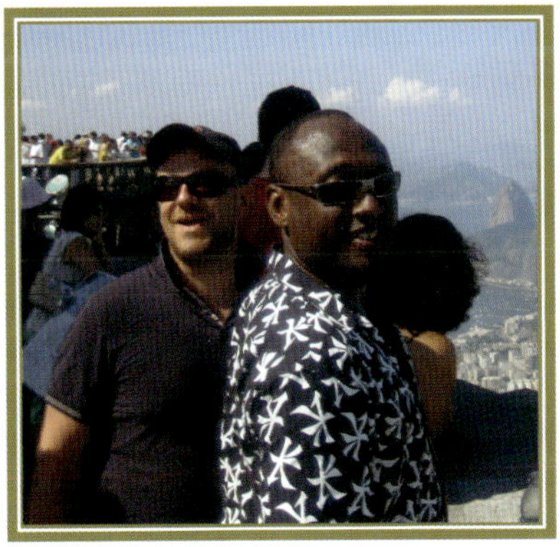

On a second cautionary note it should be mentioned that this book focuses on generally fit people who have no restrictions on their diet or a pre-existing dietary requirement. It is, therefore, probably not appropriate for patients with very advanced cancer, or for those whose tumours or treatments have affected their ability to move about, eat or digest food. In these cases patients should seek formal advice from qualified dieticians, preferably those attached to a conventional cancer centre.

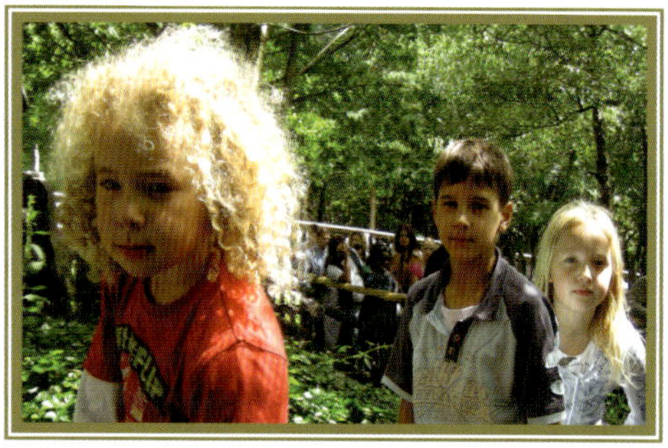

Finally, although this book focuses on lifestyle after cancer, its advice is also relevant to those interested in lowering their or their family's risk of cancer in the first place. The do's and don'ts have, in most cases, also been shown to help prevent cancer. This is particularly relevant to families with a history of cancer or those with an inherited genetic risk or those with a previous history of high carcinogen exposure or simply those who wish to *turn over a new leaf* and start leading a healthy lifestyle. Particularly as the anti-cancer advice here also has numerous other health benefits including reducing blood pressure and lowering risk of heart attacks, strokes, diabetes and dementia, to mention but a few. So the earlier you start the better.

How was this book researched and written?

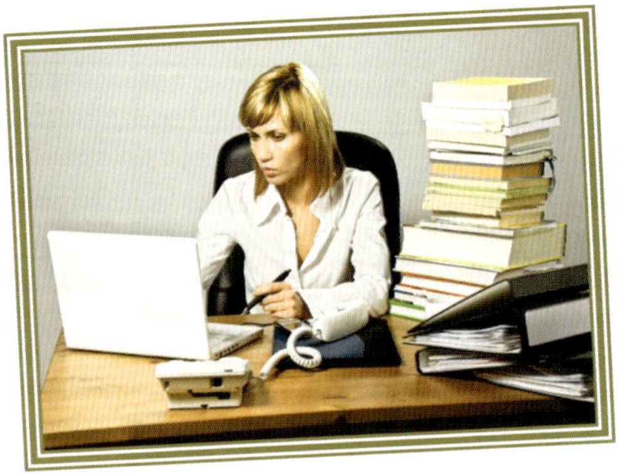

The clinical team who have supported the author have been designing and conducting lifestyle oriented clinical trials for many years. Many of these have been conducted with government funding, in conjunction with Cambridge, Cranfield and Hull Universities. They have also been designed with the help of patients themselves and include two of the only UK trials addressing lifestyle interventions among patients with progressive cancer. One of these turned out to be the largest lifestyle study on prostate cancer of its kind. Through this research we have learnt a lot about important lifestyle issues and how people interact with them. The results of these studies have been published around the world in various languages in peer-reviewed medical journals. This research, in addition to a background of first-hand experience in basic science, has created the skills to unearth and critically evaluate relevant research evidence from around the world and to summarise it into a concise, readable format - which has help with this book.

In addition, the author has written over 50 scientific papers and abstracts and also given presentations in National and International conferences – all of which require extensive background research and a summary of the latest literature. These studies are a listed in the reference section at the back of this book. He was also commissioned by Cancer Relief Macmillan to lead an editorial team to gather the world literature on cancer and lifestyle. This was then submitted as the evidence-based document for the Department of Health survivorship programme – All of this evidence has formed the background and guidance of this book - these studies are also listed in the reference section of the book. He now leads the Cancer Relief Macmillan survivorship advisory group so is continually kept up to date on the evidence for new lifestyle issues and how these can influence the cancer pathway.

Why is evidence (proof) important?

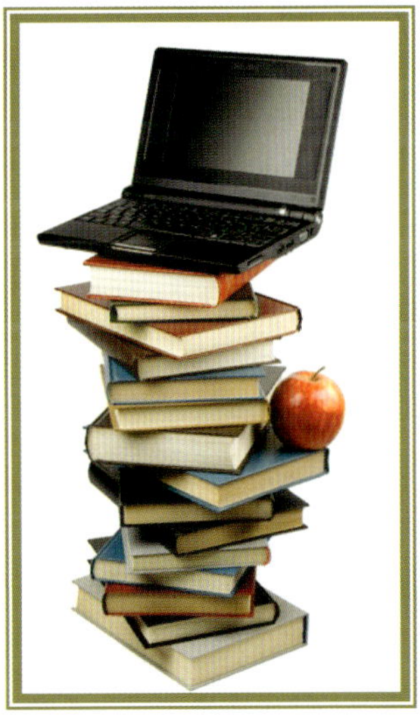

Many of the self help books on the market do not emphasise research with the same degree but any intervention given or recommended to patients should first be proven to be beneficial in clinical trials. This ensures that they are not given ineffectual treatments or exposed to side effects which may not have come to light without thorough analysis. The regulatory process may seem overly stringent at times and probably does slow the development of some drugs, but when large sums of money are involved there is an enormous commercial incentive to take short cuts to 'get to market'. This process is not however infallible – ineffective drugs still get through the strict barriers of approval or are subsequently found to have serious risks, only discovered when used more widely. Prime examples of these are thalidomide, which caused congenital abnormalities in babies born in the 1950s, and the anti-inflammatory drugs (vioxx) which were linked to increasing the likelihood of heart attacks in 2005.

It may not be a good thing that dietary supplements lie beyond the boundaries of drug regulatory authorities, although they do usually have to satisfy food standards. The justification for this is that they are less likely to directly harm the patients with the same potential as mainstream drugs and are therefore regarded as generally safer. Health professionals have concerns with this premise and suspect that supplements may be wolves, hiding from the mainstream regulatory authorities, in sheeps' clothing. Although supplements are unlikely ever to get the headline-catching adverse reactions such as the Northwick Park Hospital, in early 2006, where six unfortunate volunteers nearly died during a clinical trial, there may be insidious negative effects many years later that would be very difficult to detect. Furthermore, long term regular supplementation may counterbalance the beneficial effect of other established cancer drugs. For example, women with breast cancer may see advertisements in the back of their daily newspapers for a health supplement which concentrates plant oestrogens (phyto-oestrogens), and take them regularly for long periods of time feeling good that they are helping themselves.

However, although there is as yet no proof of harm or benefit, this supplement may inadvertently be increasing their blood oestrogen levels and thus counterbalancing the hormone drugs given by their cancer doctor. These usually afford around a 10 percent reduction in the risk of relapse and this benefit, although relatively small, may be lost or reduced with regular supplementation. In a typical UK District General Hospital, this would potentially mean 20 women a year would relapse unnecessarily. Across the world this would equate to several thousands each year! Of course, these statements are assuming a worst-case scenario, but without a trial it is impossible to put a cause or effect to the benefits or risks of supplements. Fortunately most women do not relapse and in those who do there is usually a host of other risk factors. On a reassuring note, the limited studies looking at the blood of people who have taken supplements show that they do not alter oestrogen levels by much, so they are unlikely to have such a profoundly negative affect – of course this also means they are unlikely to work! The take-home message of this example is that at the end of the day we simply do not know for sure until a clinical trial is performed.

Even if lifestyle strategies are harmless, if they don't work they are still wasting the patient's valuable time. Some strategies may also be expensive, draining patients or their carers of well-deserved financial resources by preying on their vulnerability following a diagnosis of cancer. Likewise, asking heath care providers to fork out money for new interventions from their strained budget is asking them to finance fantasy without proof.

Research can be frustrating

Some patients can find this need for credible research quite frustrating, especially if they have discovered something on the Internet themselves, which they are convinced has worked for them and they want to tell as many people as possible. I always remember an anecdote which best exemplifies this situation:

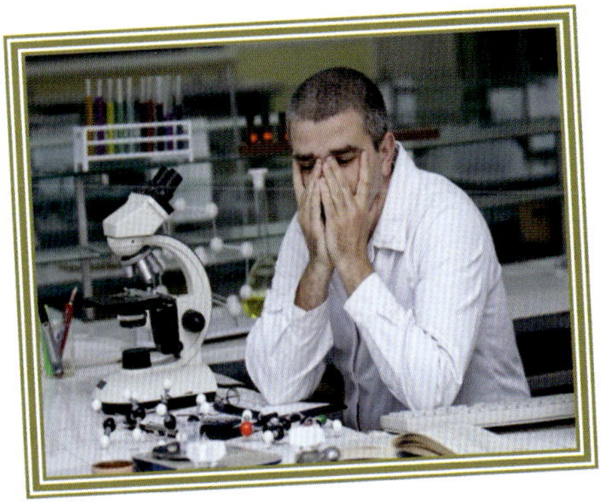

During a routine examination, I noticed a metallic object at the front of a middle aged lady's underwear. She had previously been troubled by persistent hot flushes and night sweats. Conventional medication had not helped and unfortunately lifestyle initiatives had only marginally reduced their severity. She had found, via the Internet, a magnet system that clipped to the front of her underpants. Virtually overnight, her hot flushes had subsided. Of course we were both delighted, but the jovial spirit waned when she suggested this might be offered to other patients with hot flushes. She was most distressed to hear that our clinic was unable to do so – the system had not undergone the necessary evaluation to be included in our hospital's formulary. At the patient's insistence our new drugs board reviewed the evidence which came with the product. The magnet company's interpretation of a randomised trial was to simply survey people who had bought the product and asked if it had worked! There was no information on how the people were selected or indeed who returned the questionnaires. Furthermore, there was no mention that the trial was governed by any regulatory bodies or quality control mechanisms. In short, there was no proof at all that it worked or had any side effects. It may well have helped in this case by a genuine or placebo effect and although a magnet is unlikely to do harm, it is an extra expense and inconvenience. As a strategy, it had to be placed in the 'quack category' along with thousands of other agents available across the world. Some of these may well have useful beneficial effects but simply cannot be recommended until clinical proof has been sought.

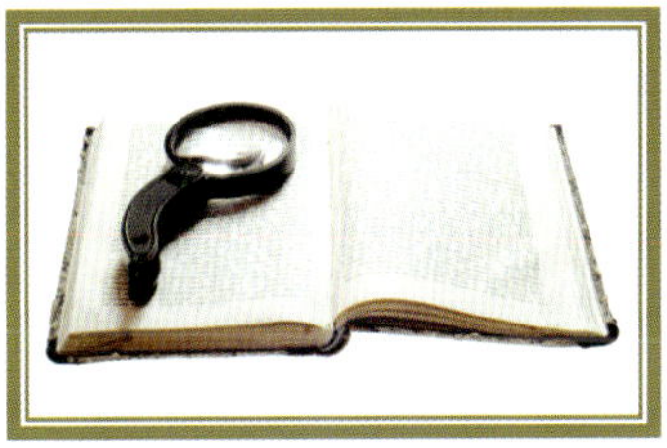

Following an explanation to the patient, who remained convinced of the benefit of the magnet, she fortunately understood the stance of the medical profession and realised that we as a profession are not intending to be narrow-minded and obstructive to 'different' ideas.

Particular challenges with lifestyle studies

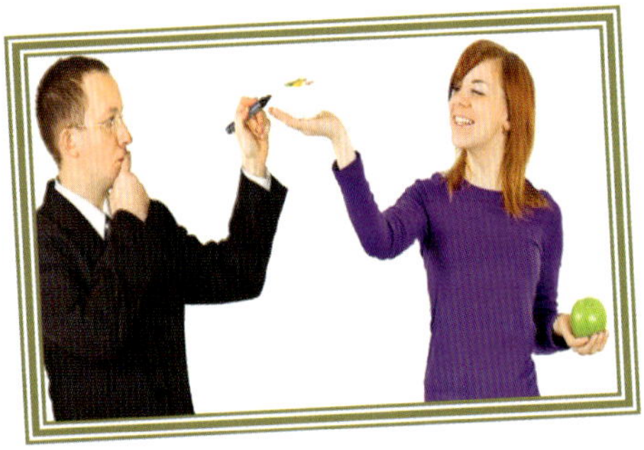

Why then, if clinical trials are so important, do we have very few in the areas of lifestyle and cancer? You would assume, with the millions of dollars pumped into clinical research each week, it would be simple for a sufficiently motivated enough research institution. In reality, however, lifestyle trials are difficult to design, lack government funding, don't attract money from pharmaceutical companies, struggle to get through the hurdles of the regulatory bodies, and have such woolly end points that the results rarely convince even the mildest of sceptics.

It is also often difficult to recruit patients into lifestyle trials as they often find their options unacceptable. Let's imagine ourselves in the shoes of a keen young doctor consulting with a patient. Let ua also imagine that a trial is an option. Dr Goodheart wants to progress his career so he takes every opportunity to show off to his peers how he can recruit patients into clinical studies. He starts with 'Now Mr Smith, as we have discussed during our consultation, I'm afraid your cancer is progressing, so I'm going to ask you whether you would like to take part in a research study'. Mr Smith, always alert to new ideas, pricks up his ears and leans forward. He thinks to himself, 'Maybe this is the break I've been looking for'. He enthusiastically responds, 'Of course – go on'. Dr Goodheart, already feeling embarrassed, starts with, 'Well we would flip a coin to randomise you. Heads you do nothing, tails you must enter a strict programme of diet, and supervised exercise'. 'But I do not want to do nothing, I'll just have the lifestyle option thank you'. 'Sorry you can't, that would not be a trial'. Of course Mr Smith leaves shortly afterwards thinking the doctor is slightly mad and, more significantly, feeling disgruntled and dissatisfied. Nevertheless, after reading the trial literature, he embarks on a major change in his lifestyle with positive effects. Regrettably, in a scientific perspective, because he was not within the formal setting of the trial, this information cannot be recorded in any worthwhile way. He becomes yet another anecdote which carries no scientific weight with the policy makers.

Not to be put off, the doctor tries a few weeks later with Mrs Jones, who admires and respects him, and doesn't want to offend him, so agrees to enter the study. She draws the control (non-intervention) arm but two weeks into the study

Mrs Jones reads in the newspaper the benefits of goji berries, a super-food containing high levels of antioxidants. She, as many others not given the intervention, changes her diet, completely distorting the trial data and making the final results unquantifiable. The trial struggles on and, like so many others, closes early without enough patients to analyse the data.

The other issues with lifestyle studies are the problems of using either a blinded comparison group or a placebo (inactive dummies). These manoeuvres are used in the most convincing clinical trials. Blinding the active from the non-active intervention ensures that subliminal bias in recording the outcomes are not inadvertently introduced, reassuring the reader of the final published paper that the differences between the two interventions were genuine. Unfortunately, it is rarely possible to include this reassurance into lifestyle studies for a variety of practical reasons. How, for example, could you disguise an apple from a donut or a salad from a burger? As for a placebo, it is easy to see how simply entering a clinical trial, with its ensuing closer human contact and attention, could improve a sense of well-being and quality of life. Although placebos in supplementary studies are possible, albeit expensive, even the most imaginative designers would struggle to devise a placebo for a diet or exercise study. Some have attempted this, for example, by massaging the wrong section of the foot in reflexology or inserting the acupuncture needles but not stimulating them. But, let's face it, disguising a lettuce leaf or sitting on an exercise bike without pedalling is ludicrous!

Because of these difficulties the published trials in this area tend to be non-comparative and have small numbers of patients. In the past the enthusiasm for their results rarely matched their scientific credibility. These comments are not a criticism of the conscientious and compassionate workers who have tried to take on the task of finding the truth through research, but it shows how difficult it is to design trials in this arena. Although it looks like this chapter appears to be defending the inertia of the medical profession, it is actually applauding those who, despite these difficulties, have managed to design trials to prove the benefits or harm of lifestyle interventions after cancer. These trials may not have the eloquent design of mainstream drugs, but have been conducted under difficult circumstances. The rest of this book reviews the evidence for the strategies that have satisfied a level of scrutiny that combined with some common sense, I would feel confident to recommend them to patients, colleagues and relatives.

Chapter Two

About cancer

What is it?

What is cancer?

In order to understand the mechanisms of how lifestyle could influence the progression or relapse of cancer, it is worth describing the fundamentals of cancer itself. The word cancer is used to describe a mass of abnormal cells that can develop in any organ of the human body. This mass of cells has markedly impaired regulatory mechanisms compared with the normal cells of the body, resulting in some fundamental differences:

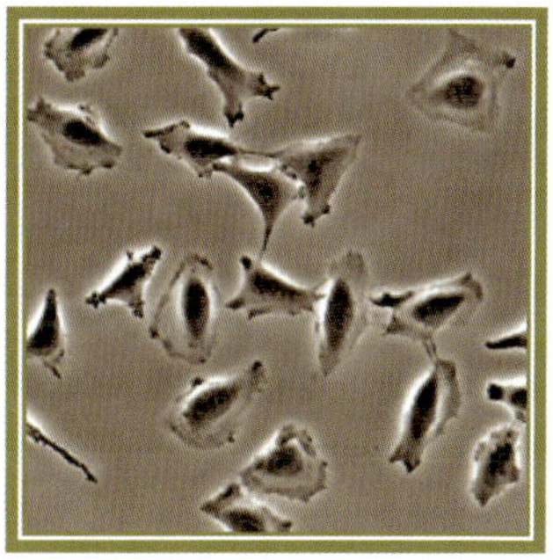

Normal cells grow to their desired size, space themselves out evenly and stick to their original and intended site – with a good respect for their neighbours. They receive and obey instructions from the regulatory systems of the body via hormones and chemicals. They do not divide or replicate unnecessarily and do so at a controlled pace Finally, they die when they are supposed to via a process called apoptosis (programmed cell death) – in order to make room for healthy young cells to take over their function.

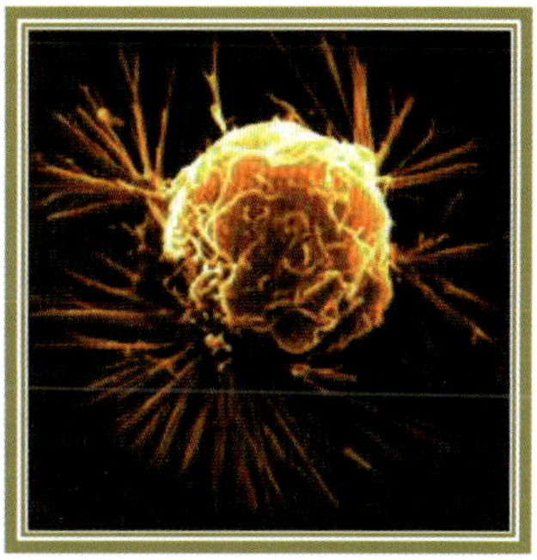

Cancer cells grow as fast as they can, don't die when they ought to, clamber on top of each other and quickly run out of space in the organ of origin. They not only expand the organ but also infiltrate and **invade** their neighbouring structures, causing considerable damage. This invasion is one of the hallmarks of cancer. The other way cancers can make room for themselves is to lose their stickiness to the organ of origin and break off and spread to another part of the body and start growing there. This is called **metastasis** or secondary deposits and is another hallmark of malignancy. Growths or tumours which have the ability to invade and metastasise are, therefore, called malignant tumours or cancer, whereas those which grow but don't invade and metastasise are called benign tumours. For the rest of this chapter we will concentrate on malignant tumours – **cancer**.

Why does cancer start?

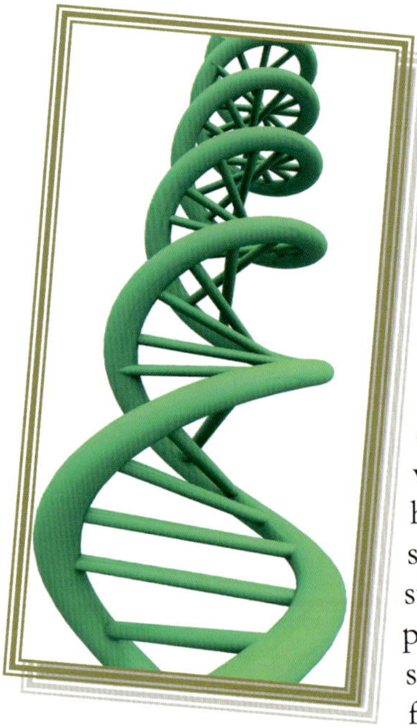

Within each cell in the human body lies a structure called a nucleus, containing strips of material called DNA. To be precise 46 strips each containing millions of packages of information called genes. These genes are the codes and templates for all the functions of the entire human body. They have evolved over the centuries through countless generations to produce the human form we know today. Over this time our genes have picked up a considerable amount of debris. Some of this debris includes strips of genes which actually cause cancer but are kept from doing harm by other genes, which lie next to them on the same strip of DNA. These *good* genes, called tumour suppressor genes, were themselves once randomly picked up through the evolutionary pathway but now serve the essential function of guarding the body from the *bad* cancer genes – we would get cancer without them. Essentially we were born with the tendency to get cancer – it is part of us!

With thousands of potential cancers already programmed in our DNA it does not come as a surprise that one in three of us will get cancer at one stage in our lives. Perhaps instead of asking **"why me?"** when we develop cancer, we should be asking **"why not me?"** when we don't.

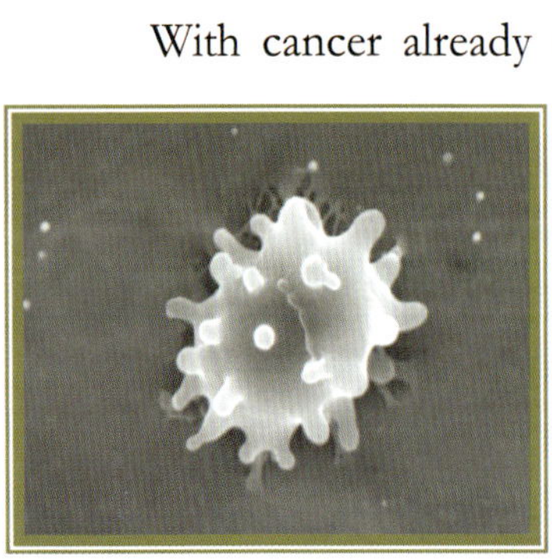

With cancer already coded in our DNA, guarded by other anti-cancer genes, any re-arrangement of the DNA can lead to the start of the malignant process. The clue as to why one person gets cancer and another does not, despite the same lifestyle, probably lies in their genetic makeup, determined at conception. Some people have been born with a rather loose arrangement between their good and bad genes, that could be separated by low carcinogen exposure within an apparently healthy lifestyle.

Alternatively, they could have an inherited defect in their suppressor genes. Examples of these conditions include the BCRA-1 or BCRA-2 gene mutation, which increases the risk of breast and ovary cancer ten-fold, and hereditary polyposis coli for bowel cancer. On the other hand, some people are fortunate to be born with their cancer genes locked in tightly by very stable suppressor genes resulting in a very robust DNA profile. It will take an awful lot of carcinogenic chemicals in these individuals to damage the DNA enough to cause cancer. These extreme cases are often quoted as excuses for hardened smokers, "He smoked 20 cigarettes a day, ate rubbish all his life and didn't get cancer". Most people, however, are somewhere in between these two extremes so, although we have an underlying risk of cancer that is outside our control, what we do to our bodies still has a great influence on our destiny.

What environmental factors trigger cancer?

The simple answer is life. Virtually any chemical in the right concentration and environment can damage the DNA and trigger cancer. Obviously some factors are more dangerous than others. This section summarises the most common categories of carcinogens (cancer forming factors). For a more comprehensive list see cancernet.co.uk.

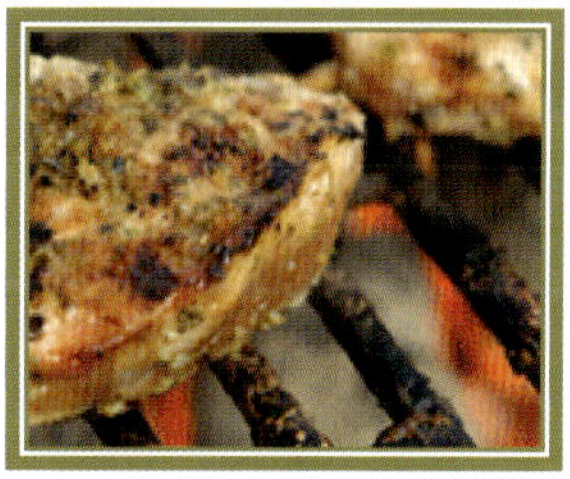

Dietary cancer-causing chemicals (carcinogens) such as polycyclic aromatic hydrocarbons and aromatic amines, found in superheated or processed foods, can directly or indirectly oxidize water or oxygen into short-lived, but highly energetic, free radicals. These damage DNA allowing cancer-promoting genes to escape from the influence of their suppressor gene guardians, forming the first cells in the cancer process.

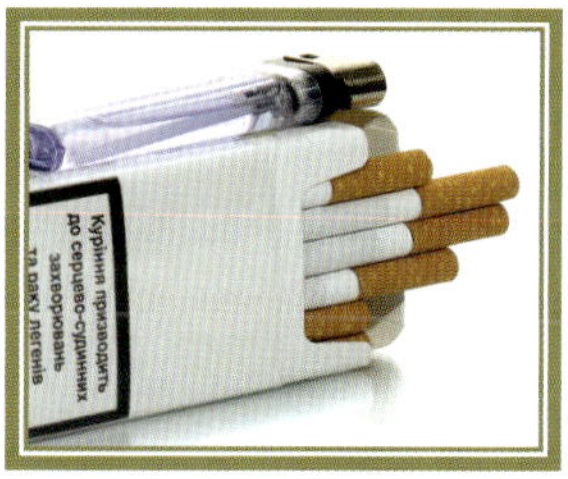

Inhaled carcinogens (smoking). Tobacco smoke contains over 4000 chemicals, many of which are carcinogenic. Culprits include the benzenes, formaldehyde, ammonia, cyanide and arsenic. These can damage the DNA of cells, causing the locked cancer genes to become active. They damage the immunity so that early cancers progress more rapidly. The chemicals also directly damage the mucous membranes, allowing other chemicals and viruses the penetrate into the body.

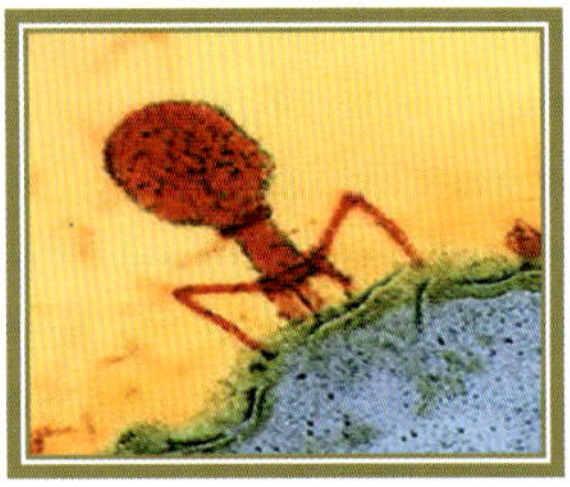

Viruses can also infect cells and damage the DNA – the most well known of these being the papilloma (wart) virus and cervical cancer, or a virus found in Africa called the Ebstein-Barr virus causing a cancer of the lymph nodes (*Burkitt's Lymphoma*). The section below explains that HIV (aids) does not trigger DNA damage but drops the immunity so early cancers are not killed by the body and therefore progress rapidly.

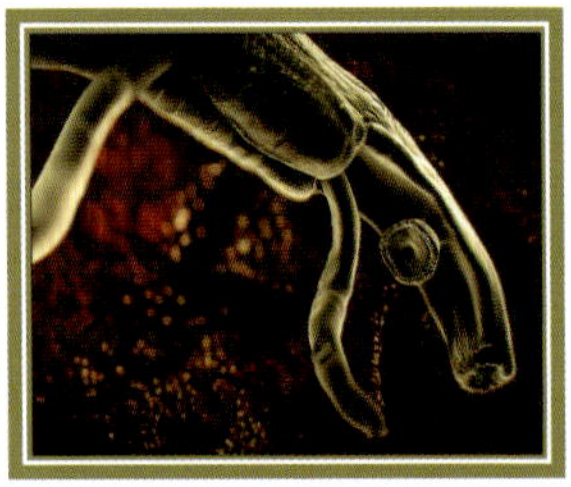

Chronic irritation from stones, acid and parasites. Repeated acid reflux in the oesophagus can cause smoothing called Barrett's oesophagus which can lead to cancer of the oesophagus. Stones in the bladder can increase the risk of bladder cancer. In Egypt and Africa a parasitic worm causing Schistosomiasis can irritate the bladder and lead to an increased risk of bladder cancer.

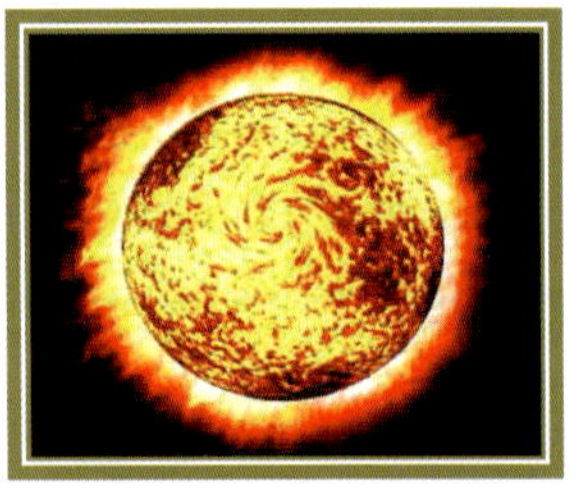

Sunlight. Although gentle regular sun exposure is healthy, prolonged exposure, particularly burning, can directly damage DNA. In fact, a few hours in the sun can result in hundreds of potential skin cancers. There is also evidence that persistent strong sun exposure can damage the proteins which repair damage caused by the sun. Exposure to other chemicals whilst sunbathing makes the sun damage worse – the classic example being cigarette smoke.

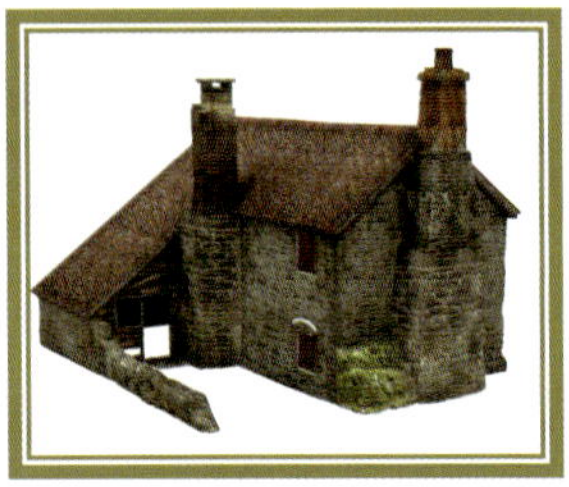

Radiation: Individuals can be exposed to radiation from a variety of sources. One of the most common are from medical X-rays, CT or nuclear medical imaging in Hospitals. Apart from nuclear power station disasters, industrial exposure can be found among submariners, nuclear power workers and even airline pilots. Radon gas is released naturally from granite rock, particularly within stone cottages built in parts of Cornwall, although some radioactive gas has been measured above kitchen work surfaces.

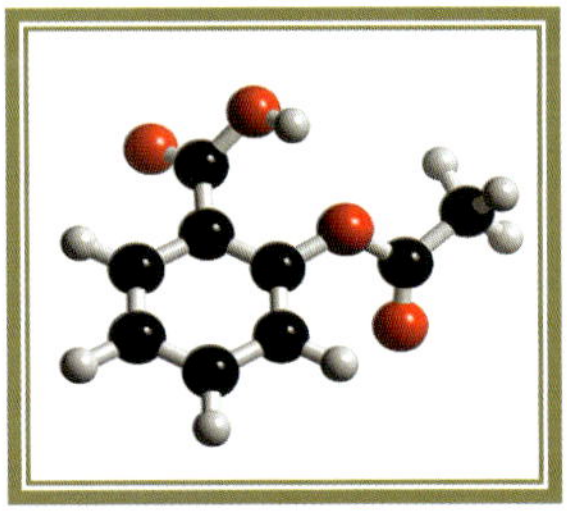

Environmental chemicals: Virtually any chemical in excess can start acting as a potential carcinogen but the main risks come from high exposure to the same group of toxins over a long period of time. The classic historical breakthrough came from the finding that the soot in the trousers of chimney sweeps caused scrotal cancer. More recent examples include workers such as electricians being exposed to asbestos causing a type of lung cancer or the exposure of workers to chemicals found in the dying and rubber industries causing bladder cancers and lymphomas.

Our body's defences against cancer:

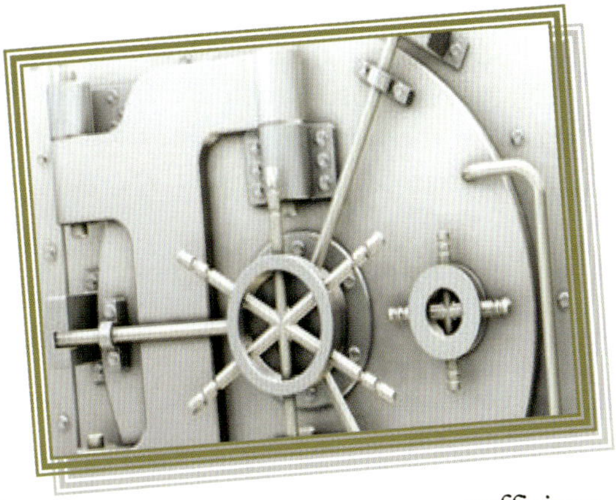

Our bodies are bombarded with cancer-forming chemicals every day, but fortunately only one in three of us get full blown cancer – and even then usually later in life. This is because the body has developed a number complex and sophisticated defence mechanisms to stop early mutations forming. Even after development of early cancer it is still important to have a healthy anti-cancer defence system as, although sufficient DNA damage has occurred in order to mutate normal healthy cells to cancer cells, the process is by no means over. Further DNA mutations encourage malignant cells to transform into more aggressive types that are more likely to progress, spread or relapse.

The enzymatic defences against super-oxide free radicals include antioxidants which wield their anti-cancer properties by mopping up carcinogenic chemicals before they get time to damage our DNA. Otherwise known as free radical scavengers, antioxidants are found in a wide variety of healthy foods. The three most commonly known are superoxide dismutase (SOD), glutathione peroxidise and catalase.

DNA repair proteins: Cellular proteins are able to repair minimal DNA damage within four hours. There are genetic conditions which impair the repair of DNA. The C-erb genes associated with breast and ovarian cancer are probably the most commonly known. Acquired disorders, such as Vitamin C deficiency, can impair the ability of DNA to repair.

The DNA policeman: A widely known protein, which protects DNA, is nicknamed DNA policeman (p53). If a cell is partially damaged, the policeman slows the cell cycle and allows DNA repair to take place. If repair is not possible it does not allow the cell to divide with damaged DNA, which could eventually cause cancer. Instead it programs the cell to commit suicide – this is called programmed cell death or apoptosis. Some people are born with a defect in this policeman gene (known as Li-Fraumeni syndrome). As you can imagine, they usually develop multiple cancers at a very early age in life.

The immunity: One of the first observations of cancer immunity was seen at the turn of the 20th century, when a women's breast cancer shrunk following a skin infection. Her body's defences were so greatly stimulated to fight the infection they also attacked the tumour. Although cancer cells originate from our own body, there are some differences in the proteins, which can make them look foreign. Only those which are able to escape the body's immunity can progress. Defects in the immune system therefore lead to more early cancers progressing. The best example of this is AIDS.

PART 2

Lifestyle affecting progression of established cancer

Evidence, mechanisms and advice

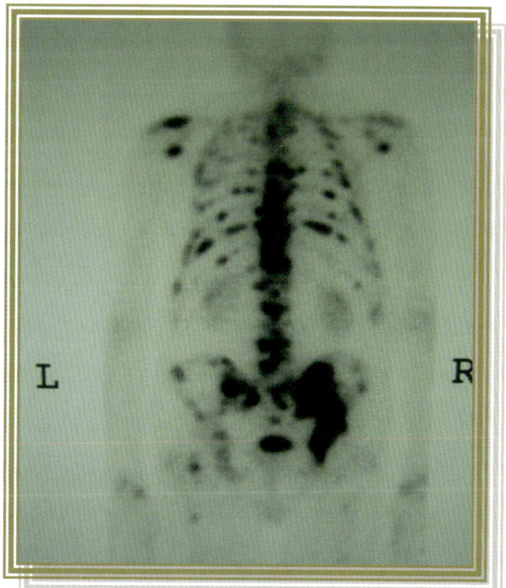

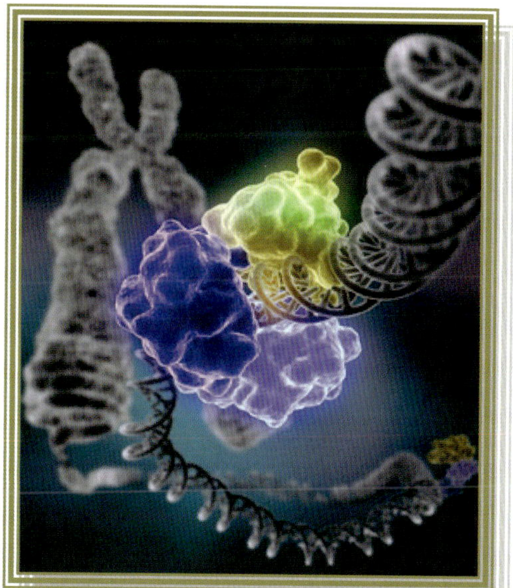

Chapter Three Evidence that lifestyle can slow the growth of cancer

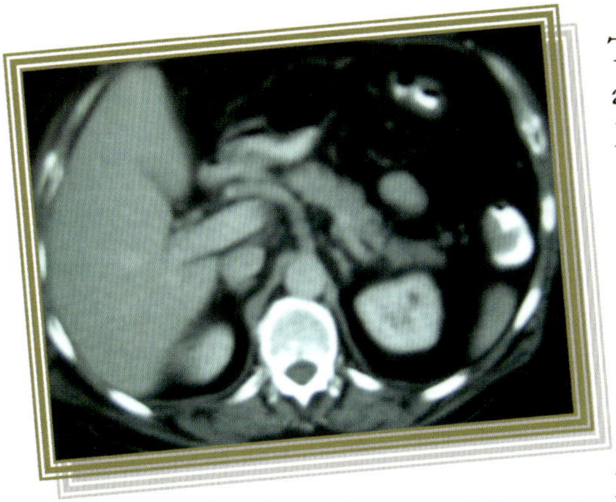

This chapter explains and discusses the available evidence showing that lifestyle can influence the rate of progression of established cancers. Before describing the good quality international clinical trials, it starts, rather mischievously, by whetting your appetite with some interesting anecdotes. These examples have been drawn from many of the patients we have had the privilege of treating over the last 20 years. These fascinating individuals of course do not prove the case, but do present an intriguing human insight into the potential benefits of a change of lifestyle:

Incredible cases - lifestyle and cancer growth.

Mr A, a 61-year-old man with a long history of chronic bronchitis, coughed up a handful of blood one day during his usual morning attack. Although scared, he went to his local doctor, who on a subsequent chest x-ray, saw a shadow consistent with lung cancer. Mr A was referred to the hospital specialist who, following a lung biopsy, diagnosed an advanced cancer on the background of marked smoking-related emphysema. Further tests on his heart, lungs and kidneys revealed he was so unfit even a haircut would be risky, let alone open chest surgery. Mr A was told treatment would be aimed at keeping him as comfortable as possible, but would do little to stem the inevitable progression of his terminal cancer. He was referred to our cancer centre to help control his symptoms.

On arrival, he was indeed in a sorry state, grey-skinned, leaning forward with thin high shoulders, gasping for short breaths between coughing attacks.

Without a doubt, standard treatments of chemotherapy or radiotherapy were out of the question so, with little else to offer, a lifestyle intervention study was optimistically considered. With some persuasion he gave up smoking, although by that stage he didn't have much breath left to light a cigarette! He had a course of chest physiotherapy clearing years of mucous and was interviewed by our research nutritionist. Even with years of experience she was shocked with the replies to her initial questions.
"You've never eaten a vegetable in your life?"
He replies between gasps "No, don't like 'em".
Thinking Mr A wasn't sure what a vegetable was, she pressed "What about peas, carrots, and cabbage?"
"No, I just told you, I don't like 'em." After further questions with a similar retort, she asked "What about chips?" Sighing with relief, she finally gets a "yes". Her notes at the time read: 'Mr A has smoked over 40 cigarettes a day since the age of 16, has never exercised recreationally and has lived on white bread, chips and poor quality meat in the form of burgers and sausages.' Not to be put off, the nutritionist persevered via a series of consultations over the next few weeks, and managed substantially to change his diet.

To our delighted surprise Mr A slowly started rallying – the physiotherapy eased his breathing, he stopped smoking, and he started enjoying assorted salads and munching on fresh berries and nuts. He later joined a gentle exercise class, and for the first time in ten years, took regular day trips to Brighton to take in the sea air. It was hard to recognise him three months later, tanned and walking upright with ease. More rewardingly his lung cancer had reduced in size and the general condition of his lungs improved.

Clearly, the sudden influx of healthy food and fresh air was enough to elicit a significant anti-tumour effect as well as a profound improvement in well-being, despite his near terminal state at presentation. This lasted for two years when he succumbed to a sudden heart attack – overall perhaps not a resounding success, but his cancer had initially shrunk and not grown over this period. During one of the later consultations Mr A had to agree with an ironic comment from a relative 'getting cancer was the best thing that had happened to him'!

Mrs B was a 52-year-old lady, who had advanced cancer of the ovary. Following a combination of surgery, chemotherapy and radiotherapy, all measurable disease disappeared from the scans. A year later a blood test (a tumour marker called CA125) unfortunately started showing cancer reactivating. Despite recommencing further chemotherapy the CA125 count continued to rise, so chemotherapy was stopped. She then decided to embark on a moderately intense programme of high anti-oxidant foods ranging from teas to herbs. The cancer count rose for one more month, then fell for three months, then stabilised for twenty-one months. Only then did it start progressing along with recurrent disease seen on scans. In this instance, despite the cancer being resistant to all chemotherapy options, the dietary change had given her almost two years of quality life.

Mr C was a very healthy, sexually active 73-year-old man. One morning, Mr C was asked by his concerned wife over breakfast "How many times did you get up to pass water last night?"
"Twice – that's normal for a man of my age. I can still do 18 rounds of golf without stopping". Not to be put off she persisted "I couldn't help noticing that it sounded more like a trickle than a stream and it takes you a lot longer to finish."

With images of his wife standing outside the bathroom door with a stopwatch he grudgingly agreed to see his local doctor. Following a blood test revealing likely prostate cancer (PSA – Prostate Specific Antigen), he had a biopsy proving the diagnosis and was referred to the oncology department for treatment. After considering the options carefully, he entered into an active surveillance programme, a useful manoeuvre to assess the tempo of disease. Over the next four months this PSA increased from 9.6 to 10.9 then 13.1; clearly cancer progression by any established criteria. The radical and probably curative treatment of radiotherapy was offered at this time. Radiotherapy is often given with hormone therapy first, for four months, which would have rendered him temporarily impotent. There was also a moderate risk that this could have been permanent after the radiotherapy. Seeing his wife's distress, and still not keen himself to rush into radical treatment, he decided to try a dietary approach, loosely based on information they had collected from the Internet. He simply took two Brazil nuts, high in the antioxidant selenium, three times a day. Three months later his PSA was 10.1, six months later it was 6.5, and to our delight – four years later, at the time of writing this book, it is less than 5. At the same time his symptoms have improved, and there is no evidence of change on examination or pelvic scans. This man's proven cancer was clearly progressing before his dietary intervention of eating Brazil nuts, and there is no doubt it has been stabilised since. Even if his cancer does start progressing in a year or two, he would still have gained a significant period of time, without the potential toxicities and side effects of treatment. In his case this may have included a lack of a loving sexual relationship with his wife.

Mr D was a 64 yrs old man with prostate cancer who started relapsing, despite successful radiotherapy some years ago. He was disappointed to see his PSA levels starting to rise but unfortunately standard tests could not find the source of the cancer recurrence (Bone and CT scans). When the PSA had risen from 0.4 to 2.5 then 6.0 he was offered hormone therapy. Instead he chose to have a lifestyle intervention aided by formal nutritional testing. This showed he had low antioxidant levels and low vitamin D. He increased his antioxidant intake by consuming broccoli soup daily, vitamin D by fish oil supplements (and increasing sensible sunlight exposure) and, at the same, time started regular exercise. To help improve his exercise regimen, he accepted an exercise referral to this local gym as part of the UK government Fit For Life programme. This involved two 1½ hours session each week supervised by a trained exercise professional. After the 12 week programme was completed he joined the gym himself and continued thereafter regularly. His PSA dropped to 3.5 within three months then 1.4 by one year. It remains less than 2.0 three years later.

Mrs E had a three month history of colicky indigestion and increasing tiredness. She was referred for a further investigation in the local hospital which included a colonoscopy (scope to look up the back passage). A large cancer was found and later removed via a lengthy operation which unfortunately found that the cancer had spread to 16 out of 21 lymph nodes and there was evidence of spread to the surface of the bowel making relapse within the abdomen or elsewhere almost inevitable. She started chemotherapy, to try and reduce this risk, but unfortunately had to stop after only 2 of 8 cycles due to side effects. Instead she accepted and exercise referral and lost 2 stone in weight and now regularly exercises 3 hours a week. She also had nutritional testing and was found to have excess zinc and selenium due to the taking of a regular supplements which she then stopped. The test also showed she had low levels of omega 3 and vitamin D. She increased her intake of fish oils and crushed linseeds to increase her omega 3 level and took more sun on her body to additionally help her vitamin D. She repeated her nutritional testing 6 months later and they were normal. She remains alive and well four years later against all the odds – a lucky co-incidence maybe but it is very likely that her significant change in lifestyle helped her stay in remission.

A cautionary note about anecdotal reports. Individual anecdotes are interesting and thought-provoking but, of course, have no scientific credibility. Although they are often published as case reports in medical journals as points of discussion, they can be misused by the lay media. These frequently over-emphasise their importance to the extent of calling them 'wonder cures'. Even worse, many of these stories are flawed, some of them even lacking a solid diagnosis of cancer in the first place. Other newspaper reports lack information of other simultaneous conventional therapies. For example, a recent British Sunday newspaper, reporting the virtues of a complementary treatment in a high profile public figure inadvertently, or maybe even deliberately, neglected to mention the concomitant administration of a mainstream conventional hormone therapy, which was almost certainly responsible for this 'amazing' therapeutic effect.

Nevertheless, sit any doctor down at a social event, and very soon most will enthusiastically embark on reams of amazing anecdotes. They are indeed relatively common but, although often captivating, unfortunately cannot be scientifically substantiated. They provide no information on the thousands of other patients who have fervently tried similar strategies only to be disappointed by the lack of response. Even so, a human story can provide a positive and emotive message, providing the seeds for the design of further clinical studies.

Studies: the effect of lifestyle on cancer growth

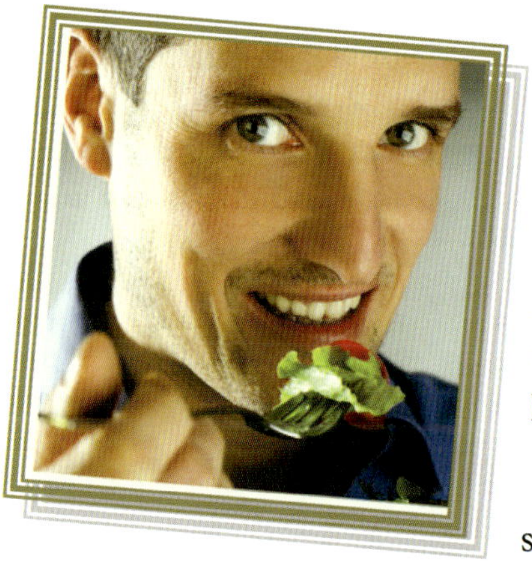

Much of the reliable evidence for the effect of lifestyle on cancer progression comes from patients with indolent or relapsing prostate cancer. The slow growth rate in many patients and availability of a simple blood test (PSA) allows time for alternative interventions, making them acceptable to both clinician and motivated patients alike.

The first category of evidence comes from studies that looked back at patients' diet and lifestyle with questionnaires and interviews. These studies, known as cohort studies, then matched patients according to their age, general health, how advanced (stage) and aggressiveness (grade) their disease was. A number of large studies, including the US health professionals study, have recorded individuals for their lifestyle history during the years before their diagnosis of prostate cancer. They then divided individuals into two groups, depending on their pre-cancer lifestyle for comparative purposes. All these studies convincingly showed that patients with a previously healthy diet had less aggressive, less advanced disease at presentation, associated with a much better prognosis. A large case-control study conducted in China demonstrated significantly lower grades of prostate cancer among individuals who regularly consumed foods containing tofu, soy and isoflavones (genistein and daidzein) compared to a matched cohort (Lee et al., 2003). By matching patients with similar types of disease at presentation another similar study confirmed that cancer progressed at a slower rate and spread less frequently (metastasised) in patients who improved their lifestyle after diagnosis, compared with those renowned for their 'salad dodging' prowess. In this last study, as both groups of patients had the same prognostic factors at diagnosis, the data clearly suggest that healthy lifestyle factors mediated the transformation of early prostate cancer into a less advanced stage.

These trials are moderately convincing and probably do accurately reflect the fact that how we lived before cancer influences our outcome afterwards, but cynics still argue that they are vulnerable to potential biases in data collection. In other words, an over-enthusiastic researcher may have inadvertently turned a blind eye to one or two patients, who have done well in the unhealthy group or not done well in the healthy group and that may have altered the results. Furthermore, studies that look back at patients' lifestyles (called retrospective studies) could simply 'cherry pick' the data that support their argument. More persuasive evidence comes from trials designed to look forward following a lifestyle intervention. These trials (called prospective studies) have predetermined, robust endpoints, which are recorded in designated trial documentation at regular intervals. It is not possible after the trial has started, unlike in retrospective studies, to change the specified endpoints. This makes the conclusions of these trials generally more reliable and convincing. Fortunately, there are two prospective studies in men with prostate cancer, which, because of the design and credible results, have quite deservedly generated copious media attention.

Vegan diet, exercise and yoga

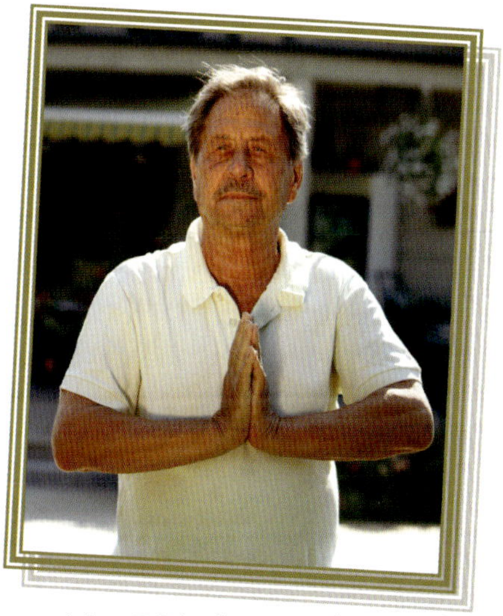

A randomised study involved 93 volunteers from the USA with early prostate cancer who, for various reasons, had opted not to undergo conventional therapies. They were randomly assigned to intensive nutritional counselling and lifestyle changes, or simple active surveillance. In the 47 patients randomly assigned to lifestyle, they switched to a vegan diet supplemented with soy, vitamin E, fish oils, selenium and vitamin C. The physiotherapist guided them into a moderate exercise program requiring at least thirty minutes of walking six days a week. They also embarked on a number of stress management techniques such as yoga and massage. The PSA decreased at twelve months in the intervention group by 4 percent, but increased in the control group by 6 percent. When this difference was analysed independently by scientific statisticians, it was shown to be highly significant. In other words it was a difference which was very unlikely to have occurred by chance (greater than 1:50 odds) – put another way, even the most cynical of scientists believed it!

The trial had another intriguing twist. A blood sample was taken from all patients at three monthly intervals. After removing the blood cells, the serum was added to sheets of living prostate cancer cells grown in culture dishes in a laboratory. Serum from the intervention group caused 70 percent of the laboratory prostate cells to stop growing, whereas serum from the control (non intervention group) only inhibited growth in 6 percent of cells. This eight-fold difference (70 percent v 6 percent) was highly significant and again statistically robust (fewer than 1:100 odds that it happened by chance). Furthermore, changes in PSA and cell line growth inhibition strongly correlated with the degree of lifestyle changes.

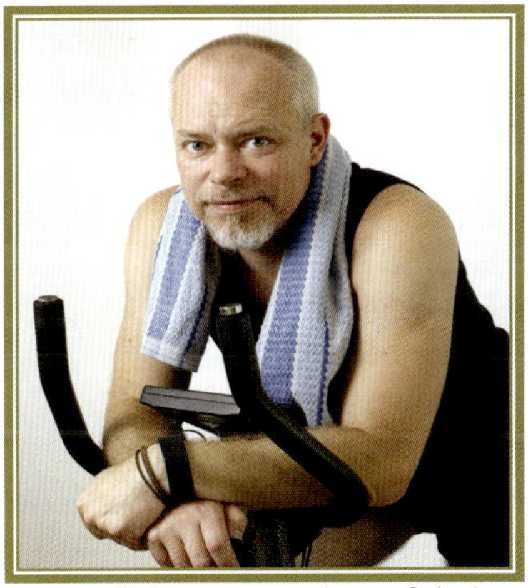

There is no doubt that these interventions had a significant benefit in slowing the growth of these men's prostate cancer. This study, however, does not tell us which intervention (diet, exercise, supplements or relaxation) was most significant. Maybe one, two or a combination of each were necessary or maybe one strategy works for one man, whilst another works for another – remember Mr C achieved the same result simply by eating Brazil nuts! Nevertheless, for these men the evidence that this lifestyle change slowed or even stopped the progression of their cancer is compelling.

A lot is said about the frame of mind and progression of cancer. There is some data suggesting meditation and yoga can alter the body's protein expression, potentially leading to a better immunity but other evidence of a direct anticancer benefit in humans is scant. There is some evidence from experiments mice – A study from Ohio State University implanted two groups of mice with cancers. The mice living in a stimulating healthy environment had a slower rate of tumour progression compared to those in a more confined environment. As well as a slower rate of tumour growth and spread in the happier mice, they had lower levels of a protein called leptin which is known to stimulate tumour growth.

Pomegranate juice

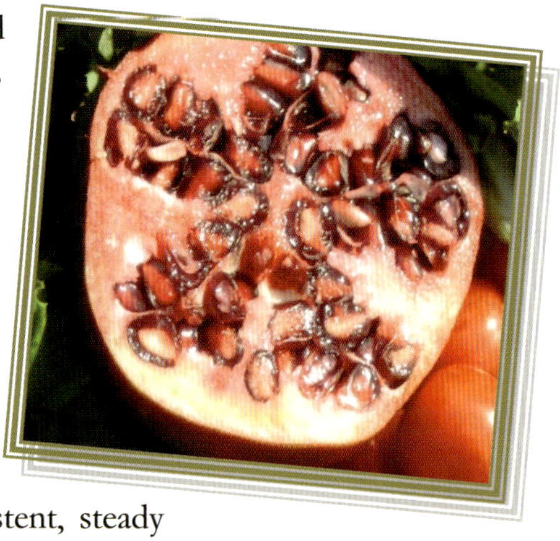

In this North American study, sponsored by the Pomegranate Growers Association, 48 men with prostate cancer were evaluated. Pomegranate juice has a particularly high concentration of antioxidants. All the patients had previously received radiotherapy or surgery but started showing evidence of their cancer returning in the form of a rising PSA blood test (generally referred to as PSA relapse). The rate of rise of the PSA for each patient was plotted on a graph and provided it rose in a consistent, steady fashion (i.e. not just a temporary increase), they were entered into the study. All men were given 200ml of pomegranate juice to drink every day. The PSA blood test was then measured for several months and again plotted on the same graph. The rate of rise of the PSA (the doubling time – PSAdt) was compared before and after consumption of the juice. There was a very significant prolongation of PSAdt, from a mean average of 15 months at baseline, to 54 months post pomegranate juice consumption. In other words this dietary intervention had slowed the growth rate of the tumour almost by a factor of four, which for men in their seventies may mean they would significantly delay or never need more aggressive hormonal intervention. For example, a man aged 74 years with a PSA of 3.5 and a PSAdt of 54 months would be 87 years old before his PSA exceeded 20.

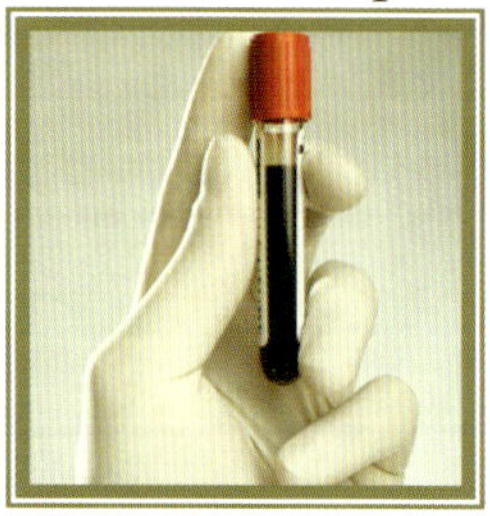

This study also had a further interesting angle. It looked at a factor known as the baseline oxidative state, which is thought to reflect the body's ability to fight off the free radicals that cause cancer or encourage slow growing existing cancers to mutate into more aggressive counterparts. These free radicals are generated by eating unhealthy foods, excessive exposure to sunlight, smoking or radiation. Anti-oxidants mop up these free radicals before they have time to exert their damage. The optimal amount of anti-oxidants needed in the diet depends on the level of exposure to carcinogens as well as the individual's own genetic makeup (i.e. vulnerability to attack). This balance of anti-oxidants and oxidative exposure can be measured in the blood with a variety of tools which in general measure the baseline oxidative stress levels in the body (BOS). The BOS was measured as a secondary end point in this study. Patients' blood BOS significantly improved following pomegranate consumption when measured at the start, then at three separate points over the next year.

Broccoli

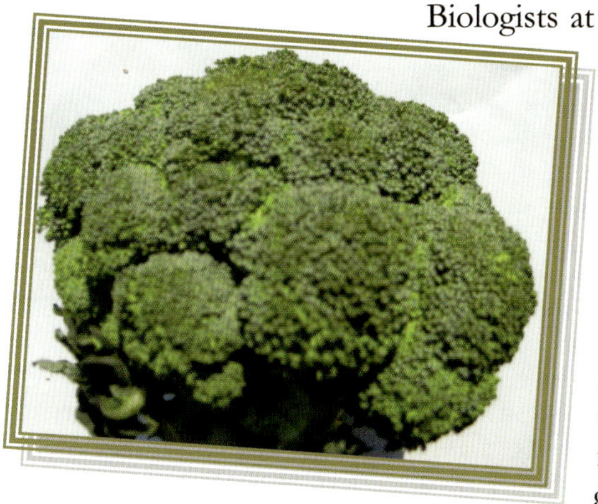

Biologists at Britain's Institute of Food Research published a study which showed that the healthy chemicals found in broccoli can prevent precancerous cells in the prostate progressing to more aggressive cancers. They found that just a few more portions of broccoli each week sparks hundreds of genetic changes, activating some genes that fight cancer and switching off others that fuel them. They split into two groups of 24 men with pre-cancerous lesions and had them eat four extra servings of either broccoli or peas each week for a year.

The researchers then took tissue samples over the course of the study and found that men who ate broccoli showed hundreds of changes in the genes known to play a role in fighting cancer. They believe the benefit would likely be the same in other cruciferous vegetables that contain a compound called isothiocyanate, including brussel sprouts, cauliflower, cabbage, rocket or arugula, watercress and horse radish. Broccoli, however, has a particularly powerful type of the compound called sulforaphane glucosinate, which the researchers think gives the green vegetable an extra cancer-fighting kick. The broccoli eaters showed about 400 to 500 of the positive genetic changes, with men carrying a gene called GSTM1 enjoying the most benefit. About half the population have this gene.

The researchers did not track the men long enough to see who got cancer but it is a very logical conclusion that just a few more vegetable portions each week can make a big difference. Furthermore it is also likely that these vegetables work the same way in other parts of the body and probably protect people against a whole range of cancers.

Diet and salicylates

In the UK, a prospective study was published in 2005, which evaluated dietary intervention, supplemented by oral sodium salicylate (an aspirin-like drug) and other anti-oxidants. A small cohort (group) of men with progressive early or relapsing prostate cancer had stabilisation of PSA, with a mean average stabilisation of 17.2 months. It was not clear which of the three components of the supplement were instrumental in this tumour stabilisation, or whether the combination was essential. Also, it was uncertain as to how much additional benefit was derived from the administered sodium salicylate or the natural salicylates found in the higher intake of fruit and vegetables. As a consequence, whether diet alone, salicylates alone or a combination of both is the optimal approach remained unanswered. For this reason our research group designed and conducted a double-blind, randomised, multi-centre controlled trial under the registration of the National Cancer Research Network (NCRN). It compared salicylates and lifestyle counselling versus salicylates, lifestyle and mineral and vitamin C supplements in patients with progressive indolent or relapsing prostate cancer. The results confirmed the suspicions from other studies that giving a "one fits all" supplement to patients has very little benefit in terms of their cancer. The results were fascinating; despite the fact that all patients were progressing at trial entry, 40 percent then stabilised for an average of 18 months. This trial was presented in the 2008 UK national research conference and gives reassurance that a change in lifestyle can slow the rate of prostate cancer progression, although the exact role of salicylates needs confirming in further studies. Further analysis suggests that if patients were selected carefully the stabilisation rate would be likely to be even higher.

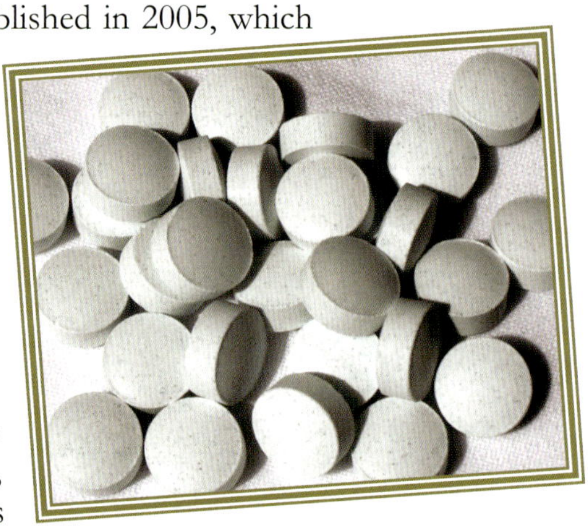

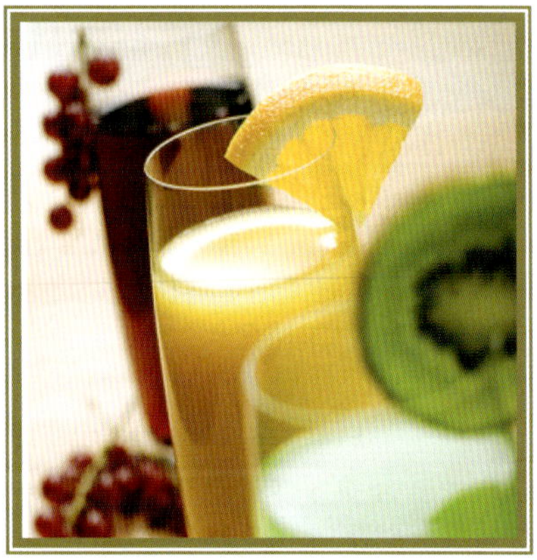

Tomatoes, chillies and lycopene

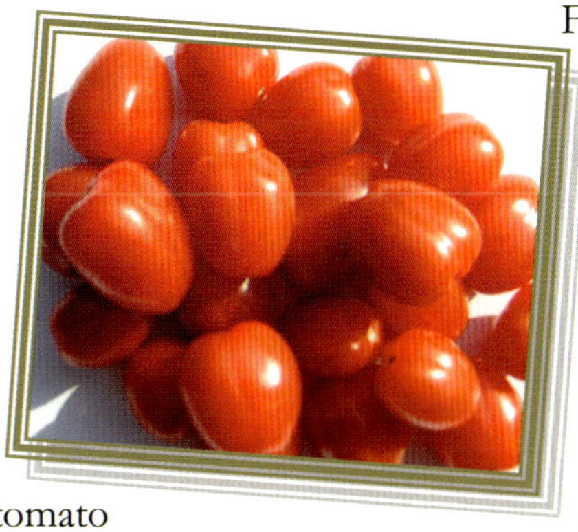

Following information gleaned from a large study of U.S. health professionals which showed that men with diets rich in lycopene (the red colour found in foods such as tomatoes and chillies), had a lower risk of prostate cancer, lycopene use was then investigated in men with established prostate cancer. Two small non-randomised studies showed that men with a high intake of natural lycopene intake in food, particularly tomato sauce, demonstrated a slowing of the rate of rise of the cancer marker, PSA.

The effect of lycopene was also evaluated in a small prospective clinical study in 26 men with localised prostate cancer awaiting prostatectomy in 2002 by the scientist Kucuk. The men were randomly assigned to receive either oleoresin or a tomato extract, containing 30mg of lycopene, or no supplementation for 3-weeks before radical prostatectomy. Biomarkers of cell proliferation and apoptosis were assessed in benign and cancerous prostate tissues. After intervention, subjects in the intervention group had smaller tumours (80 percent vs 45 percent, less than 4 ml), less involvement of surgical margins and/or extra-prostatic tissues with cancer (73% vs. 18%, organ-confined disease), and less diffuse involvement of the prostate by high-grade prostatic intraepithelial neoplasia (33% vs. 0%, focal involvement) compared with subjects in the control group. Mean plasma PSA levels were lower in the intervention group compared with the control group. This pilot study suggested that lycopene may have beneficial effects in established prostate cancer.

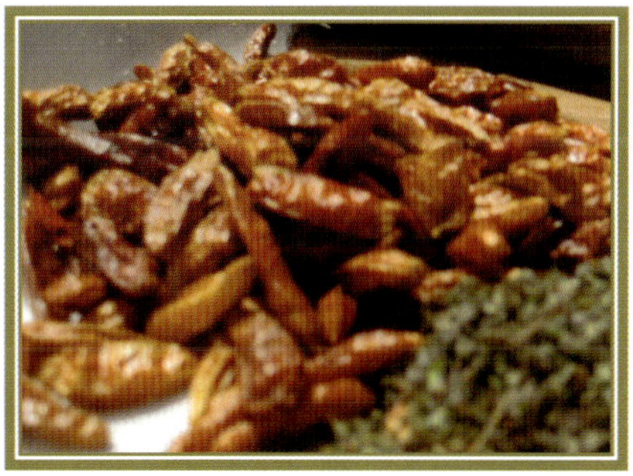

In 2008 a scientist called Schwarz reported that a randomised study demonstrated an effect on PSA in men with benign prostatic hypertrophy (BPH). These men did not have cancer at the time of the study but had an increased risk of progressing to it. This pilot study randomly compared the effects of lycopene (15mg od) supplementation in 20 elderly men (n = 20) diagnosed with BPH against another 20 who were given placebo (n = 20), both taken for 6-months. The lycopene supplementation significantly decreased PSA levels, whereas there was no change in the placebo group. The plasma lycopene concentration increased in the group taking lycopene, but other plasma carotenoids were not affected. Whereas progression of prostate enlargement occurred in the placebo group as assessed by trans-rectal ultrasound and digital rectal examination, the prostate did not enlarge in the lycopene group. Symptoms of the disease, as assessed via the International Prostate Symptom Score questionnaire, were improved in both groups with a significantly greater effect in men taking lycopene supplements. Since these two studies offer a small sample size and short intervention period, further analysis in a much larger clinical study needs to be performed before lycopene supplements can be recommended.

Green tea

A small study from Louisiana State University has found that green tea may reduce the levels of some compounds linked to prostate cancer progression. Through their study of 26 men with prostate cancer who were given a concentrated extract of tea polyphenols for an average of 34-days, they report a significant reduction in the levels of several growth factors that promote cancer as well as reductions in PSA. Furthermore, some men had reductions in growth factors of up to 30 percent.

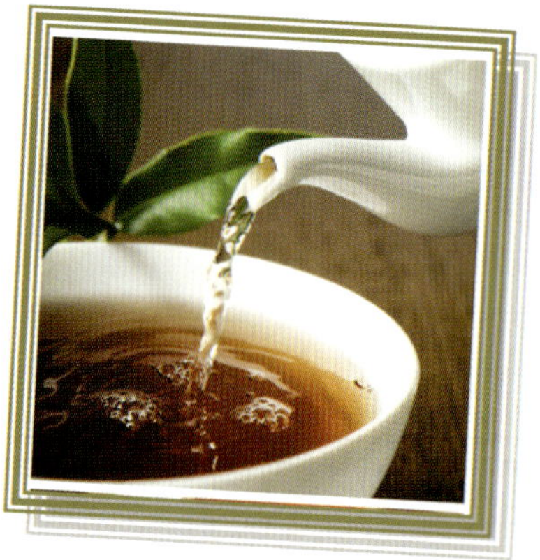

A further study from the USA looked at people with Chronic Lymphocytic Leukaemia (CLL). This condition usually affects elderly people and generally, but not always, progresses slowly. If it starts progressing rapidly, infiltrating other organs such as lymph nodes or the spleen or bone marrow or their abnormal blood count gets too high, intervention is required in the form of chemotherapy. This study looked at people's dietary intake of green tea in the chronic pre-treatment phase. Those who drank more than 4 cups a day had a significantly lower risk of their blood count deteriorating.

In conclusion, these studies confirm there is direct evidence for prostate cancer of a healthy lifestyle helping to reduce progression in those on active surveillance. Although there is a suggestion from one small study that it also helps people with Chronic Lymphocytic Leukaemia, there is still a lack of concrete evidence for other tumour types, for which it is very unlikely that trials examining lifestyle and diet alone will ever be approved through the regulatory authorities. The data is certainly not robust enough to suggest lifestyle change as an alternative to radical treatments but even if a minor percentage of individuals on active surveillance are prevented from progressing then this will save a significant amount of money for the nation and avoid the risks of intervention among the affected individuals. Clearly further randomised research is needed in this field, particularly in the areas concerning antioxidants and supplements.

As regards preventing prostate cancer relapse after treatments, these is direct evidence for obesity and exercise but the benefit of other lifestyle factors is lacking. It is not unreasonable, however, to extrapolate data from [1] Studies of prevention and incidence of prostate cancer; [2] Relapse and survival studies from other tumour types; [3] Intervention studies in active surveillance.

Summary – lifestyle and active surveillance for prostate cancer

Exercise: Aim to participate in at least 2-5 hours of vigorous exercise per week

- Incorporate more physical exercise within the activities of daily living
- Perform regular aerobic and resistance exercise in formal programmes

Diet: Aim for a healthy, varied diet avoiding fads and ensuring adequate intake of vitamins, essential minerals, fibre, essential fatty acids and antioxidants:

- Eat more
    - Green and cruciferous vegetables, fruits, berries, nuts, pulses and grains
    - Healthy oils; (unsaturated fats, omega 3 in fish, avocado, linseeds)
    - Soya based foods (beans, miso, tempeh, soy milk, tofu)
    - Ensure adequate calcium and essential minerals (nuts, dairy, shell fish)
    - Antioxdants (Green tea, pomegranate juice, goji berries)
- Eat less
    - Unhealthy fats (saturated fats)
    - Carcinogen-containing foods
    - Vitamin or mineral supplements

Other lifestyle factors:

- Avoid obesity (BMI>35 Kg/m^2) or being underweight (BMI<19 Kg/m^2)
- Limit or stop drinking alcohol,
- Stopping smoking, if relevant,
- Take regular gentle sun exposure without burning.

PART 3

Lifestyle to influence relapse rates and improve cure

"What to do more of / less of"

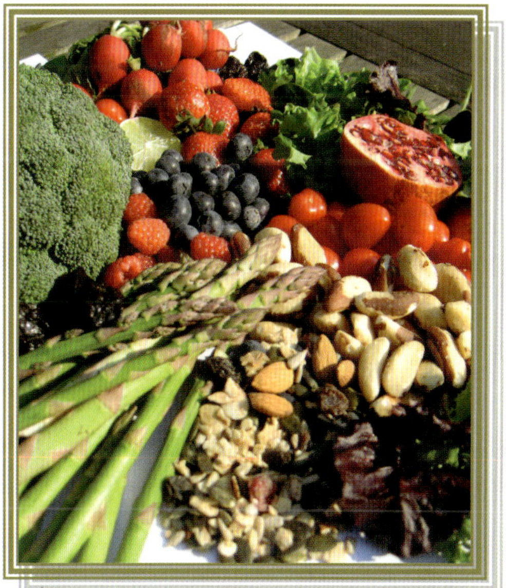

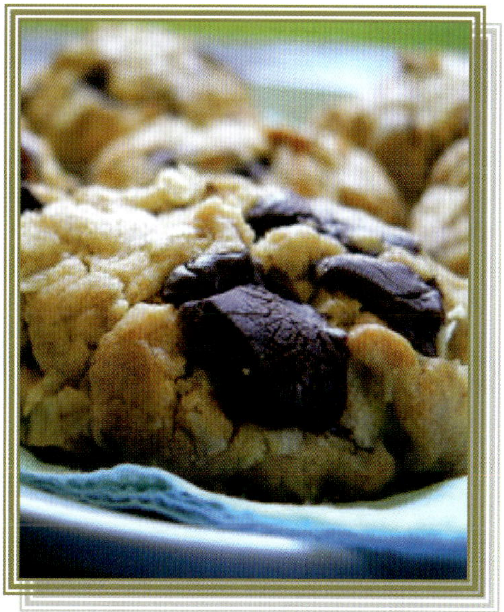

Background to this lifestyle advice

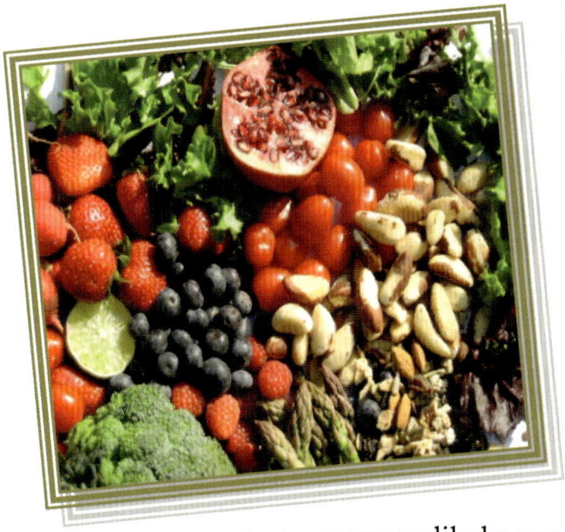

Understanding the precise mechanisms of how dietary and lifestyle factors can interact with cancer, however, is complicated by the caveat that people often follow a range of other healthy or unhealthy behavioural patterns – from exercise to smoking cessation, reducing body size, eating fat, consuming supplements and even analgesics. All these factors in varying degrees may influence the course of cancer either by making a contribution on their own or more likely combining with each other. Nevertheless, this section breaks down the constituents of lifestyle into recognised categories and describes the accepted theories of how each could either help you fight cancer or add to the risks of it growing faster, spreading and coming back after initial treatment. As mentioned in chapter one, each category in this section, as far as possible, is divided into three headings;

The Evidence This describes the evidence from published clinical trials which have satisfied high levels of scientific scrutiny and have been generally applauded by the oncology community internationally.

Underlying mechanism of benefit or harm In order to motivate you to go through the initial hardship of a lifestyle change it is also important to know why you are doing it, so the underlying mechanisms of how these factors affect the complex cancer processes are also described.

The practical lifestyle advice The two sections above are quite technical, so if you are someone who doesn't need to look under the bonnet of a car to see how it drives you may prefer to go directly to this third heading: This section describes the practical day to day tips of "what to do and what not to do" relevant to that particular topic.

The advice in this section is likely to benefit individuals at each stage of the cancer journey, as well as helping prevent cancer in the first place, as much of the evidence is overlapping. Furthermore, although separating this evidence into these neat categories helps to describe and explain the benefits of lifestyle in reality, however, food and lifestyle cannot be split into conveniently selected anti-cancer packages, since each meal or daily activity will contain a variety of unhealthy and healthy factors. The aim of course is to empower you with the knowledge to identify these factors so you increase the balance towards the healthy ones.

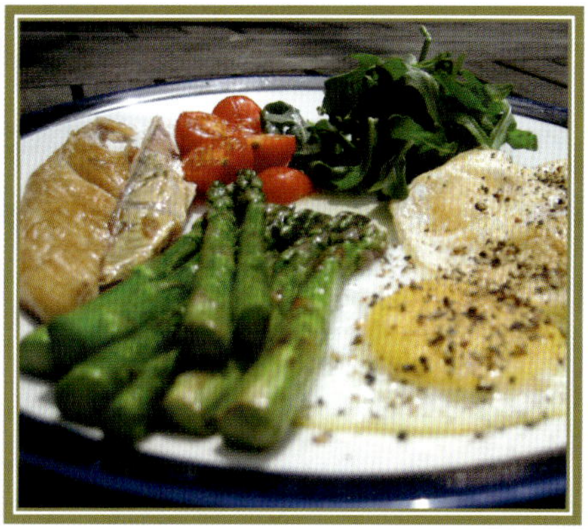

Furthermore, this advice tries not to recommend specific meals or dietary programs. Instead it aims to embody the concepts of healthy eating. Most individuals are perfectly capable of adjusting to a healthy diet within their preferences, tastes, needs or cultural parameters. This is particularly important if a lasting view of dietary change is planned. Changing to a 'faddy' diet, eating foods which are not palatable to that individual or are not freely available in their country, may lead to cravings or distress and are unlikely to succeed in the long-term.

Finally, the advice given in this book addresses people who do not have any, or have only a few, restrictions on their diet after a diagnosis of cancer. Likewise, it doesn't address any pre-existing, long standing dietary requirements. In general, therefore, it is probably not appropriate for patients with advanced cancer, or those whose tumours or treatments have affected their ability to eat or digest food. In these situations, patients should seek formal advice from qualified dieticians, preferably those attached to a mainstream cancer centre.

The prudent (healthy) diet

Before describing the evidence for the benefits and risks of the individual components of food two major studies have highlighted the impact of what they refer to as a prudent diet. This varied between individuals but in general consisted of high intake of fruit, vegetables, fish and fibre and a low intake of fat, processed meat, sugar and salt.

The biggest of these looked at the ***quality*** of the diet after a diagnosis of cancer. In this , called the Nurse's Health Study, women who had been treated for breast cancer completed a dietary questionnaire one year following radical therapy. The information was analysed into two groups. The first were those who had indicated that they had eaten what the main author, Prof Kroenke, had described as a *prudent* diet. He compared this group to the second group who had a standard USA diet, which generally had less fruit and vegetables, lower fibre and more fat. The results confirmed that the type of food women ate considerably influenced their chance of being alive years later. This difference was most spectacular when considering deaths from all causes e.g. heart attacks, strokes, other cancers, diabetes, as well as breast cancer. The main reason for this was that, fortunately, not many women in the study died of breast cancer. On further analysis however, when the highest quarter in the prudent diet group was compared with the lowest quarter in the poor diet group, particularly in women with higher risk disease (those whose cancer had spread to the local lymph nodes), the difference was marked and absolutely compelling.

A further study conducted from Illinois analysied 335 women with ovarian cancer. The results, published in the Journal of the American Dietetic Association in 2010, showed that a diet high in fruits, vegetables, and healthful grains was associated with a higher survival rate after their surgery and chemotherapy. On the other hand, the study also showed that consumption of unhealthy meats and high quantities of fatty milk-based product were associated with a shorter survival time. Their definitions of unhealthy meats were largely cheap processed meat products including pork pies, sausages, cheap burgers and processed meats. This trial was very interesting because there was no increased risk of relapse for those who ate white meats, smaller volumes of good quality red meats or fish. The trial suggests that a significant risk factor for relapse is not only the benefit of healthy food, but the danger of unhealthy foods, particularly those which are fatty and processed.

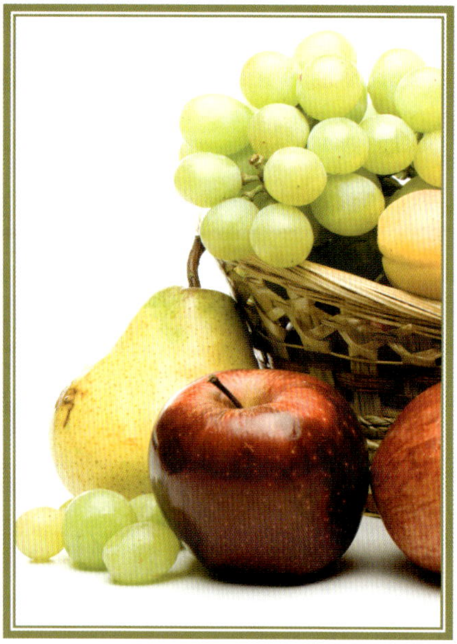

Chapter Four

Meat & fibre
Evidence, benefits, advice

Healthy and unhealthy meat

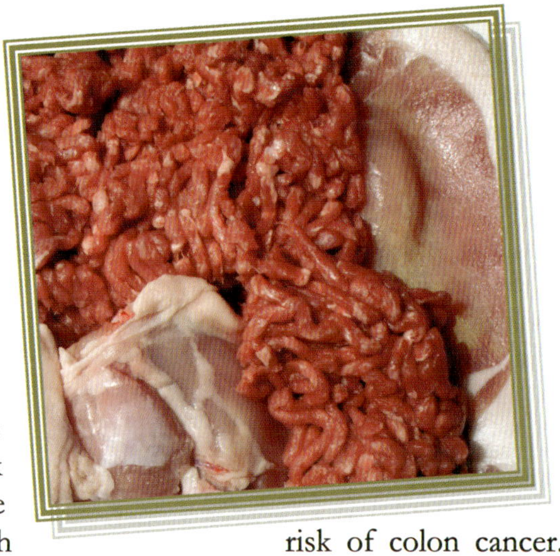

A large clinical trial called the European Prospective Investigation of Cancer (EPIC) analysed 25,000 people from Norfolk. There was a significantly higher incidence of colon cancer in those individuals who consumed a higher intake of red meat. However, on further analysis, the data showed that the meat eaters with a high vegetable and dietary fibre intake only had a moderate increased risk whereas high meat and low vegetable and fibre incurred a particularly high risk of colon cancer. As mentioned in the fibre section below, clearly the fibre protected the bowel from the effects of the meat.

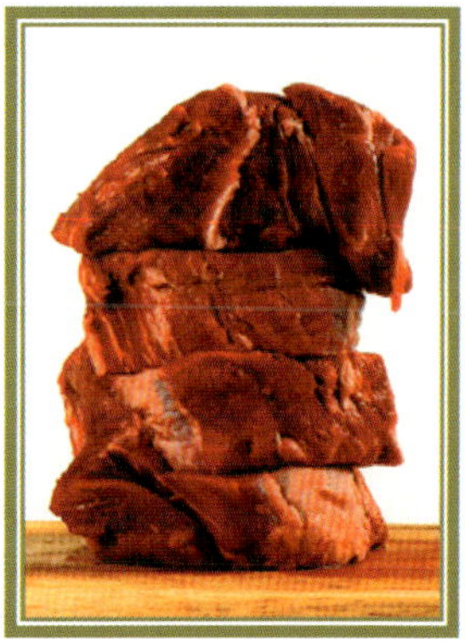

Another large study, conducted by the National Cancer Institute of California and published in the Archives of Internal Medicine, examined more than 500,000 middle-aged and elderly Americans. They also found that people with diets high in red meat had an increased risk of premature death from a range of diseases, including cancer. Researchers found that those who consumed more than four ounces of red meat per day were 30 percent more likely to die during the 10 years they were followed in the study. Men who had the highest red meat intake had a 22 percent increased risk of dying from cancer, compared to those who consumed the lowest amount of red meat. Similarly, women who reported the highest amount of red meat consumption had a 20 percent increased risk of dying from cancer, compared to those with the lowest red meat intake.

A further study from the University of Illinois already mentioned above, looked at the ***quality of the meat*** consumed in relation to the survival after ovarian cancer. Among the 335 women analysied those who ate unhealthy processed meats had a higher chance of their cancer returning after initial treatments had finished and a poorer overall survival. Their definitions of unhealthy meats were largely cheap processed meat products including pork pies, sausages, cheap burgers, processed ham and other meats. On the other hand, there was no increased risk of relapse for those who ate white meats, smaller volumes of good quality red meats or fish. Another study from the World Health Organisation (WHO) also demonstrated that the likelihood of cancer was higher among individuals who eat large quantities of meat but again found that the risk was higher in those who consumed processed, fatty varieties.

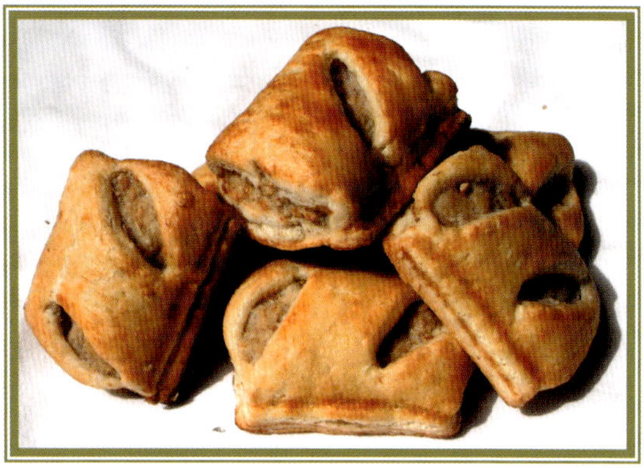

How meats are prepared can also affect the risk of their cancer potential. The carcinogen section below describes how burning or barbecuing meat increases the levels of carcinogens significantly. Even pan-frying meat with a high gas flame may be worse than a lower flame or electricity for raising the risk of cancer. Research published in the journal Occupational and Environmental Medicine showed that utagenic aldehydes and heterocyclic amines, are found in cooking fumes produced during high temperature frying of beefsteak. The hotter gas flames release more harmful chemicals from oil in the cooking process compared to lower heat.

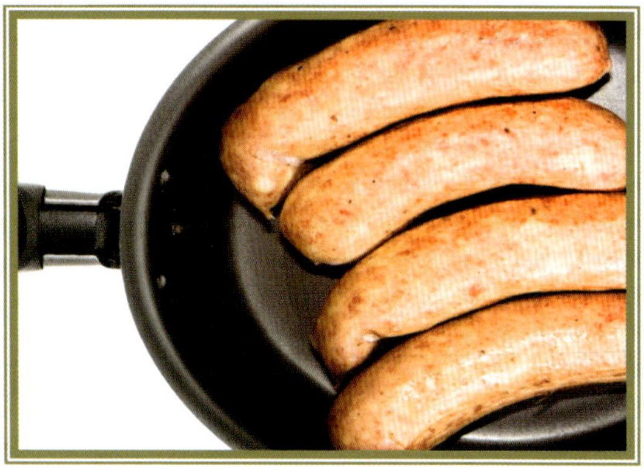

Smoking or cured meats also increases carcinogenic hydrocarbon and nitrosamide levels. One study of Taiwanese children and teenagers showed that high intake of cured meats is associated with increased risk of childhood acute leukaemia. More specifically the article reported that those who ate cured meats and fish more than once a week had a 74 percent higher risk of developing acute leukaemia than children and teens who rarely ate those foods. Furthermore, those who consumed more vegetable and soy products had an even lower risk of leukaemia. This finding supports the fibre theory in western diets. Although cured meats contain hydrocarbons and nitrites which can trigger tumour growth, the vegetables and soy contain antioxidants that neutralize these compounds.

How could excess meat be harmful?

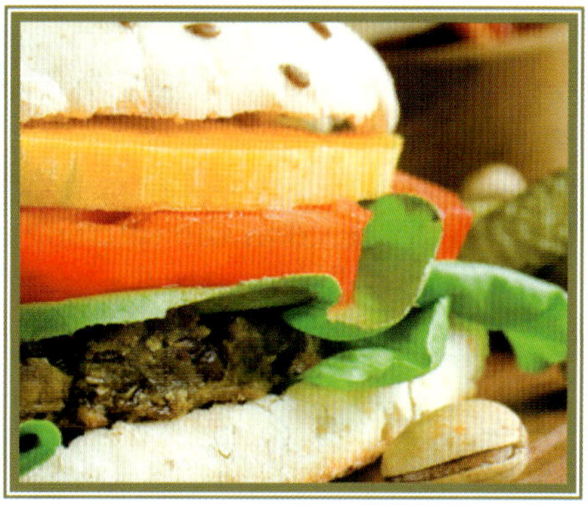

Red meat intake in excess encourages the formation of harmful carcinogenic substances called N-nitroso compounds. These form in our gut and are then absorbed into the general blood circulation. This occurs by a process called N-nitrosification which is triggered by the presence of the insoluble iron constituent of haemoglobin (the red cells found in blood). Haemoglobin present in red meat thus leads to the production of N-nitroso compounds. When people switch from a vegetarian diet to a diet rich in red meat, they experience a spike in the N-nitroso compounds. Laboratory tests have shown that N-nitroso causes DNA mutations leading to the start of the cancer process. Of special relevance is that the pattern of mutation is similar to those found in colon and stomach cancer. Curing or smoking meats also increases the hydrocarbon levels which are also carcinogenic.

Advice for healthy meat eating

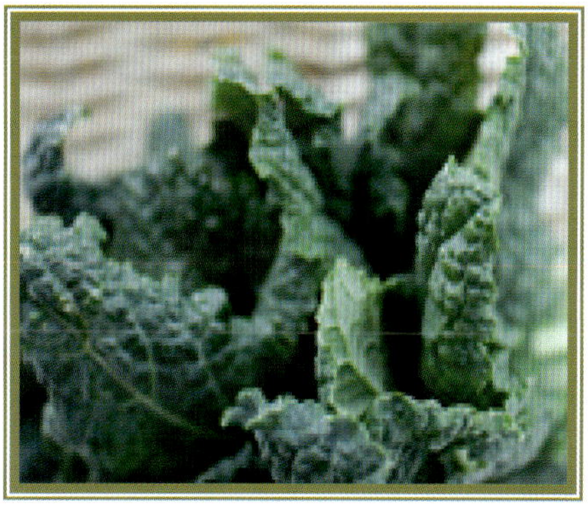

The Taiwanese study clearly showed that high intake of antioxidants in vegetables can counterbalance the carcinogen in the curing process. Likewise the EPIC trial from Norfolk showed a significantly increased risk of colon cancer in those individuals who consumed higher red meat intake, but in those who also ate good quantities of fibre the risk was lower. Other studies have confirmed that people who eat less meat are mainly benefiting from the protective effects of other foods which they eat more of – especially fruits, vegetables, whole grains and legumes found in a vegetarian diet.

Although the risk of cancer is lower in vegetarians, the evidence would suggest that eating meat in moderation is probably safe provided the diet is otherwise very healthy. There are of course some benefits to eating meat – it is the most easily absorbed source of protein and iron pre-menopausal women, teenage girls and young children, – all of whom are at high risk of iron deficiency and would benefit from regular meat in their diets. The same applies to adults with cancer if recovering from a period of malnutrition, such as a prolonged period of poor appetite, or a recent operation as, undoubtedly, meat is a good source of protein. A further study also showed that beef reared on grass as free range had good levels of omega 3 and selenium, particularly those reared organically. While the days of the 16-ounce steak are less common, a 3-ounce serving of extra-lean good quality meat, less frequently, should not be frowned upon. The extra risks of over-heating or barbequing cheap processed, fatty meats are also discussed in the carcinogen and acryalamine section and the table below gives an overall summary for healthy meat eating.

Summary – advice for healthy meat eating:

- Eat less but better quality
- Eat less red meat, particularly bloody and undercooked (rare)
- Avoid cheap meat products – sausages, burgers and pies
- Avoid processed meat products – sausage rolls, scotch eggs and cheap ham
- Aim for meat from animals which are free range, organic or feed on grass
- Consider meat 2-3 times a week rather than every day
- If exercising a lot eat more; if not eat less
- Use meat for its taste, but not as the main content of the meal
- Avoid smoked or cured meats
- Remove excess fat and skin
- Gently grill or casserole rather than fry or burn on the barbeque
- If extra oil is needed use olive oil rather than animal fat
- Use plenty of herbs and spices to counterbalance the carcinogens
- Avoid barbecued or blackened meats
- When eating meat make sure you also have plenty of fibre
- When eating meat have a higher quantity of vegetables on the plate
- Don't rely on meat as a main protein, alternate with pulses, quinoa, lentils

Fibre

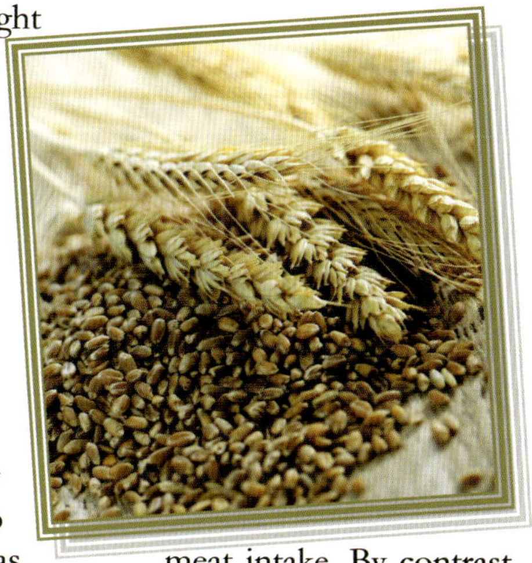

Historically, fibre has not always been thought to protect against cancer. A serious blow to dietary fibre protagonists occurred in the year 2000 when three separate clinical trials showed no significant association between fibre intake and the risk of developing polyps following cancer or polyp resection. These trials, however, were most likely to have been negative because of what they defined as a high and low fibre diet. In the USA study the difference in the quantity of fibre, between high and low intake, was fairly narrow and the trial also didn't take into account other factors such as meat intake. By contrast, the positive European EPIC study, mentioned above, had a large difference in fibre intake between the two comparative groups and also incorporated meat intake into the analysis. Furthermore, in the EPIC trial patients who had a high fibre intake also had a lower red meat intake which was unlikely to be the case in the USA where red meat intake is generally higher. It is this balance of fibre and meat which therefore seems most important rather than one or the other individually.

How is dietary fibre healthy?

Dietary fibre protects against colon cancer by binding potentially harmful bile acids and decreasing the transit time of the bulk of matter moving through the intestine, thus reducing the amount of time the colon comes in contact with dietary carcinogens, including the N-nitroso compounds produced by meat consumption.

Advice to improve your daily fibre intake

Fibre can be found in a wide range of healthy natural foods; usually processing removes the fibre. Dietary fibre traditionally is split into soluble and insoluble types. ***Insoluble fibre*** in the diet largely consists of cellulose, hemicellulose and lignin. Studies have shown that the insoluble, coarse type is good for bulking up the stool but should be combined with exercise and plenty of fluid. This fibre is good for preventing constipation related issues such as haemorrhoids (piles), diverticular disease, rectal prolapse and hernias both in the groin and stomach (hiatus hernia). This is found in whole wheat grains, bran and root vegetables.

There is however a small danger that if a lot of insoluble fibres are taken in the diet without a balance of soluble fibres the stool becomes too bulky. This can sometimes be seen on abdominal x-rays of some people, who are often surprised by the amount of stool inside them despite their high fibre diet. In some cases, for example before radiotherapy, men will be asked to change to a low residue (avoid insoluble fibre) diet because the rectum is too dilated. Regular daily exercise and drinking plenty of liquids will help to avoid this but most importantly it is wise to combine the insoluble fibres with the insoluble varieties, which tend to have a more stimulating effect.

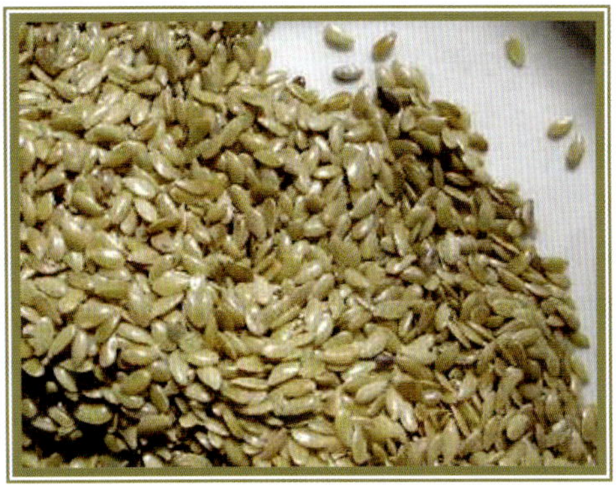

Soluble fibre largely consists of gums and pectin found more often in citrus fruit, pears, apples, guar gum and grains such as barley. The soluble type, in particular, has been shown to reduce saturated fats and cholesterol levels and to protect from diabetes. Meat eaters are particularly advised to increase both types of dietary fibre intake, as are individuals concerned about their blood fat levels. The association with blood oestrogen levels in post menopausal women is confusing – overall a high fibre diet lowers blood oestrogen levels slightly which is a good thing to reduce the risk of breast cancer or help prevent its relapse. This is thought mainly to be due to the insoluble component of fibre. Foods primarily containing the soluble fibre, however, actually increase blood oestrogen levels which potentially could be a risk for breast cancer. Fortunately, as the influence of the insoluble type completely overrides the soluble type in foods, this is only a theoretical consideration but one which one should be cautious of if the main source of fibre only comes from fruit or from guar gum products, particularly in regular laxative users. In other words, avoid

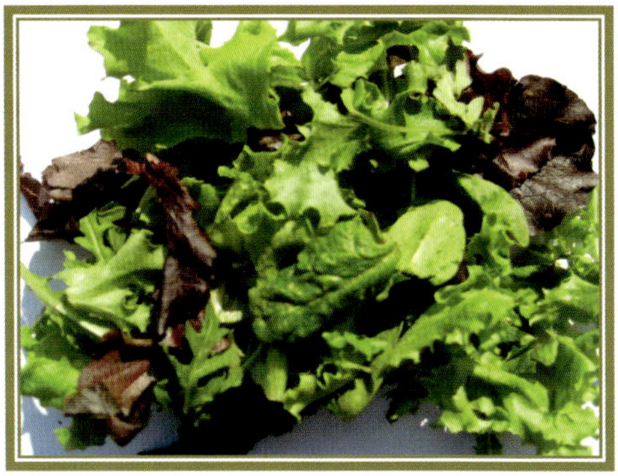

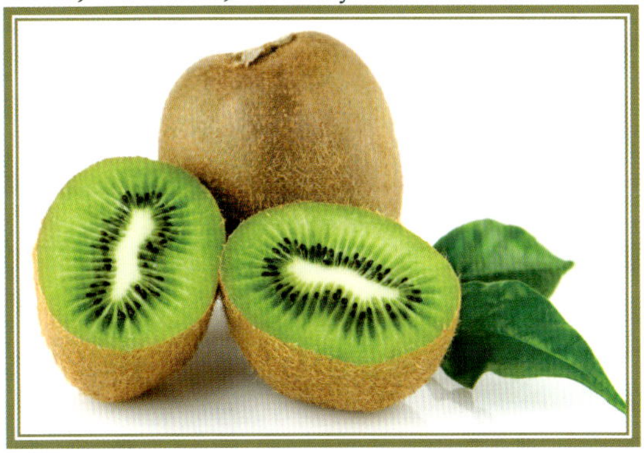

laxatives as much as possible and concentrate on foods which contain a good mix of soluble and insoluble fibre – ground linseeds, peas, beans, cereals and vegetables.

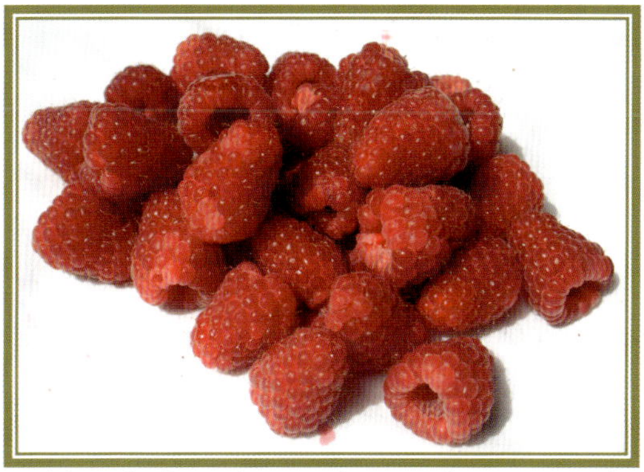

Current advice is to eat over 18g of fibre a day but remember to combine this with an adequate amount of fluids and regular exercise so the stool does not get too bulky. Most individuals who live in a western type environment eat far less than this so it is important to change the way you shop, cook and make your food. For example, stock your cupboards with wholegrain staples such as oats, bran, cereals and whole wheat flour. The only caveat to this, however, is the higher intake of wheat and gluten which can cause bloating, especially in wheat intolerant individuals. Taking pro-biotics (see supplement section) can help avoid this. There are also plenty of high fibre-containing foods which do not contain grains. For example, nuts, brown rice, seeds, fruit, lentils, brown or wild rice. As well as oats, porridge can be made from quinoa or linseeds.

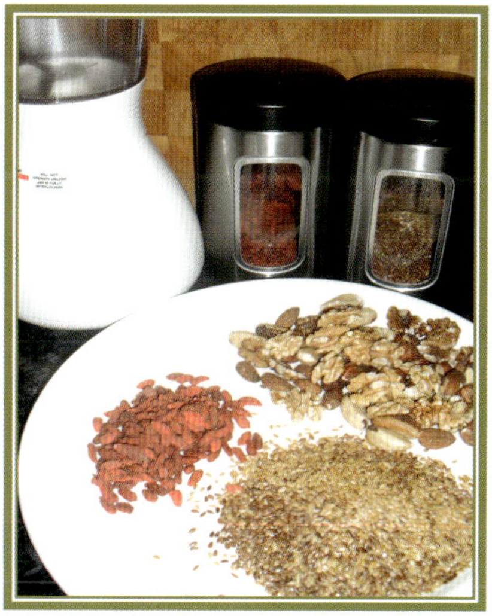

There is quinoa and linseed porridge available from health food stores which is easy to make – mix in some goji berries, raisins, nuts, bananas, dried and fresh fruit and prunes and that will set you up for the day. Instead of sweets and pastries, snack on sunflower seeds, pumpkin seeds, dried or whole fruits and mixed nuts. You can buy these in bulk and put them into small bags yourself rather than rely on the over priced tiny packets seen in coffee shops and snack bars. The chapter, on superfoods suggests grinding, nuts and grains in a food processor. These are an excellent source of daily fibre – to be eaten on its own or sprinkled on porridge or breakfast cereals.

Summary – tips to increase fibre intake, eat more:

- Whole fruits: apples, pears, pineapples, plums, bananas and prunes
- Dried fruits: prunes, raisins, dates, apricots, goji berries and figs
- Juices and smoothies: good source of soluble fibre
- Whole berries: cherries and grapes
- Legumes: beans, lentils, linseeds, chickpeas and peas
- Cereals: whole grains, bran and wholemeal oat or quinoa porridge
- Seeds: dried pumpkin, sunflower and linseeds
- Nuts: Any nut has fibre, particularly hazel nuts and almonds
- Salads: lettuce, water cress, radish and peppers
- Leafy green vegetables: cabbage, sprouts, spinach and hemp
- Vegetables: squashes, carrots, broccoli, cauliflower (better raw)
- Linseeds – soak overnight or better still crush in a food blender

Chapter Five Healthy & unhealthy fats
Evidence, benefits, advice

Dietary fats – healthy

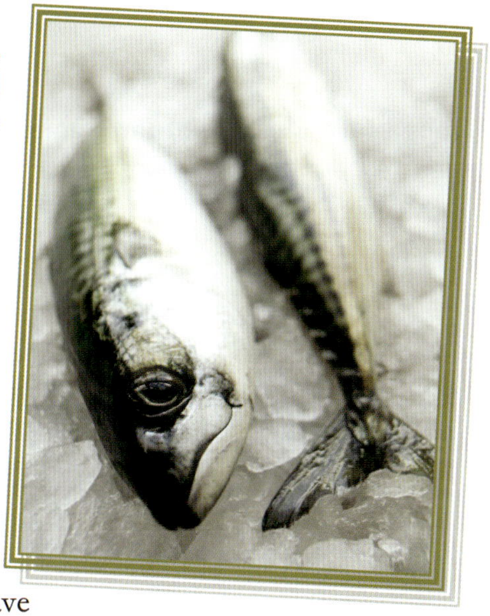

Fats are of course not all bad. Unsaturated fats (polyunsaturated and monounsaturated) and particularly the omega 3 variety are healthy. As it takes an oil to dissolve an oil, foods containing the healthy oils, high density lipoprotein (HDL) or unsaturated fats, actually reduce the unhealthy fats in the body, low density lipoproteins (LDL) or saturated fats and cholesterol. A common fault among individuals trying to reduce their cholesterol is that they reduce their healthy fats as well as the unhealthy ones. Oily foods are also a good source of the fat-soluble vitamins A, D, E and K. Population studies have shown that the cancers people develop, if they have a healthy fat intake, tend to be less aggressive and they therefore have a lower risk of dying from them.

Omega-3 (n−3 fatty acids).
Particular attention has been given to the health benefits of omega-3 fatty acids which are a family of polyunsaturated fatty acids. Clinical Cancer Research studies found that men who consume the highest amount of omega-3 fatty acids had a 63 percent lower risk of aggressive prostate cancer, compared with men who consume the lowest amount of omega-3 fatty acids. The study also noted that prostate cancer risk was also reduced in men with a genetic predisposition for the disease. As well as the anti-cancer benefits, omega-3 fatty acids have been shown to bring down triglyceride and cholesterol levels, reduce the risk of heart attacks, high blood pressure, hardened arteries and stroke. The most nutritionally important in our diets include.

- Alpha-linolenic acis (LLA)
- Eicosapentaenoic acid (EPA)
- Docosahexaenoic acid (DHA)

They are called essential fatty acids because the human body cannot synthesize omega−3 fatty acids so they need to be derived from the diet. The body can form the longer chain *n*−3 fatty acids (EPA and DHA) from the short chain omega−3 fatty acid α-linolenic acid. This is not an efficient process and these conversions occur competitively with omega−6 fatty acids, such as linolenic acid. Thus accumulation of long-chain omega−3 fatty acids in tissues is more effective when they are obtained directly from food or when competing amounts of omega−6 analogs do not greatly exceed the amounts of omega−3.

Omega-6 (n-6 essential fatty acids): These also have to be derived from the diet as they cannot be made by the human body. They are important in the formation of hormones, particularly those involved in inflammation and immunity (e.g. prostaglandins, leukotrienes, thromboxanes). As the formation of omega-6 metabolites involved in the inflammatory process competes with the formation of long chain omega-3's and visa versa, it is important that *n*−3 and *n*−6 be consumed in a balanced proportion.

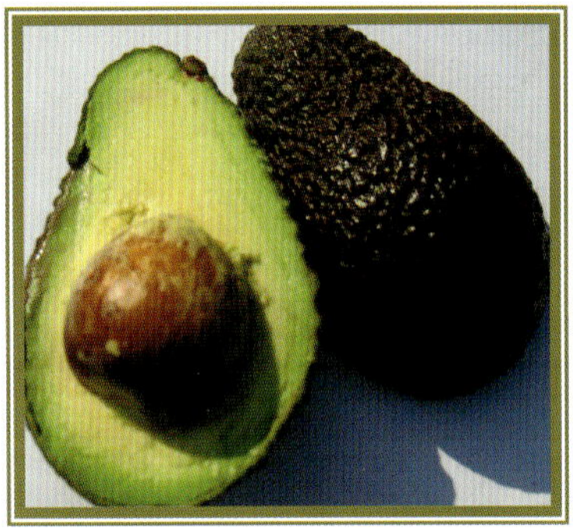

Omega-9 (n-9 fatty acids); Some *n*−9s are common components of animal fats and natural vegetable oils. They are not classed as essential because they can be made by the body from other unsaturated fats. The monounsaturated fat oleic, acid derived from olive oil, has particularly important health benefits. ***Oleic acid (olive oil)*** is a potent antioxidant and free radical scavenger. Olive oil also exhibits a number of other advantageous biological functions, including an ability to reduce blood saturated fat levels. Environmental studies have shown that higher olive oil use correlates with a lower incidence of atherosclerosis, diabetes, inflammatory and autoimmune diseases, skin wrinkling and skin aging. For centuries Greeks and Egyptians have used olive oil typically for the treatment of what they termed 'erythema' or redness, and wealthy Romans would rub it on their skin before a steam bath.

The omega 3 to 6 ratio: As mentioned above, omega -6 (linoleic acid) competes with the formation of the EPA and DAH from the shorter chain omega-3 (alpha linolenic fatty acid). Some clinical studies indicate that the ingested ratio of *n*−6 to *n*−3 (especially Linoleic vs Alpha Linolenic) fatty acids is important to maintaining health. An ideal ratio of n-3 to n-6 is 4:1 but typical Western diets provide ratios of between 10:1 and 30:1 – i.e., dramatically skewed toward *n*−6.

Mechanism of benefit

Omega fatty acids have been shown to slow the growth of cancer cells in the laboratory in Petri-dishes, as well as in mice. Human studies have suggested that marine omega fatty acids can help reduce cancer progression. The reason for this is not entirely understood, but one mechanism appeared to be the inhibition of the enzyme cyclooxygenase-2 (COX-2) which is over-expressed in some cancers (see salicylate section).

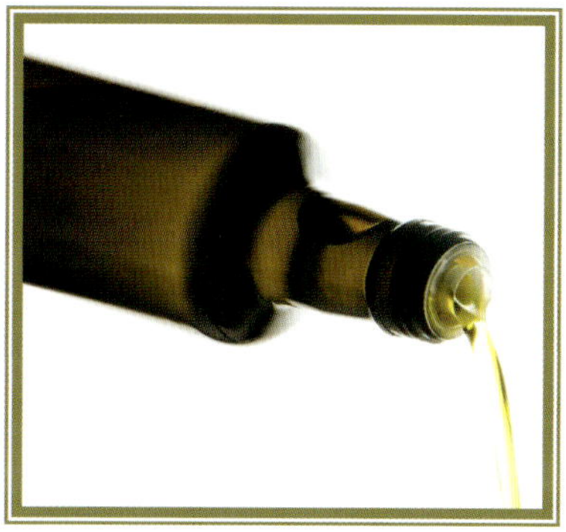

Oleic acid in laboratory experiments has been shown to repair DNA damage caused by excessive sunlight. In mice, massaging olive oil into their skin for 5 minutes every evening, after exposure to UV light, had a major effect on reducing skin damage and the number of skin cancers. Olive oil reduced the formation of 8-hydroxy-deoxyguanosine (8OhdG), a marker of DNA damage. This DNA repair effect is the reason olive oil is being used more frequently in skin care products particularly 'after sun'. Furthermore, this wonderful oil has been shown to suppress a protein in breast cancer cells called Her-2. This protein correlates with more aggressive breast cancers and is the target of the drug herceptin. Olive oil may therefore enhance the effects of herceptin. Its natural herceptin properties are very important, as a quarter of women with breast cancer overexpress the Her-2 protein. Ongoing studies are investigating whether the ***natural herceptin*** effect may help on its own or even help prevent the resistance to herceptin.

Advice to increase healthy fat intake

Plant and botanical sources:

Linseeds (flax seeds) and the healthy oil it produces has a very high percentage of unsaturated to saturated fats. It also contains a high percentage of omega-3 content, six times richer than most fish oils albeit in the short chain form (alpha-linolenic acid) with an n3:6 ratio of approximately three to one. Avocado have the highest oil content of all fruits and most of this is unsaturated, mainly monounsaturated and omega-9. Other natural sources of healthy fats include rapeseed oil, which is cheap and convenient as it can be grown in northern European countries. Most nuts contain a good percentage of unsaturated fats but walnuts are one of a few nuts that contain appreciable omega−3, with approximately a 1:4 ratio. Kiwi fruit has an even better ratio of omega-3:6 but there are only small quantities of oil in kiwis as opposed to linseeds. Pumpkin seeds have a high percentage of unsaturated fats (90 percent) and a good ratio of omega-3:6 (3:1). Other foods with a good ratio of omega3:6 include acai, butternuts, chai sage, shiso and lingonberry.

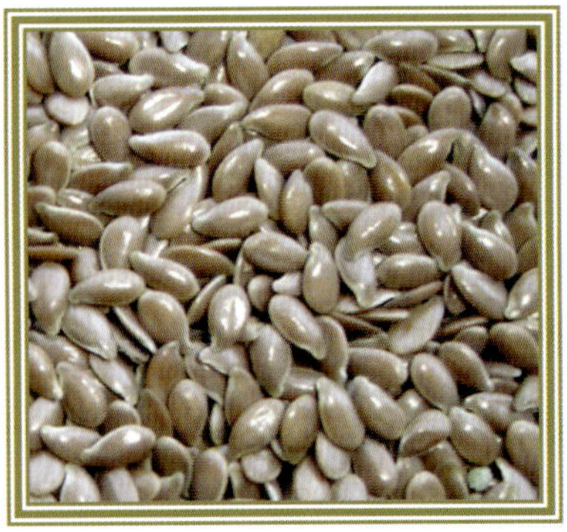

Most oils used for cooking or salads contain a mixture of unhealthy and healthy fats, as you can see in the table below. Olive and rapeseed (canola) oils have a particularly good percentage of unsaturated fats. Sunflower, soya bean and corn oil all contain mostly polyunsaturated fat so are also reasonable choices but tend to be heavily processed during manufacturing. Palm and coconuts have the worst percentage of unsaturated fats but cold pressed varieties can still be better than the healthy varieties. In terms of omega 3:6 ratio the best oils are linseeds, rapeseed (canola), soybean and olive oils (which also has omega-9). The worse oils are sunflower, palm kernel, cottonseed, grapeseed and corn oil as they contain virtually no omega-3. This obviously depends on the processing to get it onto the shelf. Heating the oil tends to damage the unsaturated fatty acids particularly the omega-3 and increases the percentage of saturated varieties not to mention increasing the levels of hydrocarbons and acrylamides. For example pumpkin seed oil contains virtually no omega-3 despite the pumpkin seeds itself being a rich source. Cold pressed oils are the best, of which olive oil is the most popular containing high quantities of omega-9 (Oleic acid) but only low to moderate amounts of omega 3 and 6. Heating this up in a frying pan, however soon damages the healthy fats.

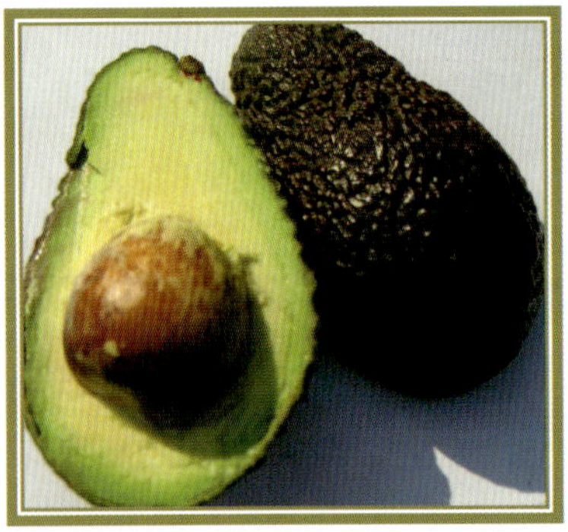

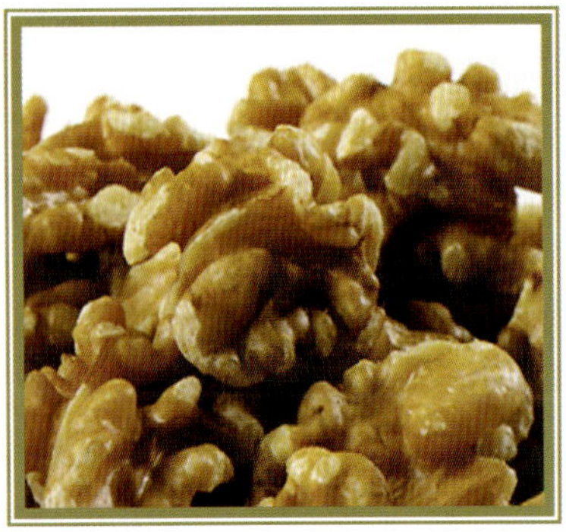

Oil	P	M	U	S
Olive	9%	77%	86%	14%
Canola	36%	58%	94%	6%
Peanut	34%	48%	82%	18%
Corn	62%	25%	87%	13%
Soybean	61%	24%	85%	15%
Sunflower	77%	14%	91%	9%
Safflower	77%	14%	91%	9%
Palm	10%	39%	49%	51%
Coconut	5%	9%	14%	86%

P = Polyunsaturated
M=Monounsaturated
U= Unsaturated
S = Saturated

As mentioned above, the microalgae are rich sources of the longer chain omega-3 fatty acid (EPA and DHA) and can be produced commercially in bioreactors. This process may be the answer to supplying the future populations of the world with enough omega-3 and is the only source of DHA acceptable to vegans. Oil from brown algae (kelp) is also an excellent source of EPA. Some vegetables and other nuts too, contain a noteworthy amount of *n*-3, particularly strawberries and broccoli.

Animal sources:

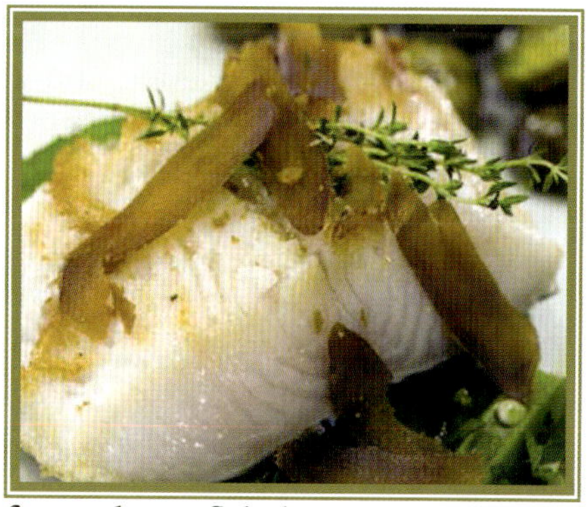

Fish: The most widely available source of unsaturated fats and the essential long chain n-3 fatty acids EPA (eicosapentaenoic acid) and DHA (docosahexaenoic acid is cold water oily fish. Interestingly, however, fish do not synthesize them; they obtain them from the algae and plankton they eat. Fish with the highest levels include mackerel, salmon, herring, anchovies, pollock, shark, swordfish and sardines. Tuna also contain *n*−3 in somewhat lesser amounts as the oils from these fish have a profile of around seven times as much *n*−3 as *n*−6. Consumers of oily fish should be aware of the potential presence of heavy metals such as mercury, cadmium (from discarded batteries) PCB's, dioxin. As these accumulate in the food chain, larger fish such as shark and sword fish have the highest levels. It is suggested that their intake should be limited to twice a week (which is still more than the majority of people currently consume in a western diet). However, in an extensive review of the evidence the Harvard School of Public Health reported in the *Journal of the American Medical Association* that the benefits of fish intake generally far outweigh the potential risks. Contamination is even lower in white sea fish such as bass and bream, and no limits have been set on their consumption, although these have lower omega-3 levels. Freshwater fish such as trout and lake varieties are almost completely free of the potential heavy metal contamination and have good levels of omega3. Some protection from mercury contamination can be gained from eating foods rich in selenium (brazil nuts, crab meat) and this metal can bind to the mercury and stop it being absorbed into the body.

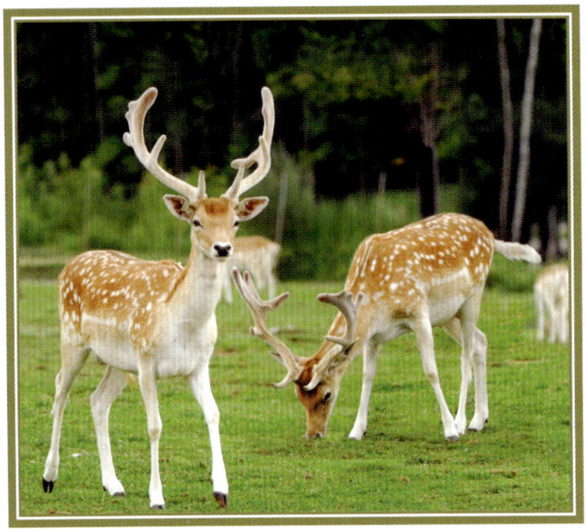

Healthy meat: Generally, grass-fed animals, particularly game, accumulate more $n-3$ than do grain-fed animals which accumulate relatively more $n-6$, healthy ratios of $n-6$:$n-3$ ranging from 1:1 to 4:1. Studies suggest that the evolutionary human diet, rich in game animals, seafood and other sources of $n-3$, may have provided such a ratio. In most countries, commercially available lamb is typically grass-fed, and thus higher in $n-3$ than other grain-fed or grain-finished meat sources. In some countries lamb is often finished (i.e. fattened before slaughter) with grain, resulting in lower $n-3$. Chickens which roam around eating grass, worms and insects as well as grain generally have much higher omega-3. Seal oil is a good source of EPA, DHA and other longer chain n-3's; however, it is not allowed for import into the European Union.

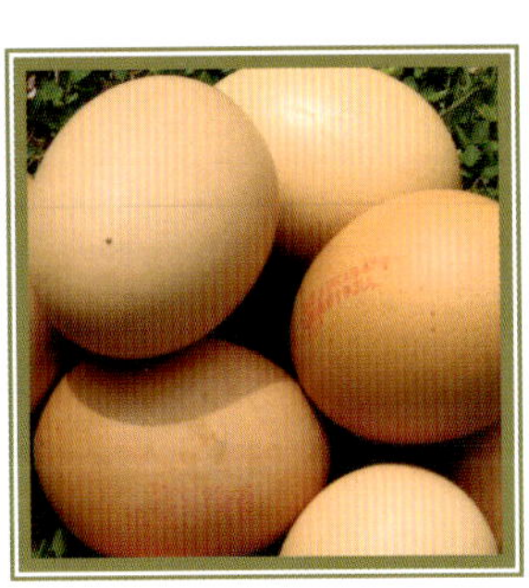

Eggs produced by chickens fed a diet of greens and insects produce higher levels of $n-3$ fatty acids (mostly ALA) than chickens fed corn or soybeans. Like the meat, in addition to feeding chickens insects and greens, fish oils may be added to their diet to increase the amount of fatty acid concentrations in eggs. The addition of flax, chia and canola seeds to the diet of chickens, both good sources of alpha-linolenic acid, increases the omega-3 content of the eggs but this is very rarely done for mass produced chicken eggs.

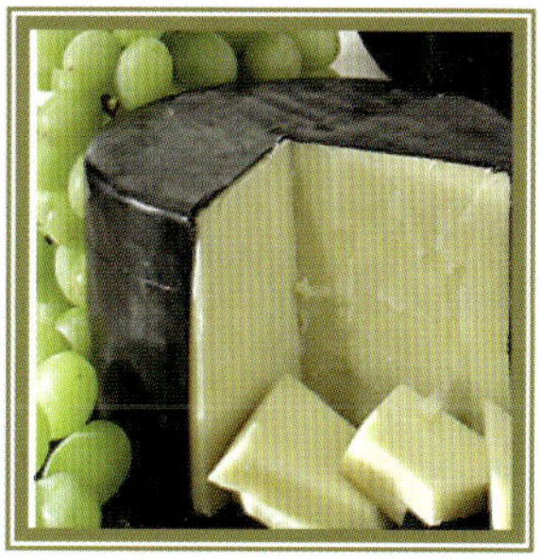

Milk and cheese from grass-fed cows may also be good sources of omega-3. One UK study showed that half a pint of milk from grass feed cows provides 10 percent of the recommended daily intake (RDI) of ALA, while a piece of organic cheese the size of a matchbox may provide up to 88 percent. One UK company is now producing premier cheese which is made only from milk from cows which have grazes on the first spring grass – packed with natural fats and nutrients.

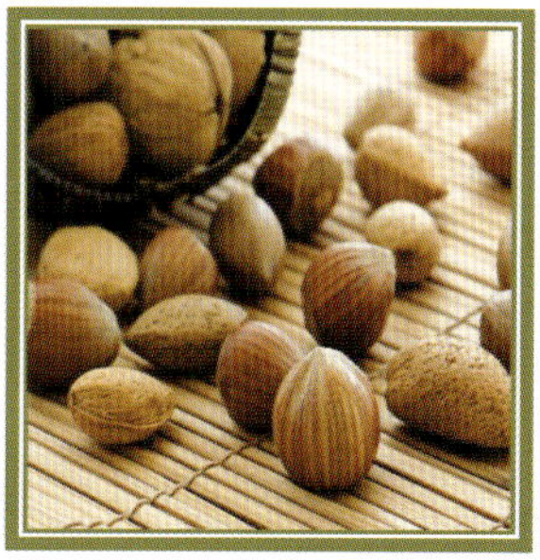

In conclusion: foods which contain lower levels of saturated fats and higher levels of unsaturated facts are beneficial to one's health because they reduce the risk of cancer, reduce cholesterol and low density lipoprotein (LDL-bad fats) and also reduce blood pressure and the risk of cardiovascular disease including strokes and heart attacks. Foods which contain higher levels of omega-3 (particularly the longer chain varieties EPA and DHA) are thought to also protect individuals from degenerative disorders such as dementia, poor eye sight and Parkinson's disease. It would be very wise to ask your doctor to measure your lipid profile with a fasting blood test. If your cholesterol or LDL is high it is time to change the type of fat you eat, to reduce the risk of cancer relapse and improve your chances of survival, not only from cancer but heart disease and stroke.

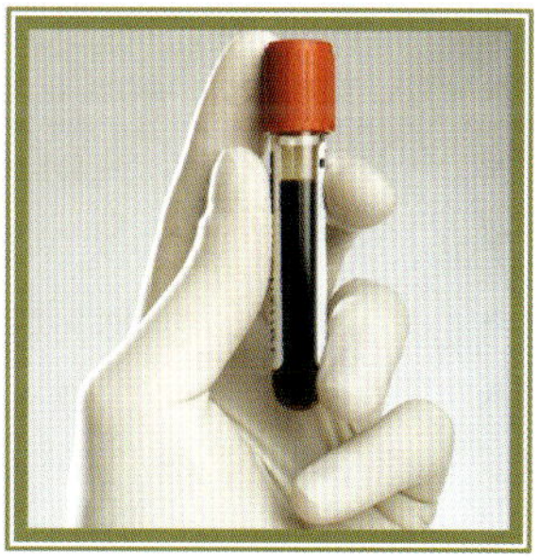

The ratio of omega 3 to 6 is also important as too much 6 blocks the conversion of shorter chain omega 3's into the more healthy longer chain omega 3's. Excessive omega 6 may also increase the body's inflammatory process and concerns have been raised for hyper-immune type illnesses such as asthma and rheumatoid arthritis. Humans in the west have omega 3:6 ratios in the region of 10-20:1 when ideally they should be 3-4:1. The best way to improve this ratio is to eat oily fish 2-3 times a week as part of a regular balanced diet. This and other advice tips are highlighted in the table below but the problem is that it is hard to know for sure our body's levels of omega 3 and 6 as dietary sources vary between foods even of the same varieties and certainly by different methods of food processing. The only way to know for sure is to measure the levels of essential fatty acids with a blood test. This will not only highlight the body's levels of omega 3, 6 and 9, but it will also tell you the ratio of 3:6. Unfortunately, this test is not available in most hospitals but only in specialist nutritional laboratories and can be rather expensive. Nevertheless, it is money well spent because if an imbalance is found correction with a change in the diet could have major long term health benefits (For more information see cancernet.co.uk/nutritional-tests.htm).

Summary – dietary sources of healthy oils:

Unsaturated (polyunsaturated and monounsaturated) fatty acids:

- Oily sea fish – mackerel, herring, tuna, swordfish, salmon, sardine, fish oils
- Other white sea fish – cod, sea bass and bream
- Fresh water fish – lake varieties, trout and river salmon
- Olive oils and others; rapeseed (canola), soya and sunflower
- Avocados
- Cold pressed vegetable oils particularly olive and rapeseed (Canola)
- Root vegetables, carrots, squashes
- Walnuts in particular
- Other nuts; almonds, Brazils, peanuts, pine, cashews, hazel and macadamia
- Seeds – dried pumpkin, sunflower, sesame and linseeds
- Legumes – lentils, quinoa and beans
- Leafy green vegetables and hemp

Sources of omega 3 (n-3) essential fatty acids:

- Algae, krill and brown algae (kelp)
- Oily sea fish – mackerel, herring, tuna, swordfish, salmon, shark, sardine
- Fish oil supplements
- Other white sea fish – sea bass and bream
- Fresh water fish – lake varieties, trout and river salmon
- Linseeds and pumpkin seeds
- Walnuts
- Meat from wild game or animals fed on grass
- Dairy and eggs from free range animals fed on grass or natural foraging
- Kiwi fruit, strawberries and lingonberries
- Vegetables – leafy greens and broccoli
- Herbs – Chai sage and perilla

Dietary fats – Unhealthy

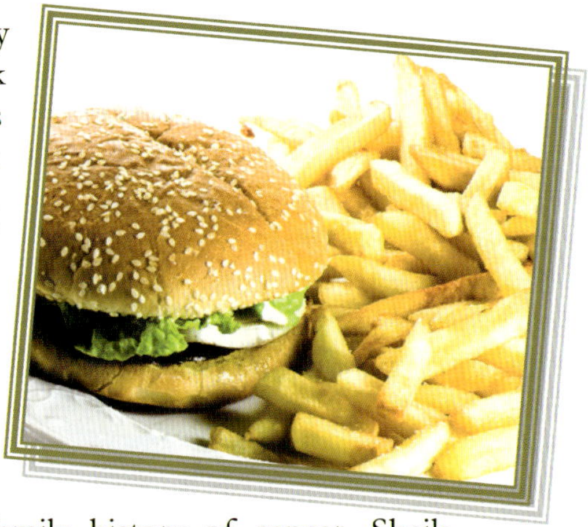

There is strong evidence that unhealthy fat and calorie excess adds to the risk of developing cancer. Evidence is particularly strong with saturated fat acid, high intakes of which have been associated with a poorer prognosis of cancer. The Health Professionals Study revealed that health professionals who had a high energy and fat intake had an increased risk of advanced prostate cancer, especially in those who presented at a young age or who had a positive family history of cancer. Sheila Bingham of the Medical Research Council, UK, presented data in 2003 to show that women who ate more than 90g of fat a day had twice the risk of developing breast cancer than those eating 40g per day.

The most convincing data so far addressing diet ***after*** a diagnosis of cancer has been derived from a recent prospective trial that looked at both the quantity and quality of what patients ate. Professor Chlebowski presented the world's first randomised interventional trial at the American Society of Clinical Oncology conference in 2005, and immediately triggered a wave of international media attention. He and his team approached 2,437 postmenopausal women with early breast cancer to give consent and enter this study, after they had completed their initial therapy. With a metaphorical flip of a coin (randomisation) half the women received nutritional counselling based on getting patients to eat less, and particularly less fatty foods. The other half carried on eating what they wished. The dietary intervention counselling for the first group was given by a qualified nutritionalist and included eight bi-weekly individual sessions. The first result of this trial may seem obvious was fundamental to any intervention programme but had not actually been demonstrated before in a trial of this magnitude. The dietary fat intake reduction was significantly greater in the dietary group. In other words lifestyle intervention works – and this was not just in a highly selected subgroup of

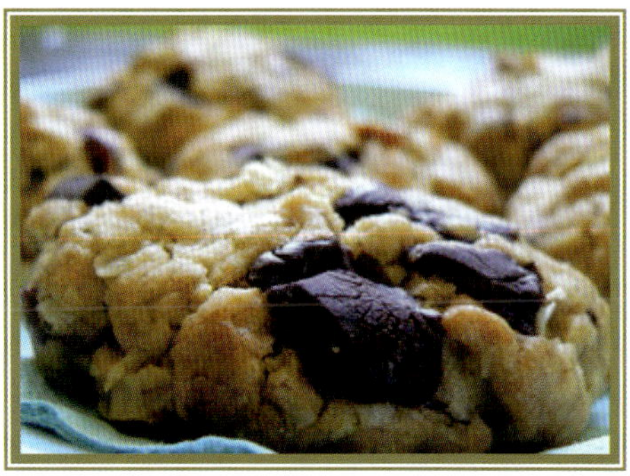

motivated individuals, this was in a group selected at random. This fact alone will pave the way to a host of interventional studies over the next few years, using some of the dietary and exercise strategies described in the next few chapters. The second important point of this study refers to the relapse rate and overall survival after their initial breast cancer treatments. After 60 months follow-up, the number of patients whose cancer had relapsed was significantly lower in the intervention group and this was statistically significant (less than a 1:30 probability this could have been a chance finding). This difference was even greater in patients with more aggressive cancers and those whose tumours were not sensitive to oestrogen – the ER negative subgroup, where there was less than a 1:50 probability this could have been a chance finding. As in Prof Kroenke's study described above, in terms of overall survival, the benefits of encouraging patients to eat a low fat diet applied to all causes of death from heart attacks to breast cancer.

Other evidence for the risks of unhealthy fats comes from studies using statins, which are now commonly used to reduce blood fat levels by reducing absorption from the gut. Five early randomised trials suggested fewer breast, colon and melanoma cancers in long-term users of statins compared to controls. The data for prostate cancer, however, is inconclusive as two large clinical cohort studies did not demonstrate a reduced risk with statin intake. Although a further cohort study of 16,976 subjects showed a reduction of prostate cancer, this did not stand up to robust statistical analysis. The consensus conclusion from these studies is that the lifestyle for reducing the fat levels, in terms of cancer, is significantly healthier than simply reducing the levels with a statin. There are also concerns that statins may restrict the absorption of the healthy fats as well as the unhealthy ones, actually increasing the risk of some chronic illnesses such as dementia.

Underlying mechanism of harm

The underlying mechanism by which bad, saturated fatty acids influence cancer is not completely clear but several mechanisms are implicated. A dietary experiment in men with prostate cancer suggested that a saturated fat diet correlated with higher testosterone and Insulin-like Growth Factor-I levels – a hormone also linked with obesity and lack of exercise, which has been shown to influence breast cancer development and progression. Higher consumption of saturated fats increases blood cholesterol levels which have been linked to a higher risk of cancer and a higher risk of its relapse. The most important factor, however, is that individuals who eat a lot of saturated fats tend not to eat the healthy unsaturated fats and hence do not get the benefit from adequate omega fatty acid levels.

Advice to reduce unhealthy fat intake

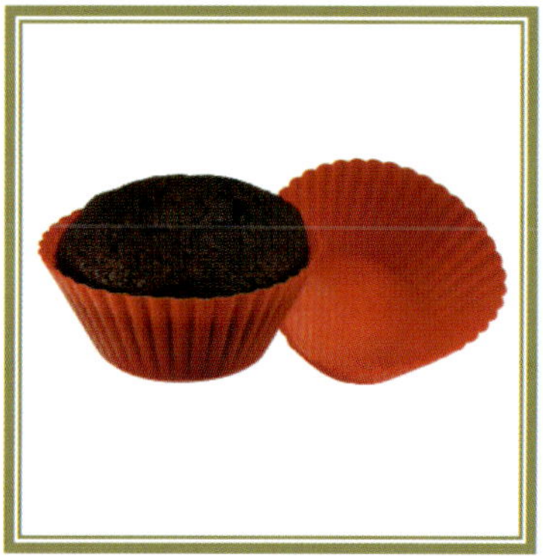

We should be aiming to cut down on unhealthy fats, particularly trying to replace saturates with unsaturated fats. A particularly harmful group of fats are the trans-fats or hydrogenated fats. Hydrogenation is one of the processes that can be used to turn liquid oil into solid fat. The end product of this process is called hydrogenated vegetable oil. It is used in some biscuits, cakes, pastry, margarine, processed foods, and particularly the fast food industry. The trans-fats found in food have no known nutritional benefits, and emerging evidence suggests that they may be worse than saturated fats. As a result Denmark, Canada and the USA have started labelling foods with their trans-fat content.

It is worth asking your family doctor to check your blood fat levels. If your cholesterol and unhealthy fat level are high it is very likely you are eating the wrong types of fat and an extra effort needs to be made. As mentioned above, the lifestyle to reduce the serum fat level is more important than simply reducing the fats with a statin, so a trial of lifestyle is always worth a go before starting statins. Repeating the blood test after 6 months of healthy living is a good measurable benchmark to see how well you are doing. If the cholesterol still remains high, even with improved diet and exercise, there is evidence for the benefits of statins to reduce blood cholesterol to help lessen the incidence of heart disease and stroke, so it is certainly worth considering them. The evidence that they reduce the incidence of cancer is less sound. Almost certainly the lifestyle measures to bring the cholesterol down are more important than the level itself.

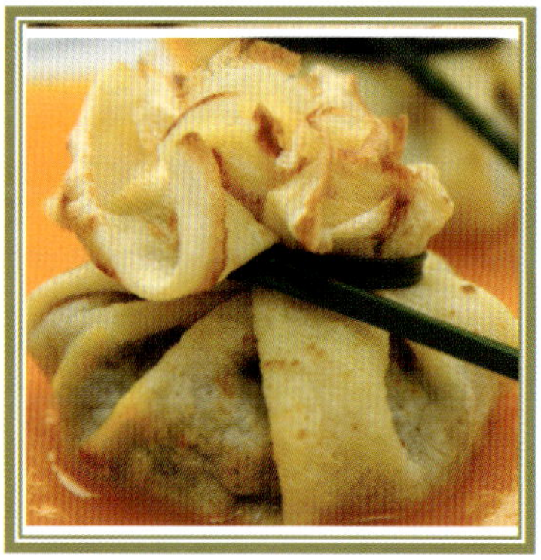

A common mistake when embarking on a low fat diet is that individuals tend to reduce all fat intake. It is only the unhealthy fats which need reducing. In fact the intake of healthy fats should be increased. It takes a healthy fat to dissolve an unhealthy fat, so cutting out all fats will lead to a tasteless diet with no change in the cholesterol levels. The other thing to remember is that fats are stored in the body, as they are a good source of energy. Very useful if you are a caveman off to catch your next meal but hardly relevant in our society where most of us have well-stocked fridges and fast food outlets are found on every street corner. To stop fats being stored we therefore need to increase our energy consumption by exercising regularly, more strenuously and more frequently.

Summary – advice to reduce saturated and trans-fat intake:

- Avoid biscuits
- Avoid cakes and muffins
- Avoid pastries
- Avoid hard cheese, cream and butter
- Avoid processed meat pies, sausages and burgers
- Avoid processed fatty foods containing coconut or palm oil
- Choose lean cuts of meat and chicken without skin
- Cut the fat off meat
- Use semi-skimmed or skimmed milk, rather than full-fat or condensed
- Choose low-fat yoghurt and cheese
- Cut down on deep-fried snacks – crisps, pakoras, samosas, bhajis,
- Cut down on fatty chips
- Don't eat hash browns or batter on the fish from fish & chip shops
- Cut down on sweets, desserts, creamy foods and chocolates
- Avoid curry dishes containing ghee
- Stick to drier (less fatty) dishes, rather than dishes with rich creamy sauces

Obesity or gaining weight

Before describing the human studies summarised below it is worthwhile recounting a much quoted laboratory experiment with mice that demonstrated a simple but powerful take-home message.

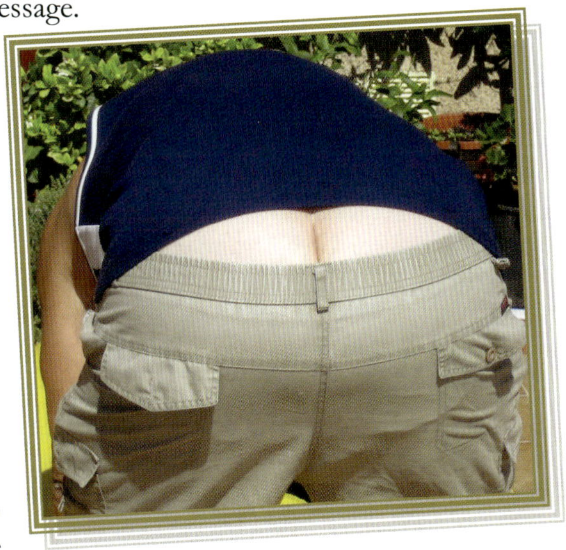

A healthy colony of mice was split into two groups and kept in a safe, comfortable, stimulating and warm environment. The only difference between them was that one group had as much food as they wanted at all times, and the other group had their food withdrawn for a few days every fortnight. The group that endured a modest degree of regular fasting lived almost twice as long as the others. It is not clear how this relates to humans, but it is fair to say most of us would not tolerate missing a meal let alone going without food for more than a day. Maybe the fasting practices in some reliions are based on a fundamental wish to improve the health of their followers, rather than the more commonly held belief that it is a penance to demonstrate their faith.

The largest trial in humans, again from the USA, evaluated 4,310 patients between 1989-94, who had successfully been treated for breast and bowel cancer. They had all undergone surgery to remove their cancer, most had received six months additional chemotherapy and all had no evidence of residual cancer at the starting point of the survey. The analysis performed under the prestigious auspices of the National Surgical Adjuvant Breast and Bowel Project (NSABP) showed that obese patients with colon cancer (BMI > 35) had worse overall survival than normal weight patients, due to both greater recurrence risk and non-cancer deaths. On a cautionary note however, patients who were very underweight (Body Mass Index < 19) also had a worse outcome.

A study from Cedars-Sinai Medical centre in Los Angeles, published in 2006, analysied 1069 men treated with prostate cancer between 1994 and 2002. They had either received surgery or radiotherapy. The cure rate for either was the same but overall obese men had a significantly higher rate of early disease recurrence.

A study published in 2009 examined a cohort of 365 women with ER+ve breast cancer who had later developed a contralateral breast cancer. He compared their lifestyles with 726 matched controls. Obesity (BMI > 30kg/m^2), consumption of >7 alcoholic beverages a week, and smoking were all positivity associated with the risk of a contralateral cancer. A further analysis of the Nurses' Health Study looking at weight gain after breast cancer treatment. 5204 registered nurses participated in the questionnaire survey between 1976 and 2000. There were 860 deaths (553 from breast cancer) on subsequent follow up. A high BMI at diagnosis correlated with an overall worse survival but a correlation with breast cancer relapse was only seen in non-smokers. Of more clinical relevance was weight gain after breast cancer treatments had finished. Weight gain more than 0.5kg/m^2 at 1year correlated both with overall survival and breast cancer specific survival. This effect was strongest in women who gained the most (>2kg/m^2).

Overweight women also had an increased risk of breast cancer irrespective of their daily saturated fat intake. In other studies, obese men were shown to be 33 percent more likely to die of cancer compared to those of a normal weight and obese women had a staggering 55 percent increased risk of dying from cancer. Associations of fat distribution in the body, and outcomes after cancer treatments, have been substantially observed for bowel cancer but also for breast and prostate cancer, with the improvement in survival being a result of decreased cancer deaths as well as reduced deaths from all causes.

Why is obesity harmful?

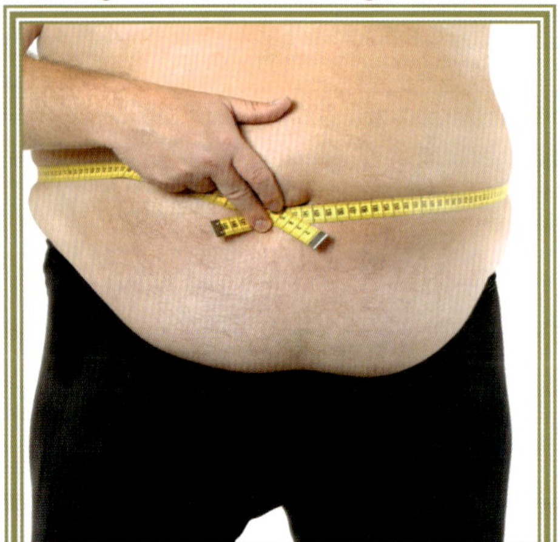

For bowel and prostate cancer the direct mechanism of being overweight is not completely certain, but for breast and endometrial cancer, the evidence is clearer. Irrespective of their daily saturated fat intake, overweight women have higher levels of the female sex hormone oestrogen and these higher levels have been reported to lower following weight reduction programmes. Of course, overweight people tend to lead more unhealthy lifestyles because they are overweight so in terms of cause there is a self-fulfilling prophesy. Furthermore, underlying mechanisms are likely to be multifactorial and linked to other lifestyle factors. These are summarised into the following categories:

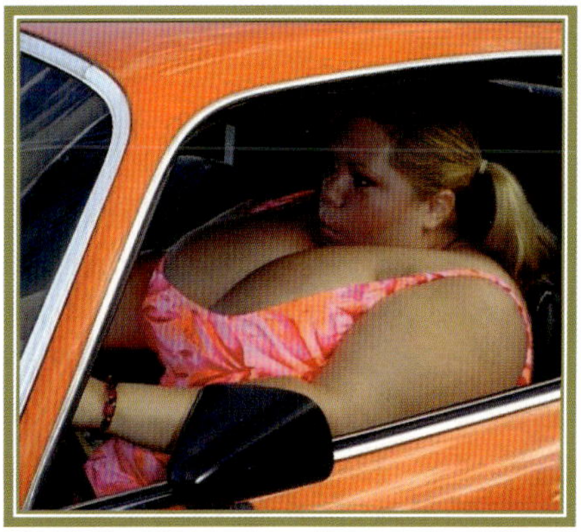

Oestrogen levels – Adiposity influences the production and availability of the body's sex hormones including oestrogen, androgens and progesterone. In post-menopausal women oestrogen is made in the peripheral body fat whilst in pre-menopausal women it is produced primarily in the ovary. This may explain a higher risk of breast and endometrial cancer for overweight post-menopausal women but not pre-menopausal women. Fortunately, oestrogen levels have been shown to reduce, following weight reduction programmes. Dietary fats may have an influence on oestrogen by a direct effect, and not via obesity. Animal and case-controlled studies have shown that diets low in fat and high in fibre are associated with a high excretion of oestrogen in the urine, which lowers blood levels irrespective of the adiposity.

Insulin and Insulin-like growth factor receptor (IGF-1) – The increased risk of cancer, or its rate of progression, is not just hormone related. We know this because overweight women have a worse prognosis after cancer, regardless of whether their cancers were sensitive to oestrogen (ER+ve) or not (ER-ve). One mechanism for a non-hormone related increased risk of cancer progression is via IGF-1, which is higher in overweight people. Higher levels have also been associated with breast, ovary and prostate cancer. This protein, also higher in sedentary individuals, has been shown to promote cancer cell division (encouraging proliferation), to inhibit apoptosis (cells not dying when they should) and encouraging cancer cells to spread. Fortunately, this cancer promoting protein drops in the blood stream if individuals lose weight or exercise.

Leptin – This is a multifunctional neuro-endocrine hormone generated primarily from fat cells. There is a direct correlation with the amount of body fat levels and circulating blood levels of leptin. There is also a correlation between leptin and serum insulin, IGF-1 and progesterone levels. Leptin has been shown in several laboratory experiments to promote proliferation, reduce apoptosis and reduce the 'stickiness' of cancer cells, encouraging them to spread and metastasise. Higher leptin levels are associated with higher expression of Cycloxidase 2 which also, as described below, encourages cancers to grow faster and to spread. An experiment with mice published in 2010 also showed that leptin is associated with a greater sense of well-being. Mice with cancer where spilt into two groups. One group had a normal cage the other had a five star version with more room, more toys and gadgets. The tumours of the mice in the second group grew significantly slower and these mice had lower leptin levels.

Progesterone – Another important hormone affecting women who are overweight is progesterone. Compared to women with pre-menopausal 'normal' weight, obese women in particular have reduced serum progesterone. There is a significant body of evidence demonstrating that progesterone plays a protective role in cancer progression, particularly in the ovaries. Progesterone increases in pregnancy, which also adds some protection against breast and ovarian cancer. In post- menopausal women who are not overweight (BMI < $35kg/m^2$), the evidence is less clear. The risk of breast cancer, in one large study from Sweden, was higher in women taking HRT containing progestin than those containing oestrogen alone. On the other hand, another study of post-menopausal women with breast cancer from Boston, USA, women with higher blood levels of oestrogen and androgens had a worse prognosis, but no such correlation was found with progesterone. It may well be therefore, that the protective effect of progesterone is greater in pre-menopausal women.

Advice how to lose weight

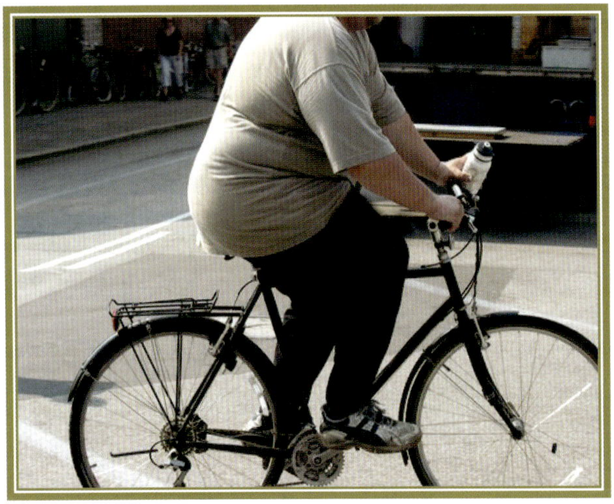

It is hard enough to lose weight at the best of times, but it is even harder after cancer, both physically and emotionally. There are several reasons why there is a very common tendency to gain weight after a diagnosis of cancer, particularly breast cancer in the early stages. It may be useful to be aware of these causes to help with the motivation and understanding to resist gaining weight:

Chemotherapy tends to cause some mild nausea, which many patients report getting worse on an empty stomach, resulting in regular snacking. With modern anti-sickness medications, unlike in the past, nausea is seldom enough to stop people eating, apart from the first few days. Many oncology units and information materials, however, still encourage patients to eat more as a throw-back to days where vomiting and weight loss was normal.

Steroids are usually given with chemotherapy drugs which encourage a strong appetite and tend to cause increased fat deposition. They also cause wakefulness at night and when they are stopped, withdrawal fatigue.

Fatigue causes disruption of a daily routine; regular activity is inevitably affected, putting further pressure on the pounds!

Hormone therapies such as tamoxifen, aromatase inhibitors and zoladex can also cause weight gain and, unlike chemotherapy, are usually given for many years after initial surgery.

Attitude, finally, but of equal importance, is the attitude of patients to food during treatments. Many people have had to be careful with their calories before they even get their diagnosis. Unfortunately, these good intentions often go out the window after their diagnosis – "dammed if I'm going to diet now I've got cancer!"

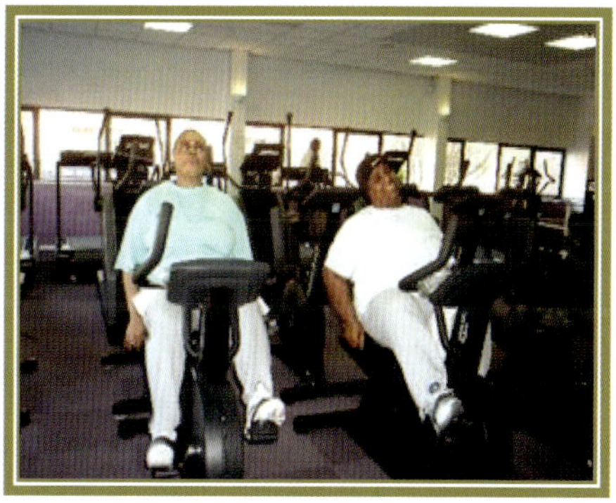

The trick is not to put on weight in the first place. This, as many people know too well, is easier said than done and if we were all perfect we would not be human. Nevertheless, despite the inevitable daunting task ahead, whatever the reasons, it is never too late to slim down. Fat is the storage of energy. When we have more energy coming in than being used it is stored under our skin and around our organs. The only answer to losing weight is to:

- Decrease the energy intake in our diet below the level we need to use.
- Increase the amount of energy we are using above that provided in our diet.

In either way the body will have to find the extra energy from our reserves. Fat will be broken down and weight will be lost. Fat is a very efficient energy source so in most cases this would have to continue for several months in order to make any difference. Unfortunately, this means that you will have to feel hungry most of the time. There really is no easy short cut! Furthermore, once the weight has been lost, the energy intake then has to match the energy requirement – so even then you cannot relax and start overeating.

Summary – tips for eating less calories and losing weight:

- Avoid faddy diets
- Don't worry about feeling hungry
- Distract yourself from thinking about food
- Avoid processed food (high fat, sugar)
- Eat less food cooked in fat e.g. deep fried batter, chips, crisps
- Avoid pastries, pies,
- Avoid biscuits and cakes (a muffin has more fat than a bacon sandwich!)
- Trim fat off meat
- Eat less meat and more fish
- Eat a large salad with every meal
- Reduce alcohol intake
- Try not to eat 3 hours before bed
- Try not to snack between meals, especially sweet snacks
- Avoid food between lunch and evening meal
- Increase exercise levels (see exercise chapter)

Chapter Six

Antioxidants
Evidence, benefits, advice

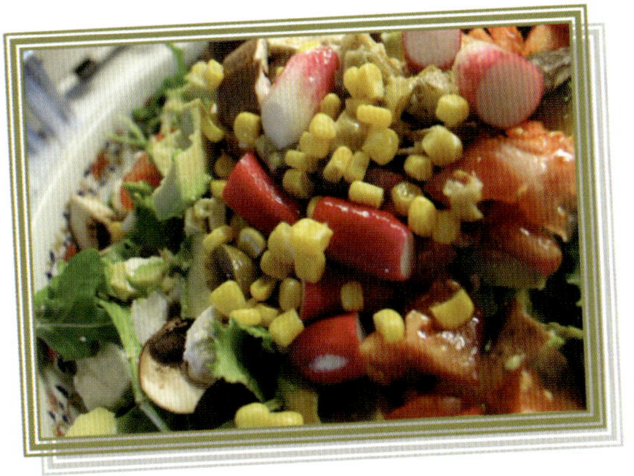

Antioxidants are natural chemicals found in healthy foods which protect us from the effects of unhealthy chemicals which damage our DNA by a chemical process called oxidation (see more below). There have been many studies linking the consumption of foods containing antioxidants with the lower risk of developing cancer. There is also evidence from the chapter above that antioxidants in foods or juices such as pomegranate and green tea could slow the rate of cancer progression. There is also evidence that their regular consumption helps prevent cancers relapsing or new similar cancers forming. For example, a study from Queensland Australia analysed over a thousand individuals who had been treated for skin cancer – a common occurrence in fair-skinned migrants to hot climates. They estimated their intake of dietary antioxidants via interviews and questionnaires over the next eight years. The results showed there was a significantly lower rate of subsequent skin cancers in those who had a high level of dietary antioxidants compared to those who did not. This was particularly associated with foods which contained lutein and xeaxanthin found commonly in leafy green vegetables. Interestingly, individuals who took supplements of vitamin E actually had a higher rate of recurrent skin cancers – there are clearly no short cuts to a healthy diet.

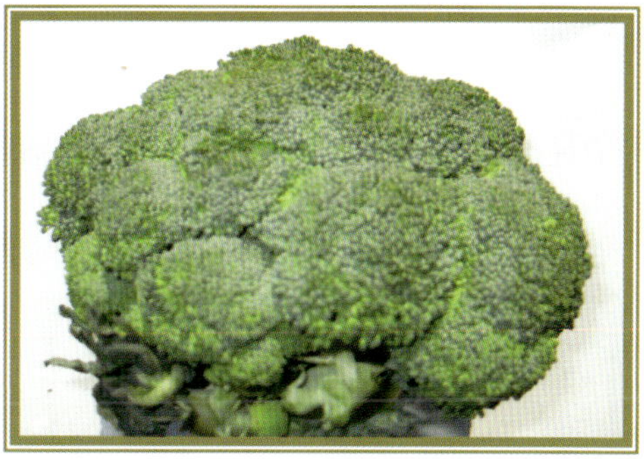

Phytochemicals are naturally occurring dietary antioxidants, otherwise referred to as polyphenols, which come from plants. They are usually classified as either non-oestrogenic, including the carotenoids (pigments) or oestrogenic (phytoestrogen), which have a similar structure or function to the body's own female hormone oestrogen.

Non-oestrogenic phytochemicals or polyphenols include the phenolic acids namely benzoic acid (hydroxybenzoic acid, gallic acid) and cinnamic acid (caffeic and quinic acid), together with the non-oestrogenic flavanoids, including anthocyanidins, the flavanols (catechins and proanthocyanidins), lignans and stilbens. These phytochemicals do not act via a hormonal route but have been shown to have a direct anti-cancer effect. Kaempferol, found in broccoli, asparagus and kale, in particular, has been shown to reduce the risks of ovary, prostate and breast cancer within a large study of dietary patterns among nurses. Green tea, for example, contains a variety of phytochemicals of which the epigallocatechin gallate is the most abundant. This antioxidant has been extensively investigated in the laboratory. When added to cancer cells grown in a laboratory, it has been shown to induce apoptosis (i.e. tells the cancer cells to die when they ought). Tumour arrest and prevention of metastases were also demonstrated following injection into mice bearing prostate cancers. In humans, both green and black tea consumption has been associated with lower risks of developing cancer, and those with established cancer have better prognostic features.

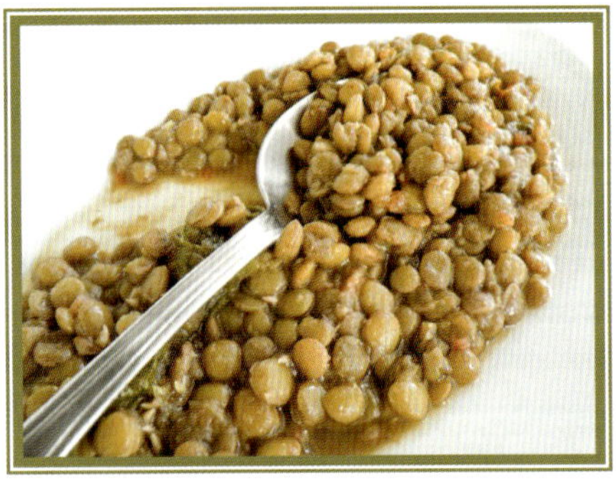

Legumes: such as beans, pulses, nuts and cereals have been shown to be rich in the phytochemical inositol pentakisphosphate (InsP5). Lentils are a particularly good source. This chemical has been shown in mouse models to significantly inhibit the growth of cancer cells. It also appears to enhance the beneficial effects of chemotherapy without increasing their side effects and further development of this compound is being investigated for future clinical use.

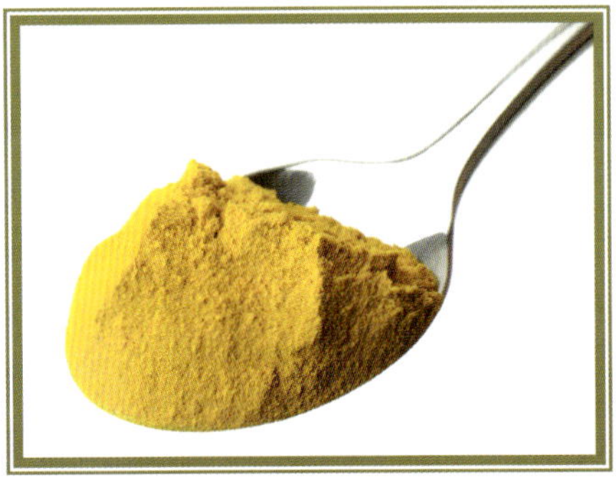

Curcumin (turmeric) and pepper: A number of lab studies have demonstrated the benefits of these spices. Research conducted at the University of Michigan Comprehensive Cancer Centre found that compounds in black pepper and curry powder help halt the growth of stem cells that give rise to breast cancer. After applying piperine, found in black pepper, and curcumin, the main ingredient in the curry spice turmeric, to breast cancer cells in a laboratory dish, researchers found that the combination reduced the number of cancer cells, but did not harm normal breast cells. A team from Columbia University found that curcumin and ginger reduced prostate cancer cell growth and increased the rate of programmed cell death. They are now investigating a combination of turmeric and ginger in humans. In support of this, following an environmental study of the local population, researchers at Leicester University have postulated that the antioxidants found in spices such as capsaicin, the chemical responsible for the heat in chillies, and curcumin, the chemical that gives turmeric its yellow colour, could be responsible for the low levels of colon cancer in the Asian community.

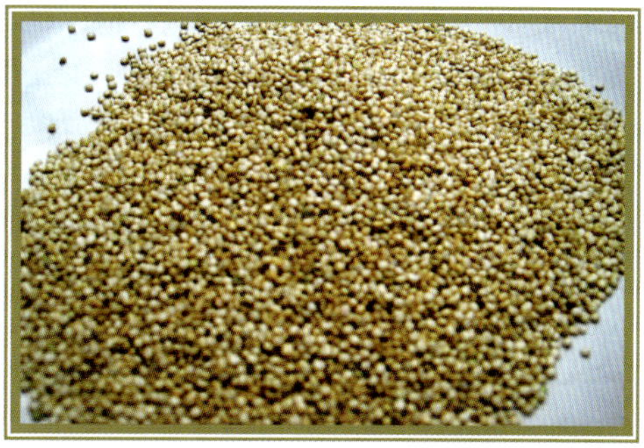

Oestrogenic phytochemicals; Although many of these substances also have antioxidant properties they are classed separately from antioxidants because they also have weak female hormone (oestrogenic) properties. Collectively they are referred to as phytoestrogens, and include flavones, isoflavones, flavanones (genistein, daidzein, glycitein and equaol) derived, in human diets, mainly from soybeans. The other type called lignans (mainly enterolactone) are derived mainly from legumes, including peas, lentils, quinoa and other beans.

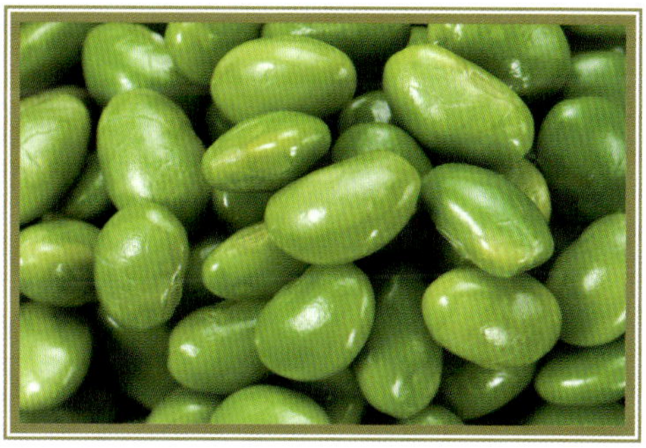

The phytoestrogens and cancer story is becoming clearer as good scientific data is emerging. Dietary intake potentially creates a more favourable hormonal milieu for men with prostate cancer by inhibiting 5-alpha-reductase, the enzyme responsible for converting testosterone to the more active metabolite dihydrotestosterone. The benefit in men was also highlighted in a study from the USA which found that a natural compound found in hop plants might help to prevent prostate cancer. This supports previous lab research which revealed that xanthohumol can effectively bind to oestrogen receptors, and may work similarly with testosterone, potentially interrupting the development of prostate cancer proliferation and spread.

In women, historically, the implication of benefit stems from the finding that populations and cultures that have had a high dietary intake of phytoestrogenic foods, such as those from the Far East, have the lowest incidence of breast cancer and menopausal symptoms such as hot flushes and osteoporosis. After cancer, soya products, particularly those which are fermented (miso, tofu, tempura) which are more easily digested, are also likely to be beneficial in terms of reducing the risk of osteoporosis, relapse rate and improving the overall survival. In sensible amounts phytoestrogens in these foods attach to the ER but only have weak oestrogenic activity. They therefore dilute the effect of their own body's oestrogen. Genestein attaches to the ER in the same way as tamoxifen – inhibiting the oestrogen effect on tumours, but stimulating the bones and uterus. The largest population study in the world so far was called the Shanghai Breast Cancer Survival Study and involved Chinese women patients who had completed treatments for breast cancer. Published in 2009, it demonstrated that soy foods are very likely to be safe, and probably beneficial, for breast cancer survivors. They looked at the intake of soy products such as soy milk, tofu, edamame, pad thai, or miso soup. Researchers at Vanderbilt University analysed 5,042 Chinese women aged 20 to 75. The investigators found that patients with the highest intake had a 29 percent lower risk of death during the study period and a 32 percent lower risk of breast cancer recurrence compared to patients with the lowest intake of soy foods, which was measured by either soy protein or soy isoflavone intake. What's more, the association between soy and a reduced risk of death held true even for women with oestrogen receptor-positive cancers and women taking tamoxifen. The study was however done in China, where soy intake tends to be up to tens times higher than in the west. The anti-cancer benefit may also be via the antioxidant effect of the healthier food rather than the oestrogenic action, and some suggest there may be other factors in the East which are beneficial, so simply taking high phytoestrogen-containing foods such as soya products may not translate into a western diet.

The benefits of phytoestrogen foods may not translate into phytoestrogen chemicals extracted into a supplement form. In this case the oestrogenic effect can become too strong and the oestrogen receptor can start to be stimulated so as to cause potential tumour growth. This was highlighted in an experiment with monkeys who were given a high dose phytoestrogen extract. After several months the uterus started to thicken, indicating a negative oestrogenic affect. Other animal studies have also showed that strong phytoestrogen supplements could potentially stimulating tumour cell growth as well as having effects on the body's normal cells sensitive to oestrogen. Furthermore a well conducted placebo-controlled study of phytoestrogen supplements among patients with breast cancer showed no benefit regarding hot flushes.

Despite these potential concerns it appears that phytoestrogen-containing foods after breast cancer and prostate cancer are safe and may be beneficial in terms of relapse rates. A large dietary and lifestyle study, currently underway in the UK, will hopefully confirm this conclusion. The DietCompLfy trial is studying women who have been successfully treated with breast cancer, and over the following years will measure levels of phytoestrogens in their blood stream, as well as analysing a detailed dietary history. The study will compare the phytoestrogen exposure between those who have relapsed and those who have survived. The results are not likely to be available until 2015.

How could antioxidants help?

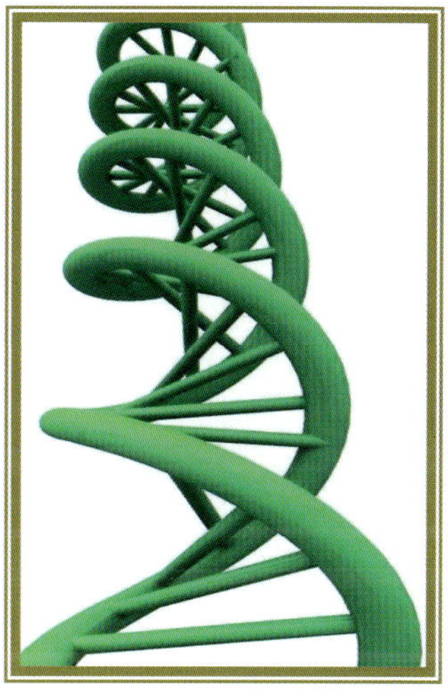

Antioxidants are thought to wield their anti-cancer properties by directly or indirectly counterbalancing the superoxide free radicals generated from our diet or environment. They stop free radical damage to the DNA, as described, before it can rearrange the genes within the cells leading to the development of cancer. Although patients with established cancer have already sustained sufficient DNA damage in order to mutate from normal healthy cells to cancer cells, the process is by no means over. Avoiding further DNA insults prevents further mutation that can encourage less aggressive malignant cells or pre-malignant cells to transform into more aggressive types that are more likely to grow and spread faster.

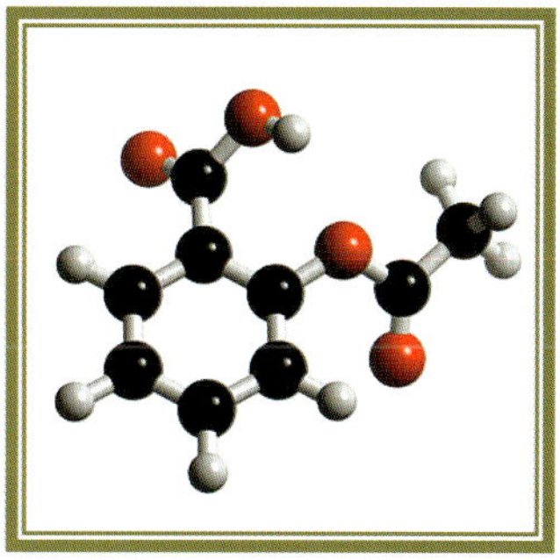

Antioxidants, otherwise known as free radical scavengers, are likely to also have further anti-cancer mechanisms of action; they have been shown to stop cancer cells progressing to a more aggressive form (becoming less differentiated). They slow the rate at which cancer cells divide and multiply (reduce proliferation), and each of these actions may be independent of their free radical scavenging benefits. Studies involving antioxidants have shown how they can fight cancer by reducing cells' propensity to spread (metastasise) and also encourage them to die when they ought to (like normal cells) in a process called apoptosis. Antioxidants are commonly found in foods which also have oestrogenic properties and visa versa, although these have completely separate influences on the cancer process. These are called phytoestrogens and the issues related to cancer are discussed above.

Dietary advice for a healthy antioxidant intake

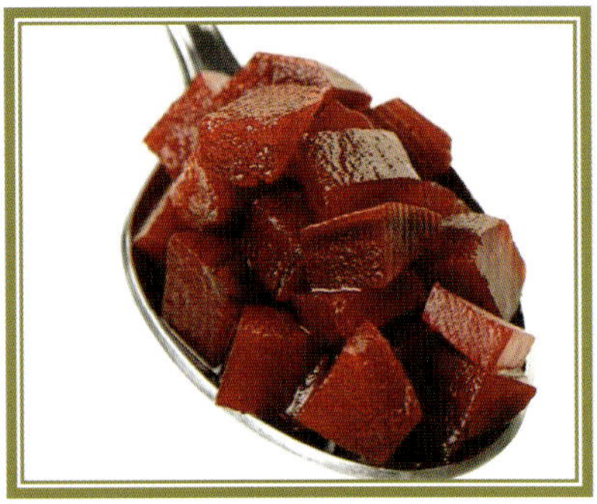

Antioxidants are found naturally in a wide variety of healthy foods. As luck would have it, these foods are generally tasty and are healthy for a wide variety of reasons other than cancer. They are particularly abundant in spices, dark green leafy vegetables, herbs, calciferous vegetables, colourful fruits, beetroot, herbs, legumes, nuts and berries. Drinks such as traditional green and black tea contain a variety of phytochemicals and many other fruit and herbal teas are also now readily available. Phytochemicals can also be found in less obvious sources such as honey, coffee, chocolate, the apples used for cider, beers and the tannin component of red wine, although the benefits of these later drinks are diluted by the other harmful ingredients such as alcohol, fat, carcinogens and sugar. The level of antioxidant may also vary between brands and varieties, where and how the food is grown and how it is prepared. Dry fruits, for example tend to concentrate the anti-oxidant content compared to the fresh original but this does not necessary make them healthier overall.

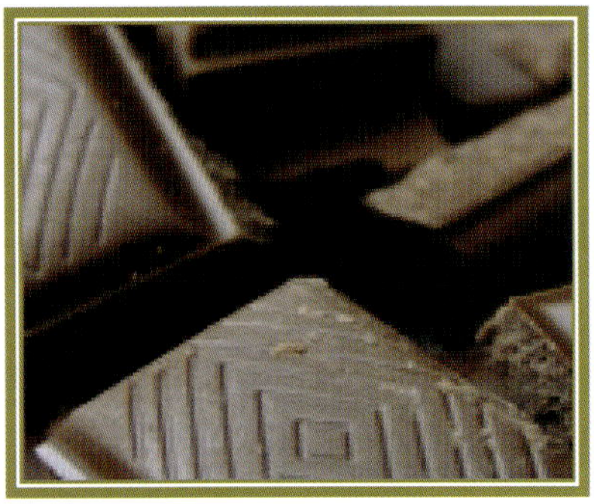

In an attempt to introduce some science to the discussion, the USA Food and Drug Administration (FDA) have published league tables of various foods' ability to scavenge and remove DNA-damaging free radicals. They rank food according to their Oxygen Radical Absorbance Capacity (ORAC). The FDA has recommended over 3,000 ORAC units a day and the ideal amount in the diet. The tables below list some examples of common foods in terms of their AC rating derived from the 2010 FDA analysis: When viewing these tables, remember that these figures are concentrations so, for example a few hazels nuts may have the same absolute quantity of antioxidants as an apple which has a bigger volume.

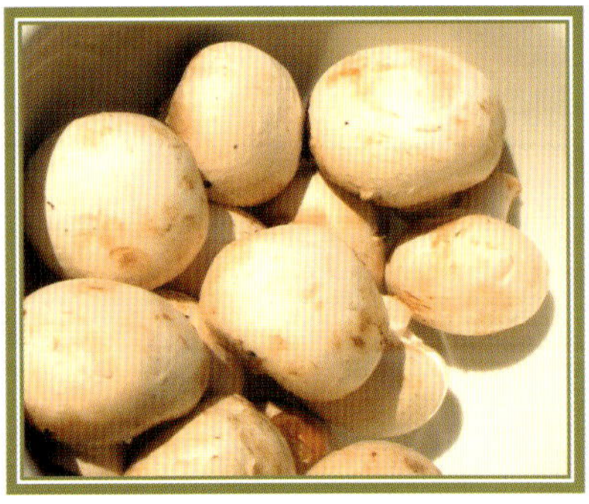

Table - the ORAC rating over 2000 micromol TE/ 100g of popular foods:

FOOD	**ORAC (units /100 g)**
Wide Tibetan goji berries	>20,000
Vietnamese gac	>20,000
Quinoa	>20,000
Sorghum	>20,000
Pecan nuts	17,000
Elderberries	14,600
Walnuts	13,000
Dried pears	9,500
Cranberries	9,000
Currents & raisins	8000-10,000
Hazelnuts	9,600
Artichokes boiled	9,500
Blueberries wild	9,000
Pistachio nuts	7,500
Chocolate (bars)	7,200
Lentils	7,200
Artichokes - raw	6,500
Blackberries	5,900
Prunes	5,770
Raspberries	5,000
Fresh pomegranate	4,500
Almonds	4,500
Blueberries farmed	4,200
Peaches dried	4,000
Apples – red delicious	4,000
Strawberries	3,700
Cherries	3,700
Commercially farmed goji berries	3,300
Dried apricots	3,200
Broccoli - raw	3,100
Cabbage - red	3,100
Peanuts	3,100
Apples – granny smith	3,000
Savoy cabbage - boiled	2,100
Whole pears	2,000
Asparagus - raw	2,000

Table: ORAC of popular foods 500-2000 units/100g

FOOD	ORAC (units/100g)
Spinach	1,700
Popcorn	1,700
Kale	1,700
Radishes	1,700
Asparagus - boiled	1,600
Broccoli - boiled	1,600
Lettuce – green raw	1,500
Avocado	1,370
Brussels sprouts	980
Mushrooms	950
Alfalfa sprouts	930
Broccoli florets	890
White onion	860
Beets	840
Tomato	770
Oranges	750
Red grapes	739
Red bell peppers	710
Carrots	650
Peas	500

Antioxidant-rich foods?

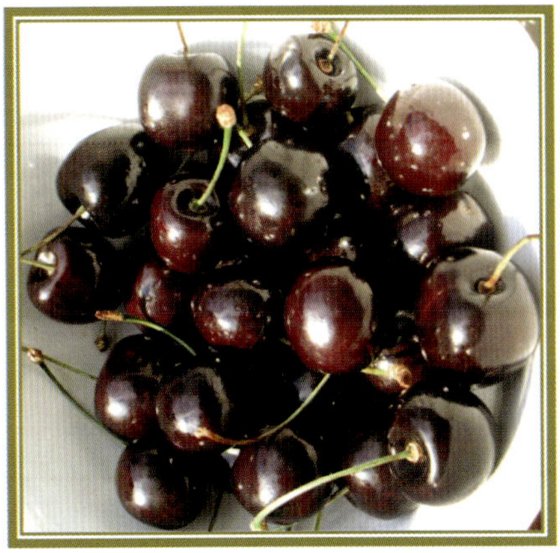

The expression "superfood" is commonly used in the media and health magazines, generally referring to foods which contain high levels of antioxidants although no particular threshold of ORAC has been chosen for a food to be designated "super". For a food to be particularly healthy, of course, it should contain a high content of a variety of health elements ranging from vitamins, essential fatty acids, minerals, fibre and well as antioxidants. Examples, of such foods are described at the end of this section under the heading "Superfoods".

More recently an increasing number of foods, more uncommon in the Western World, have been discovered, which have extremely high antioxidant concentrations. These are generally originating from Asia, China and the Far East. Many of these more exotic fruits are often more conveniently available in the dried form, in supplements or available in juices. That is not to say that some foods commonly grown in The West can also have good levels of antioxidants with the level of intake depending on the quantity eaten, the type and how they are prepared and farmed.

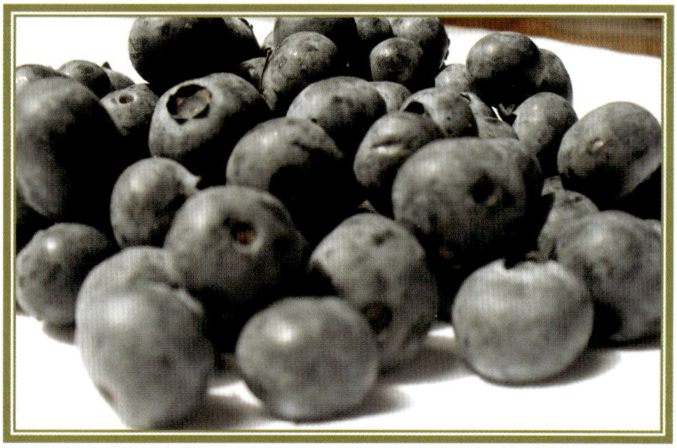

Berries, for example, such as strawberries, blueberries and blackberries have a high antioxidant content if eaten in sufficient quantities, as do colourful vegetables such as beetroot and radishes. Fruit which is dried has a higher ORAC rating because the flesh is more concentrated. Raw calciferous vegetables have more antioxidants than those boiled. Colourful varieties of any fruit (red apples) and vegetables (red cabbage) have a higher ORAC than less colourful varieties. The ORAC is not the whole story; broccoli green tea and pomegranate, for example, appear to have anticancer properties over and above their antioxidant activities. Also be careful how these foods are produced. Some are now intensively farmed and are sprayed with large amounts of pesticides and herbicides and as they have a high surface area they may not be as healthy as they seem. Also, probably because of intensive farming methods the antioxidant level may change from country to country or over time. For example, look how the ORAC rating of goji berries has dropped over the years. The wild varieties always have more antioxidants and by definition are organic. Blackberry picking is therefore a very healthy activity and is strongly encouraged.

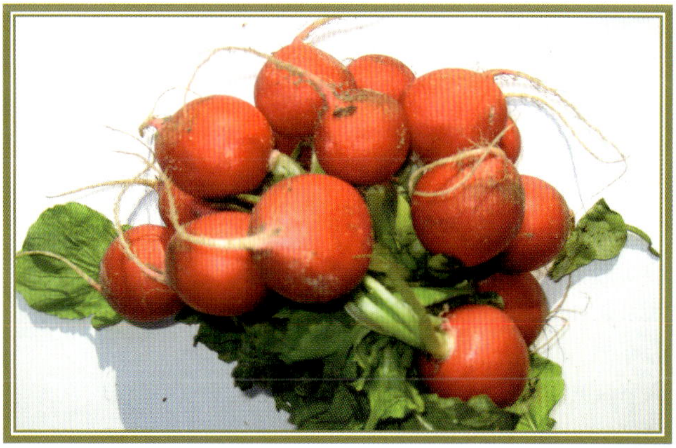

Spices

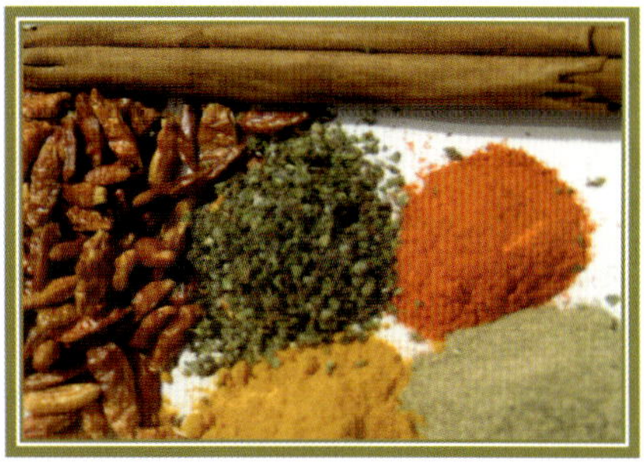

Spices have more antioxidants than any other foods but tend only to be consumed in small amounts. Unlike vitamins and other nutrients, antioxidants are not destroyed by cooking processes; in fact the table below demonstrates how the drying concentrates the levels. If spices are added regularly to meals they are likely to significantly increase the antioxidant power of the diet. In support of this, researchers at Leicester University, as mentioned above, have postulated following an environmental study of the local population that the antioxidants found in spices such as capsaicin, the chemical responsible for the heat in chillies, and curcumin, the chemical that gives turmeric its yellow colour are thought to be responsible for the low levels of colon cancer in the Asian community.

Spice	**ORAC (units /100 grams)**
Basil, fresh	4,805
Dried basil	61,063
Marjoram, fresh	27,297
Coriander leaves	5,141
Ground dried cloves	290,283
Fresh Sage	119,900
Fresh peppermint	13,978
Ground cinnamon	131,420
Cumin seed	50,372
Garlic powder	6,665
Dried sage	119,929
Fresh thyme	27,426
Dried thyme	157,380
Dried turmeric	127,068
Dried vanilla beans	122,400
Dried rosemary	165,280
Black pepper	34,053
Dried parsley	73,670
Pepper, red or Cayenne source	19,671
Dried chilli powder	23,636
Raw ginger	14840
Ground ginger	39,041
Dried ground oregano	175,295

Green tea

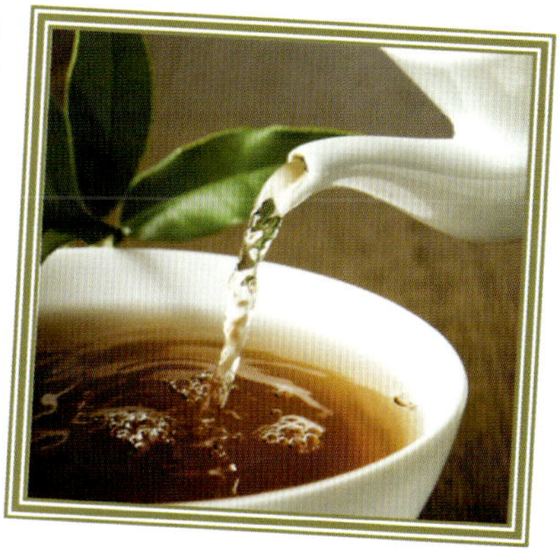

It may surprise some people that both green tea and the black stuff we've been drinking in the UK for several hundred years come from the same plant, Camelia Sinensis, found in tropical and sub-tropical regions like India and China. When dried, black tea is fermented and oxidised. Green tea is left unfermented, and then merely steamed. Many experts now believe that green tea is thus a better, more whole, source of natural chemicals like proteins, sugars and vitamins and, in particular, natural polyphenols and antioxidants.

The polyphenol, epigallocatechin gallate (EGCG), seems to be the most active antioxidant within green tea. In terms of reducing the risk of developing cancer, research from Perth University in 2002 showed drinking just one cup per day reduced ovarian cancer risk by 60 per cent, and in 2003 the same group showed it reduced prostate cancer risk by 33 per cent. As well as the antioxidant properties, Green tea´s active ingredients are also thought to be anti-oestrogenic. This was confirmed in a further study in 2009, which showed that Green Tea could reduce breast cancer rates by 40 per cent. And if women ate mushrooms daily as well as drinking green tea, only 1 in ten of them would get breast cancer compared to those who consumed neither. Furthermore, EGCG has been found to block an enzyme, ornithine decarboxylase, which tells cells to proliferate faster. As well as slowing cell growth by blocking this enzyme, has also been shown to cause cancer cell death or apoptosis.

Research from the Shanghai Cancer Institute looked at the risk of oesophageal cancer among those who neither drank alcohol nor smoked (two of the main causes). They found drinking green tea further and significantly reduced their risk, starting at 57 per cent in the no alcohol group and 60 per cent amongst the non-smokers. Overall the more green tea drunk, the better the results.

After the development of cancer, green tea has also been shown to be beneficial. The prestigious Mayo Clinic in the USA researched green tea in patients with chronic lymphocytic leukaemia and concluded that over 4 cups per day prevented leukaemia cells developing. In fact the Phase I Clinical Trials showed that high doses of tea helped decrease the white cell count by one third in CLL patients. Those people with enlarged lymph nodes showed a 50 per cent reduction.

Other studies have suggested that green tea has a beneficial effect in breast cancer, liver cancer and colon cancer prevention, and there is also work showing it improves the positive effects and reduces the negative effects with people undergoing radiotherapy. On a cautionary note, it is not wise to drink excessive amounts during chemotherapy as the powerful antioxidants can repair the chemotherapy damage on the cancer cells and therefore actually prevent the chemotherapy doing its job. Of course one or two cups is fine.

As mentioned above, a small study from Louisiana State University has found that green tea may reduce the levels of some compounds linked to prostate cancer progression. Through their study of prostate of 26 men with prostate cancer who were given a concentrated extract of tea polyphenols for an average of 34-days, they report a significant reduction in the levels of several growth factors that promote cancer as well as reductions in PSA.

Other factors to consider when drinking green tea: It does contain relatively high levels of caffeine so be careful not to drink it in the evenings; also tremors and agitation can occur at high levels of consumption. Other side effects such as diarrhoea and stomach irritation have been reported. The main objection to green tea is its taste but the bitter taste can be offset in other blends, for example green tea with jasmine or with lemongrass, or by sweetening with honey. The Japanese in particular have a whole range of soft drinks based on green tea but these do have quite a high sugar content. Another downside of green tea is that it can cause discolouration of the teeth, turning them yellow or even green. The polyphenols in green tea are potent antioxidants and have also been shown to protect against heart disease, as they can prevent the oxidation of LDL into cholesterol.

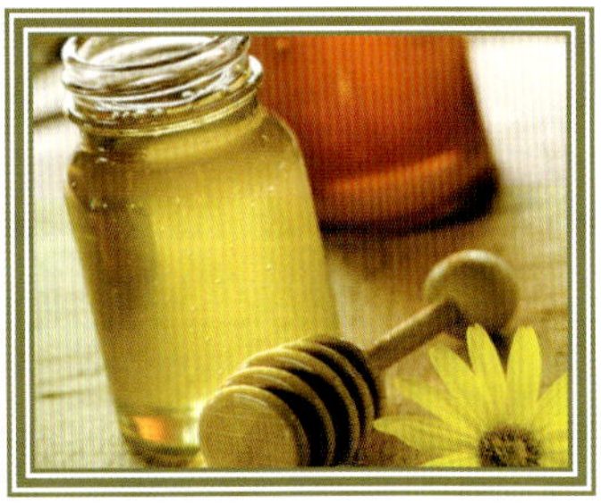

Researchers from the University of Pennsylvania and Boston Biomedical Institute have also shown that EGCG helps protect the brain from the build up of amyloid proteins. They concluded that Green Tea would help prevent Parkinson´s and Alzheimer's, and could also be used in treatment. Other 2009 researches from the American College of Nutrition found that regular Green Tea consumption could prevent colds and flu. The study compared people taking a green tea supplement with those taking a placebo and showed one third less colds and flu in the green tea supplement group. Green tea is also alleged to improve skin tone, smooth out wrinkles and even to help you slim. EGCG is also known to cause good bacteria in the intestine to flourish, thus aiding recovery after antibiotics or chemotherapy.

Calciferous vegetables

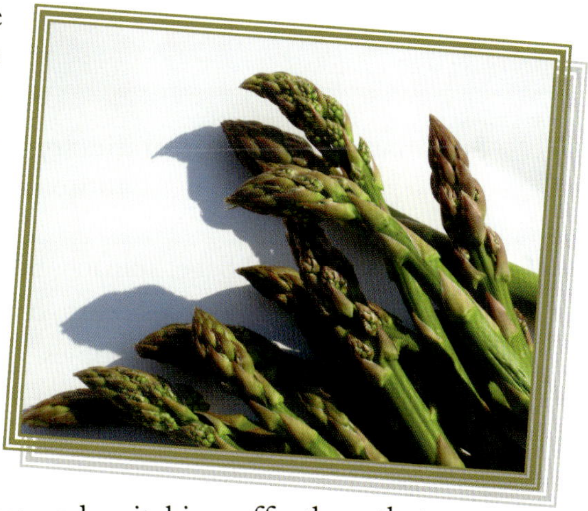

Not all superfoods have to come from tropical climates or remote locations. Biologists at Britain's Institute of Food Research published a study which showed that the healthy chemicals found in asparagus and broccoli can prevent precancerous cells in the prostate progressing to more aggressive cancers. They found that just a few more portions of these calciferous vegetables each week initiates hundreds of genetic changes, activating some genes that fight cancer and switching off others that fuel them. These vegetables contain a variety of healthy antioxidants but the group most touted as significant are called isothiocyanates (indole-3-carbinol and sulforophane). The trial split participants into two groups of 24 men with pre-cancerous lesions and had them eat four extra servings of either broccoli, asparagus or peas each week for a year. The researchers then took tissue samples over the course of the study and found that men who ate broccoli showed hundreds of changes in genes known to play a role in fighting cancer.

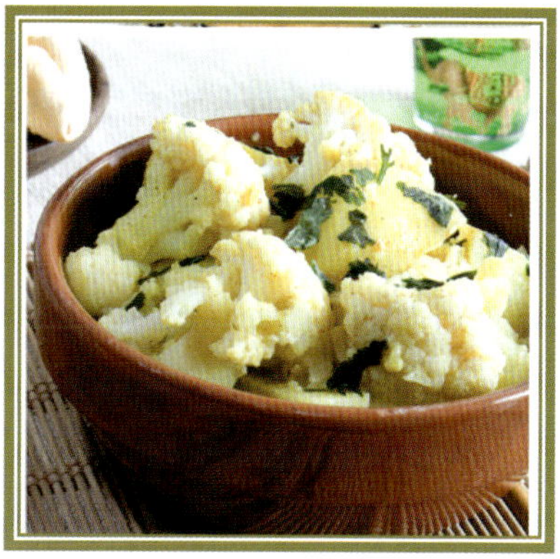

The researchers believe this benefit would likely be the same for other cruciferous vegetables including brussels sprouts, watercress, cauliflower, rocket or argula, kohl rabi, turnips, daikon, cabbage or kale, pak choy and radish. Broccoli and asparagus, however, has a particularly powerful type of isothiocyanate – sulforaphane glucosinate, which the researchers think gives the green vegetable an extra cancer-fighting kick. The broccoli and asparagus eaters showed about 400 to 500 of the positive genetic changes with men carrying a gene called GSTM1 enjoying the most benefit. About half the population have this gene.

The researchers did not observe the men long enough to see who got cancer but it is a very logical conclusion that just a few more vegetable portions each week can make a big difference. Furthermore it is also likely that these vegetables work the same way in other parts of the body and probably protect people against a whole range of cancers.

Summary – Examples of dietary sources of phytochemicals and antioxidants:

- Green vegetables – cabbage, spinach, broccoli,
- Salad – dark green salad leaves, leeks, onions, celery
- Fruits (especially ripe) – plums, apples, apricots, pears, oranges, grapes
- Tropical fruits – pomegranates, kiwis, oranges, nectarines, bananas, gac
- Mushrooms – white and wild varieties
- Dried fruits – raisin, prunes, apricots
- Berries – cherries, blueberries, strawberries, cranberries, chocolate, goji berries
- Legumes – beans, peas, lentils, quinoa, chick peas
- Nuts – hazelnuts, almonds, walnuts, peanuts, cashews, brazils
- Herbs – garlic, parsley, mint, coriander, thyme, rosemary,.
- Spices – turmeric, chilli, cumin, curcumin
- Drinks – white, green and black teas, red wine

Food phytochemicals also classed as carotenoids (pigments):

- Vegetables – carrots, red and yellow peppers
- Fruits – red grapes, tomatoes and strawberries
- Berries – blackberries, blackcurrant, goji berries, cherries and cranberries
- Herbs and spices – chillies, paprika and turmeric

Food phytochemicals which are phytoestrogens (oestrogenic properties):

- Soy products – tofu, soya milk and yoghurt, miso soup
- Legumes – soy, lentils, red kidney bean and pinto (baked beans)
- Seeds and grains – flaxseed, linseeds and cereals
- Herbs – sage, parsley, thyme, rosemary, saw pallmentto

Chapter Seven

Dietary vitamin intake

Evidence, benefits, advice

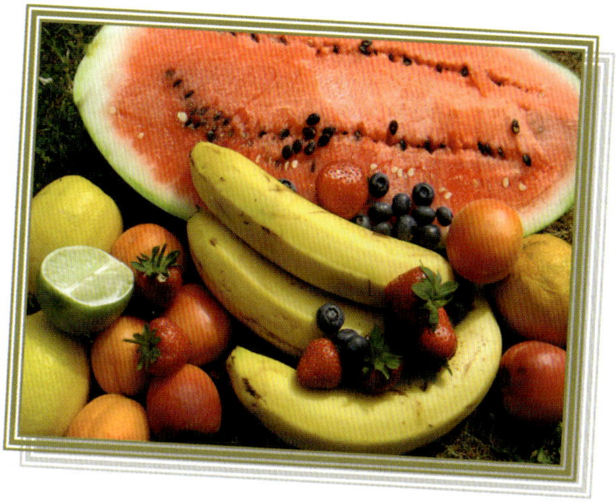

These are chemicals which are essential to the normal biochemical function of our body's metabolism. They cannot be made internally and without them we can contract disease and illness. The most notable historical example of vitamin deficiency was scurvy among British sailors, which was corrected by consuming vitamin C through eating limes (earning their nick-name: 'Limeys').

In South and Central America the reliance on corn as a main carbohydrate caused a deficiency in vitamin B_6 resulting in a disease called pellagra. The manifestation of rashes, weakness and malabsorption devastated large communities until it was discovered that adding limes to corn enabled the vitamin B_6 to be absorbed – hence the propensity for limes with tortilla and other corn dishes to this day.

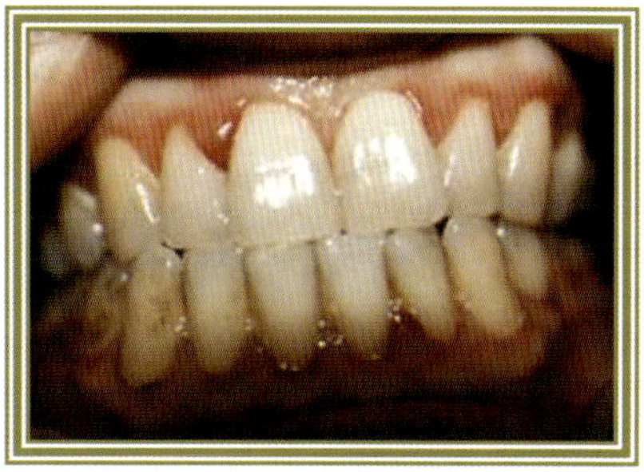

In the Far East the reliance on rice only as a stable carbohydrate source, low in thiamine, caused vitamin B_1 deficiency resulting in nerve damage and a disease known as beriberi. Asians, particularly women and children immigrating to the UK in the 60's, had a high incidence of the bone diseases osteomalacia and rickets due to vitamin D and calcium deficiency brought on by the lack of sunshine and low dairy diet.

In modern society, however, with the wide choices of food available to us, overt vitamin deficiencies are unlikely. These historical examples do nevertheless serve as a good lesson that it is important to vary food sources. Too much reliance of one source could lead to sub-clinical deficiencies which, although unlikely to manifest themselves as the full blown syndrome, may impair the body's ability to fight cancer. The most important vitamins implicated in the cancer process, described in the last chapter, include vitamins A, C, D and E, but it would wise to aim for a diet which provided adequate amounts of *all* the vitamins as well as the essential fatty acids and minerals.

Vitamin A and carotenoids

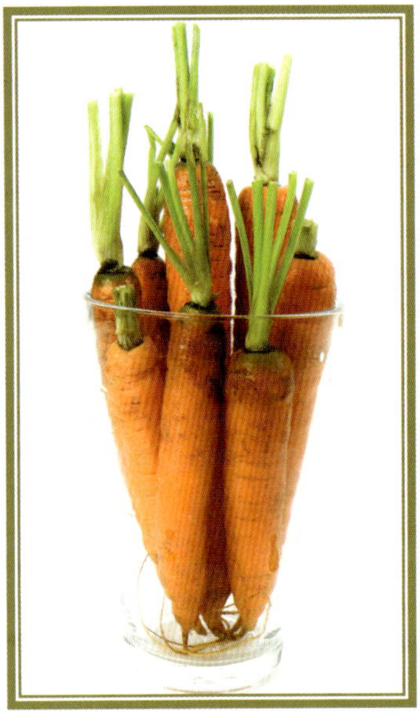

Vitamin A is a fat-soluble essential vitamin found in fish and dairy food in the isoform retinol. It can also be ingested in fruits and vegetables that contain carotenoid provitamins such as beta-carotene which is then metabolised to vitamin A. Prostate cancer cells grown in the laboratory have demonstrated an increased apoptosis (programmed cell death) and reduced proliferation (growth) when exposed to synthetic retinoids such as fenretinide. Likewise in genetically susceptible mice, fenretinide reduced the incidence of prostate cancer by 49 per cent. Carotenoids, particularly the beta-carotene called lycopene, are naturally occurring pigments found in Vietnamese gac, chillies, palm oil, papayas, mangoes, tomatoes, peppers, carrots, leafy vegetables and other colourful foods. Unlike other antioxidants, carotenoids such as lycopene are not destroyed by the cooking process, so although they are only found in relatively small quantities in tomatoes, higher concentrations can be found in tomato sauces and pastes. However caution should be exercised regarding taking purified carotenoids in the form of supplemented tablets (lycopene, xeaxanthin and lutein). In a laboratory experiment, this time in rats with cancer, half had their diet supplemented with dried tomato powder and the other half with the carotenoid lycopene. After only a few weeks there was a measurable difference in the growth rate of their tumour in favour of the natural tomato powder but not the pure lycopene. The processed pure lycopene had not worked but the tomatoes had!

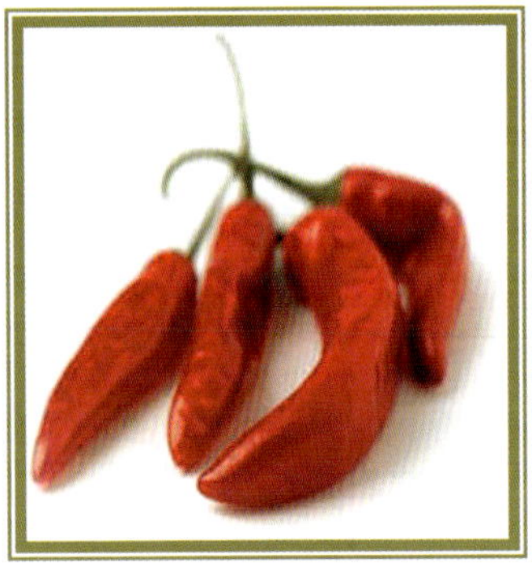

Even more concerning is that they may actually cause harm. A landmark European study evaluated a large group of individuals who had a high risk of developing lung cancer (previous cancer of the throat or heavy smokers). They were given carotenoid supplements in the form of beta carotene and vitamin E in the form of alpha-tocopherol. After several years, involving thousands of participants, the trial was stopped because the results were showing an elevated risk of both lung and prostate cancer!

Another large human dietary prevention study combined beta-carotene with retinol (Vitamin A), and showed complex but fascinating results which probably provide the best insight to date on the whole supplementation story. In this eloquent study, people who started the trial with naturally low blood levels of beta-carotene had lower levels of prostate cancer after years of beta-carotene supplementation. Those people who had high initial levels of beta-carotene, following supplementation, ended up with a higher risk of cancer, particularly prostate. This trial provides a clear take-home message – correcting a natural or acquired deficit is beneficial, but too much of a good thing, as in this case of a single anti-oxidant, is harmful.

However, in a subsequent prospective study involving 10,472 U.S. men, no reduction in prostate cancer incidence has yet been demonstrated, although there have only been 93 events so far in the 5-year follow-up period. The other trials of the carotenoid lycopene are reviewed above as are the preventative studies combined with Vitamin E. Evidence of a benefit for extra supplements in humans with an adequate diet has therefore not yet been established.

Vitamin B

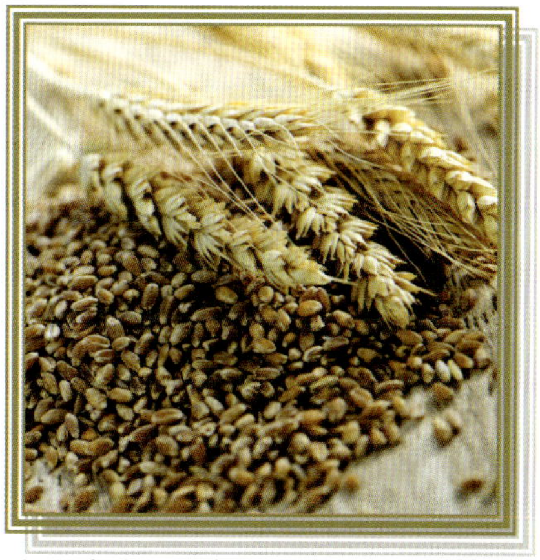

These are water soluble vitamins which have several subtypes, the most important being vitamin B1 (thiamine) Folic acid, vitamin B6 and Vitamin B12. Vitamin B_{12} is found in meat and, to a lesser extent, legumes, although alternative sources include seaweed. The other B vitamins are generally found in grains such as wheat, barley and oats, so usual sources in western diets come from bread and cereals. There are no studies suggesting that vitamin B_1, folic acid or $Vitamin_{12}$ deficiency can increase the risk of cancer but there are concerns that an excess can increase the risk. A Swedish study published in 2009 suggested that Vitamin B_6 appeared to play a role in preventing colon cancer. After reviewing data from 13 dietary studies, they concluded that individuals with adequate blood levels of pyridoxal-phosphate (PLP), the main active coenzyme form of vitamin B_6, had a lower incidence of colon cancer, whereas those with low levels had a higher risk. They also showed that it was important to have adequate levels through a healthy diet rather than Vitamin B_6 supplement because those who took them did not have a lower risk of cancer.

Other studies have demonstrated more sinister concerns with Vitamin B supplements. A study from Norway published in 2009 investigated whether giving vitamin B supplements to patients with angina or following a heart attack could reduce the incidence of another cardiac event. In total 6,837 patients between 1998-2005 were included in the trial; half were given placebo and half oral treatment with either folic acid (0.8 mg/d) alone or folic acid plus vitamin B_{12} and vitamin B_6 or vitamin B_{12} and vitamin B_6 alone. After three years there was no cardiac benefit but a significant increase in cancer (mainly lung cancer) in participants who received folic acid either alone or with Vitamin B_{12} although vitamin B_{12} alone did not increase the risk.

These results were confirmed in a separate post heart-attack study also published in 2009. Men who took folic acid supplements were more than twice as likely to develop prostate cancer compared with men who took a placebo. Researchers noted that the estimated prostate cancer risk was 9.7 per cent for participants in the folic acid group and 3.3 per cent for the placebo group. This study made another interesting observation: it also found that, independent of whether they took a supplement or not, the prostate cancer incidence was slightly lower in men who had adequate amounts of folate in their diet.

These trials tell us that individuals eating diets with inadequate Vitamin B_6 and folic acid may have a higher incidence of cancer. Taking supplements of Vitamin B_6 has no benefit and supplements of folic acid increase the risk of cancer particularly prostate and lung.

Vitamin C

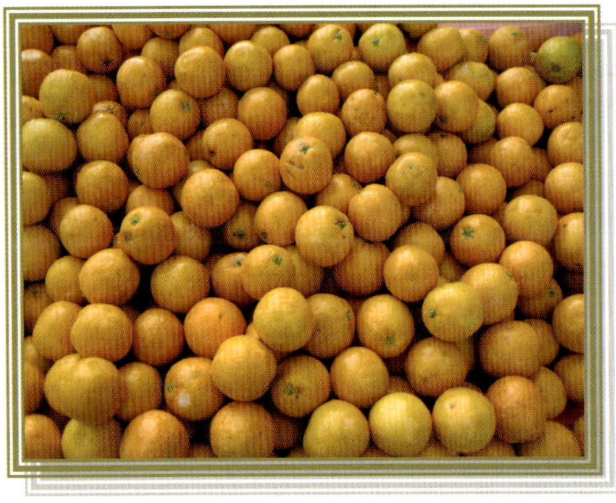

A water soluble vitamin found in citrus fruits, berries, nuts and leafy green vegetables. *Vitamin C* is involved in the mechanism which enables DNA to 'sense' the damage done by free radicals, by integrating with the iron imbedded in DNA. This process facilitates DNA repair and is therefore a significant aspect of immune surveillance. This is an important factor in the first stage of cancer development, which takes place in the seconds between the DNA damage to the subsequent mutation, gene rearrangement and then cancer. This protection is needed every minute of every day as, according to estimates, each cell in the body can be expected to suffer approximately 100,000 potentially DNA-damaging events daily. So a healthy DNA repair system is imperative. Vitamin C has also been shown to protect the intracellular component cell from toxic products such as hydrogen peroxide. This is thought to be via a mechanism which prevents inhibition of gap-junction intercellular communication (GJIC). Inhibition of GJIC is related to carcinogenesis and tumour promotion. Convincing experiments in humans in relation to cancer have not been carried out, but in very large doses vitamin C could to be harmful.

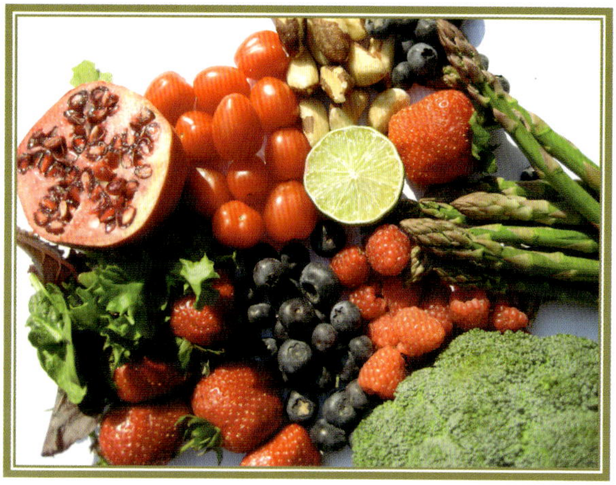

Vitamin C only lasts in the body for a short time, so fruits and berries have to be eaten regularly. Improvements in food logistics have ensured that the availability of fruits from around the world has never been so good. Both conventional fruits and exotic varieties often have very high levels of vitamin C. As fruit ripens the vitamin C content increases, so don't be put off by a few soft bits! Fruit juices are a great way to increase your fruit intake. If you are thirsty on a hot summer day consider a freshly squeezed orange juice mixed with water and ice. One lemon squeezed into a pitcher with a spoon of honey topped up with sparkling water makes healthy lemonade for children. These natural drinks, although requiring a little effort, are healthy, cheap, tasty and a great alternative to the sugary, chemical-rich drinks found in the majority of cans and bottles. Ideally, fruit juices should also be drunk fresh. After squeezing, juice changes its chemical composition quickly becoming more acidic and losing its nutritional content. The juices within cartons have generally been heavily processed and often need the vitamin C re-added to keep the levels up. Most plastic bottled 'freshly squeezed' juices and smoothies have been pasteurised to prolong their shelf life. Although there is little evidence that this is harmful, heating and cooling a food to extreme temperatures is not particularly natural – it also affects the taste. If possible look for unpasteurised juices or, better still, eat the real fruit, make your own smoothies or squeeze them yourself.

Extra note: Fruit intake and indigestion.

People often say – "I can't eat fruit because I have indigestion or heartburn". Although it is true that initially fruit can result in a little irritation in vulnerable individuals, it is not the root cause of the problem and in the long term fruit will improve the health of the stomach and oesophagus (gullet). The underlying cause is usually an unhealthy balance of fat, meats and sugar which the stomach has to work harder to digest – i.e. produce more of its own hydrochloric acid. To make matters worse, sufferers often turn to antacids for immediate relief. The stomach then senses a more alkaline environment and responds by producing yet more acid, perpetuating the problem. On the other hand, consumption of mildly acidic fruit sends signals to the stomach lining to produce less of its own acid. After a while, with perseverance, eating fruit and other less gastric-irritating foods will therefore reduce the acid levels and improve the health of gastric lining, and thus prevent indigestion.

Vitamin D and sun exposure

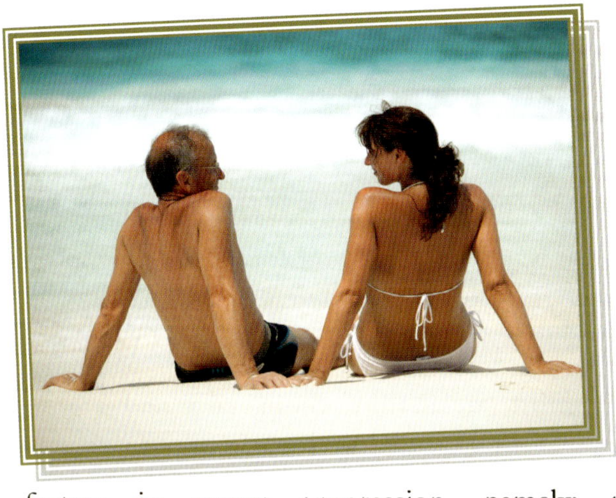

Vitamin D is converted to the active metabolite calciferol in the kidney. Over 80 per cent of the body's Vitamin D actually comes from the skin following exposure to sunlight. This was the reason why Asian immigrants in the early seventies were vulnerable to the bone disease rickets. Cancer cells exposed to calciferol in the laboratory have been shown to help key factors in cancer progression, namely; reduce proliferation, promote differentiation, inhibit invasion, prevent loss of adhesion and promote apoptosis. It has also be shown to interact with the androgen-signalling pathway in animals, inhibiting the production of factors which stimulate new blood vessels growing into cancers – stopping them growing (angiogenesis).

Two retrospective studies have highlighted the benefits of vitamin D after cancer. The first showed that those survivors of bowel cancer with regular exposure to sunlight had a lower incidence of subsequent relapse. The most surprising study involved people who had been treated for the skin cancer melanoma. Obviously, as the risk of this disease increases with sun-burning patients are told to keep out of the sun afterwards. However the study demonstrated that those patients who ignored this advice and continued to have regular sun exposure actually had a lower risk of the melanoma spreading to another part of the body. This study was supported by another observational evaluation of men with jobs involving exposure to high levels of sunlight. They found that they were less likely to develop kidney cancer than those with little or no sunlight exposure at work. More specifically, the study appearing in the journal "Cancer" showed men with the highest level of work-related exposure to sunlight were 24 percent to 38 percent less likely to have kidney cancer than other men. Interestingly, the association between job-related sunlight exposure and kidney cancer risk was not apparent in women. On the other hand a further survey showed that men who had sedentary desk jobs had a higher rate of prostate cancer.

The benefits of sunlight in these studies are almost certainly due to higher blood vitamin D levels. In view of the other dangers of sunlight, scientist have been endeavouring to develop tablets which could mimic vitamin D. Unfortunately so far clinical studies of oral calciferol tablets had to be abandoned because it dangerously increased serum calcium. Pharmaceutical companies have, however, now developed new vitamin D analogues which it is hoped have anti-cancer properties, but without the risk of raised calcium and these are currently being investigated in a large ongoing multi-centre study.

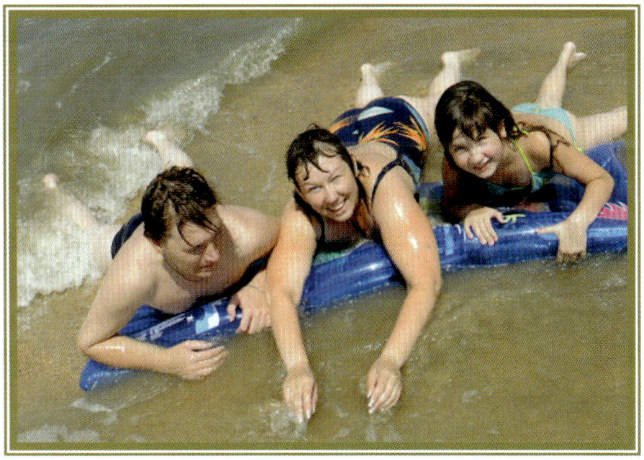

The problem is that the rate of skin cancer caused by sun burning is significantly increasing in Northern Europe and the USA, despite the general lack of sun over the long winter months (causing Vitamin D deficiency). Increasing numbers of the population then take short holidays in the sun and inevitably burn their skin especially in vulnerable areas such as the face shoulders, hands and neck.

The benefits and risks of tanning beds remain controversial. Sensible use over the winter months may be a good way to keep up the vitamin D levels. However, in a recent study The Lancet Oncology commented that sun beds pose as big a risk as tobacco and asbestos. It reported a new analysis of about 20 studies which concluded the risk of skin cancer jumps by 75 percent when people start using tanning beds before the age of 30. In addition, researchers from the International Agency for Research on Cancer (IARC), the "cancer arm" of the World Health Organization, found that all types of ultraviolet radiation (UVB) caused worrying mutations in mice. The IARC team found the same mutation in the skin of mice treated with UVA. Therefore the agency decided to reclassify all types of ultraviolet radiation – UVA, UVB, and UVC – as carcinogenic to humans, or Group 1 carcinogens. They have therefore now issued a warning that people younger than 18 years should avoid tanning beds.

Advice: vitamin D intake & healthy sun exposure

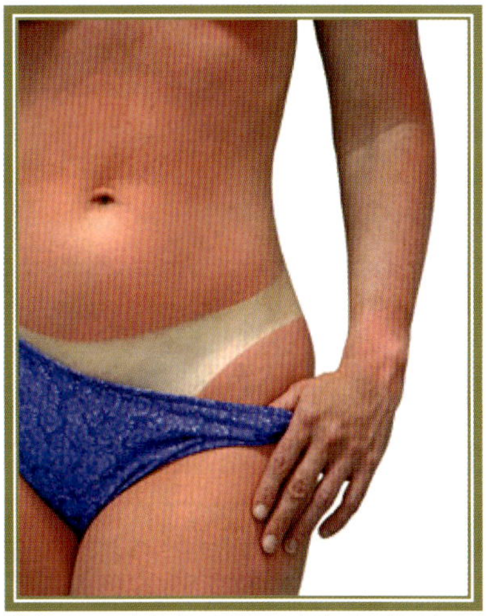

Vitamin D is an oil present in nuts, fish, fish oils, fresh vegetables, grains and cereals. A steady regular but controlled exposure to sun is the best way to increase your blood vitamin D levels. Vitamin D will help you maintain healthy bones, particularly important after chemotherapy if a premature menopause has occurred, or if you are taking certain breast cancer hormone drugs such as femara, Arimidex or Aromasin. While sunbathing is recommended, try to expose area of the skin which get the least sun normally, avoiding the face, hands and upper chest. Burning is particularly hazardous as not only will this cause thin, sun-damaged skin, it particularly increases the risk of skin cancers.

Smoking whilst sunbathing If you want to look ten years older smoke – if you want to look 20 years older smoke while sunbathing. The carcinogenic chemical in cigarette smoke enhances the harmful aspects of sun. Stop smoking altogether – if you can't, at least don't smoke whilst in the sun. For the opposite reasons it is worth increasing the antioxidant intake if high sun exposure is anticipated, such as during a summer holiday or skiing.

Sun exposure and chemotherapy During and shortly after chemotherapy, the skin can be more sensitive to the sun. All chemotherapy drugs can photosensitise the skin but particularly florouracil type drugs for bowel and breast cancer. Sensitivity to chemotherapy agents usually wears off after three months.

Sun exposure and radiotherapy Be very careful with skin specifically treated with radiotherapy; although better with modern techniques, the skin can still be damaged. For example, with breast cancer the upper cleavage area is treated so take care when wearing a v-shaped top. The sensitivity to radiotherapy will be life-long. Wear a high factor sunscreen or preferably barrier cream on irradiated tissue. Also ask your oncologist where the radiotherapy field started and finished so you know exactly where to apply the sun block and cover adequately with sensible clothing when in the sun.

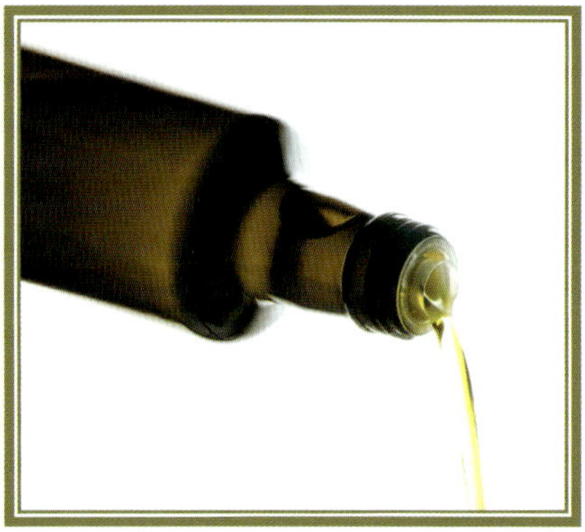

After sun lotions Massaging lotion into skin after sun exposure is not just a way to avoid peeling, to make the skin feel better or to trigger a romantic early evening holiday frolicking; there is evidence that some products could reduce the risk of skin cancer. Although not included in the usual after-sun lotions, two natural products have been shown to reduce the risk of sun damage via two separate mechanisms. In one experiment, olive oil was massaged into the skin of hairless mice for 5 minutes every evening, after exposure to UV light. Another group had the same UV exposure but no olive oil. There was a major difference in the number of subsequent skin cancers between the two groups. They discovered that the oleic acid within olive oil had reduced the formation of 8-hydroxy-deoxyguanosine (8OhdG), a marker of DNA damage. In other words the olive oil had helped repair the damage the sun had inflicted on the DNA within the cells of the skin, preventing the mutations which go on to cause cancer. In another experiment involving sunbathing mice, scientists applied the antioxidant resveratrol before and after the UVB exposure. As described in the alcohol section this polyphenol is found in grapes and red wine and its strong antioxidant properties mop up the free radicals before they damage the DNA. The study found that this chemical inhibited skin damage and decreased skin cancer incidence. It would make sense to regularly use olive oil based lotion after sun exposure or, failing that, olive oil itself. It also makes sense not to apply lotions which are packed with hydrocarbons and potentially carcinogen chemicals just when the skin is most vulnerable to DNA attack so use a product with as pure and natural ingredients as possible. Due to their expense in manufacturing, these creams are rarely available, but one which uses olive oil as its main oil base, has only natural essential oils and has no hydrocarbons, artificial chemicals or preservatives is made by Nature-medical (see keep-healthy.com for more details).

Fake tanning agents

There is no direct evidence that fake tanning creams and lotions are harmful, but regular exposure of your skin to dyes and chemicals is generally not advisable. A few times a year, for special occasions, it is probably not harmful, although there is little convincing evidence either way.

Summary – advice for careful sun exposure:

- Gentle regular sun exposure is healthy but excess in harmful
- It is particularly important not to get burnt
- Do not sit in the sun when it is hottest – between noon and three p.m.
- Avoid prolonged or regular use of artificial sun-beds
- Cover up particularly if you are out in the sun when it is midSummer.
- Wear a hat, long sleeved shirt covering the neck
- When sunbathing, aim for the gentle sun exposure late in the afternoon
- Particularly cover vulnerable areas of the body; face, chest, shoulders, hands
- In the evening apply after sun lotions
- Use an after sun lotion based on olive oil
- If none available apply olive oil to all sun exposed areas then shower
- Eat sensibly – lots of antioxidants after-sun exposure
- Chemotherapy sensitises the sun – take extra care
- The skin within the radiotherapy field is more sensitive – take extra care
- Smoking enhances the negative effects of the sun

Vitamin E

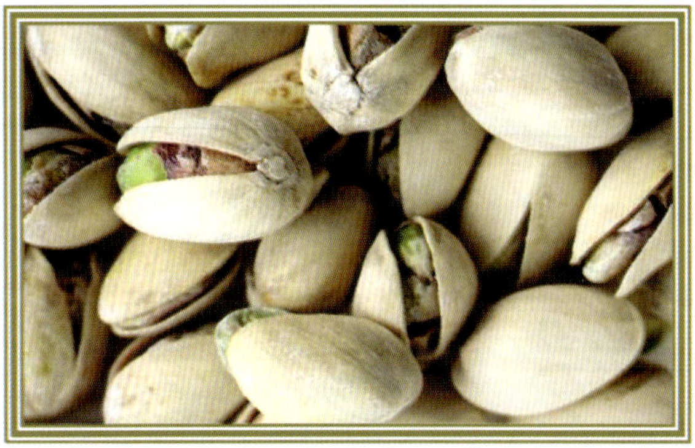

Vitamin E has eight naturally occurring isoforms. This correlation was particularly high with the isoform of vitamin E called gamma-tocopherol, which is the main vitamin E found in healthy foods as opposed to the alpha-tocopherol found in man-made supplements. he tocopherols isophorms of vitamin E have been thought to be linked to the cancer process mainly via an antioxidant effect. Tocopherols have also been shown to prevent less aggressive tumours changing to a more aggressive type (differentiation). In humans a number of leading trials have provided an excellent insight into the relationship between vitamin E and cancer. The Alpha-Tocopherol, Beta-Carotene cancer prevention trial (ATBC), involved 29,133 male smokers taking vitamin E (alpha-tocopherol) and vitamin A (Beta-carotene) or a placebo. After several years follow-up the treatment group had a statistically significant reduction in the incidence of prostate cancer. At last, a positive supplement trial, you may be saying to yourself, but before you applaud too loudly there was a sting in the tail. The incidence of lung cancer, the main trial end point, was higher in the treatment group than the placebo group. The beneficial effect on prostate cancer is probably genuine because it was supported by a further large trial involving male health workers called the Health Professional Follow-up Study (HPFS). In this study, vitamin E intake was also associated with a decreased risk of prostate cancer, but only in smokers and not overall. The relationship between smokers, the risk of prostate cancer and vitamin E was then investigated in the Cancer Prevention II (CPII) Nutrition Cohort study. As well as a detailed dietary history, this study also measured participants' blood levels for vitamin E. It showed that blood vitamin E was lower in smokers, and that there was a correlation between low blood vitamin E levels and higher incidence of prostate cancer. This correlation was particularly high with the isoform of vitamin E called gamma-tocopherol which is the main vitamin E found in health foods, as opposed to the alpha-tocopherol found in man-made supplements. A further trial involving 5000 patients with diabetes or cardiovascular disease was undertaken, this time in women (The Women's Health Study). Supplementation with alpha tocopherol demonstrated no reduction in cancer, and the incidence of heart disease was slightly worse. Likewise, in the ATBC study, cerebral haemorrhage risk was also higher in smokers with hypertension who took alpha-tocopherol.

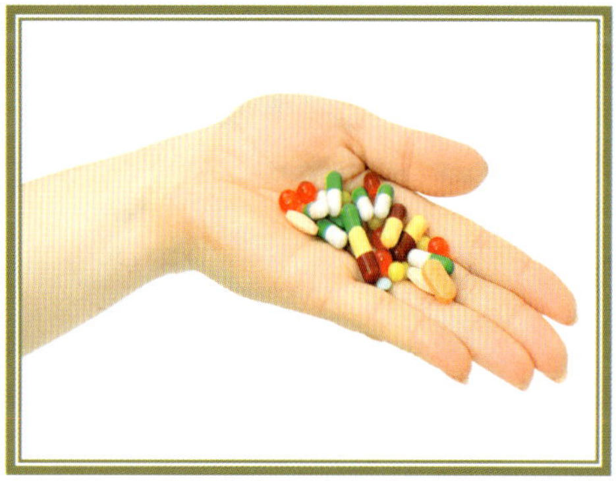

As mentioned above, a study from Queensland Australia analysed over a thousand individuals who had been treated for skin cancer. The risk of a further cancer was reduced if individuals ate foods with a high level of dietary antioxidants compared to those who did not, but individuals who took supplements of vitamin E actually had a higher rate of recurrent skin cancers.

The USA National Cancer Institute sponsored double-blind, randomised SELECT study comparing selenium and vitamin E supplementation against placebo, published in 2009, did not show any benefit in cancer prevention.

Summary: Advice for adequate vitamin intake

A repeated theme emerging form the evidence about vitamins is that a marked deficiency leads to severer disease and a mild deficiency over a long period of time could increase the risk of cancer. Taking supplements regularly either has no beneficial effect or increases the risk of cancer. The general advice to ensure adequate but not too much intake is, not surprisingly, a varied well-balanced diet – especially concentrating on the foods summarised in the table below. The difficultly comes when individuals have had a recent illness such as cancer, poor appetite or intense treatments. In these situations short term supplementation may be appropriate. The question is what to take, the only way to know for sure is to measure individual vitamin levels then correct accordingly, either through diet or tablets. These tests tend to be rather expensive but may be money well spent if a deficiency or excess is found. More information is written about nutritional testing later in this book (or see www.cancernet.co.uk.)

Summary – dietary tips to increase natural vitamin intake:

Vitamin A – The retinol isoform is found in all types of fish and many dairy foods such a cheese and yoghurt. The pro-vitamin beta-carotene, which is then metabolised to vitamin A, can also be ingested from fruits and vegetables such as carrots, spinach, cabbage, beetroot, peppers, goji berries, gac and tomatoes

Vitamin B – Barley, wheat, rye and other grains, whole meal and fresh vegetables

Vitamin C – Citrus fruits: limes, oranges, apples and lemons. Exotic fruits: kiwi, pineapple, mango, papaya, bananas and star fruit. ***Berries***: blackberries, cranberries, cherries, strawberries, goji berries etc. Nuts: almonds, brazils, walnuts, hazel nuts, etc.
Vegetables: green, red peppers, lettuce. Spices: chillies, black peppers

Vitamin D and K – Nuts, fish, fish oils such as cod liver oil, fresh vegetables, grains and cereals. Most of our vitamin D is generated by sunlight on our skin

Vitamin E – nuts particularly pistachio**,** fresh fruit, raw and calciferous vegetables, grains, oily fish, and salads

Superfoods

The expression "superfood" is commonly used in the media and health magazines, generally referring to foods which contain high levels of healthy vitamins and antioxidants although no particular threshold of ORAC has been chosen for a food to be designated "super". There is a tendency for foods to go out of fashion as "New" foods are discovered in far-flung, exotic places of the world. This section provides some examples of these and also describes how you can make superb "superfood" mixes simply and cheaply in your own kitchen with readily available, often local, products.

The Goji berry

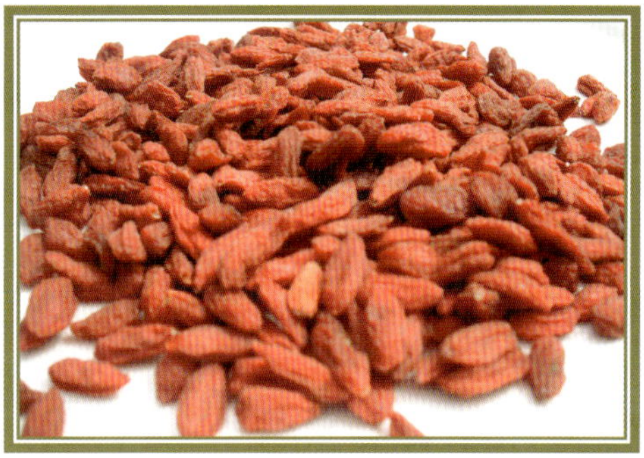

A good example of one of the better known superfoods. The best variety originates from Tibetan (Lycium Barbarum). The goji berry has been used in traditional Tibetan medicine for centuries. In the past, the berries are said to be never touched by hand when picked, no pesticides are used in their production and the high-altitude, ancient soils are free of pollutants. More recently and they are now mass produced in lowland areas using intensive farming techniques including herbicides and pesticides. Also the similar Chinese ground berry (wolfberry) tends to be highly sulphured as a preservative. The 2007 FDA rating put goji berries at over 25,000 units/but by 2010 they dropped the rating of commercially produced berries to 3,500 units/g. Nevertheless, the goji berry also has other healthy nutrients; they it contains 25 mg of vitamin C per gram of fruit, making it one of the world's richest sources of vitamin C, just behind the Australian billy goat plum and the South American camu camu. It is packed with more beta-carotene than carrots, has more iron than spinach, plus B vitamins, vitamin E, 18 amino acids and 21 trace minerals. As this little secret is being increasingly discovered across the western world they are becoming expensive as demand is superseding supplies.

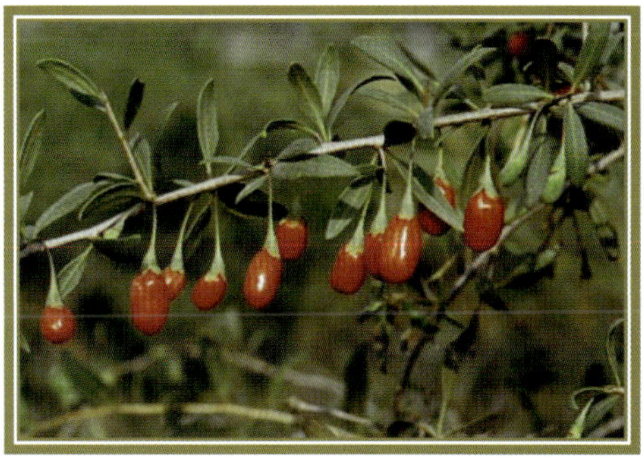

At the time of writing this book, the popularity of the little Goji berry has outstripped demand and it is becoming expensive in the UK. A little known fact, however, is that they grow well in the UK and particularly can be found in hedgerows around Gloucester. Unfortunately, there is currently a ban on live bush imports but for the more adventurous of the readers there is no restriction to picking the wild seeds growing your own harvest.

Quinoa

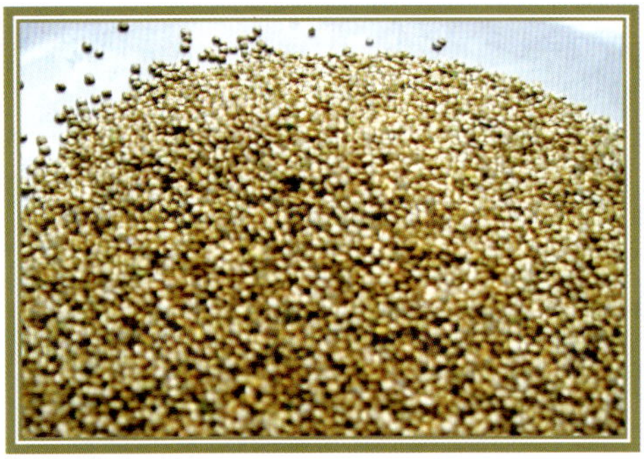

Quinoa originated in South and Central America, in the pre-Columbian era, where it was known to be of great nutritional importance and grown as a cereal. It is not, however, part of the cereal family such as wheat and barley as it not a grass. Quinoa is more closely related to species such as beets and spinach. In contemporary times, this crop has become highly appreciated for its nutritional value, as its protein content is very high (12%–18%). Unlike wheat or rice, which are low in lysine, quinoa contains a balanced set of essential amino acids, making it an unusually complete protein source among plant foods. It is a good source of dietray fibre, phosphorous, magnesium, iron and magnesium. It is gluten feed and hence easy to digest. It is also high in antioxidants and omega health fats, particularly linoleic acid. NASA have reported that they would use quinoa as a plant in a future space station because of its universal nutritional benefits.

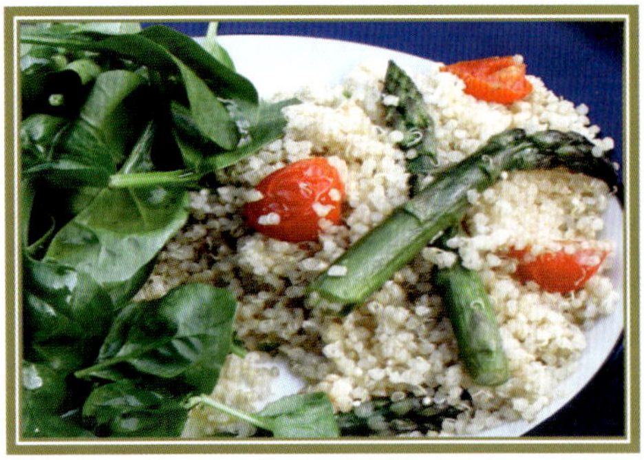

Quinoa has a light, fluffy texture when cooked, and its mild, slightly nutty flavor makes it an alternative to rice or couscous. In the UK, it is available from health food stores and more recently supermarket,s pre-rinsed with the husks (saponins) removed. A common cooking method is to treat quinoa much like rice, bringing two cups of water to a boil with one cup of grain, covering at a low simmer and cooking for 14–18 minutes or until the germ separates from the seed. The cooked germ looks like a tiny curl and should have a slight bite to it. As an alternative, one can use a rice cooker to prepare quinoa, treating it just like white rice.

Vegetables such as asparagus and spinach along with and seasonings can be added to make a wide range of dishes. Chicken or vegetable stock can be substituted for water during cooking, adding flavor. Lean chicken or bacon can be added for additional taste if desired. The dish above, for example, took 10 minutes in total to make. (Boil the quinoa with a touch of olive oil and herb salt. Gently fry the asparagus in a wok and later add cherry tomatoes and pepper for taste. When cooked, mix with the quinoa, add feta cheese and serve with spinach salad) – superfood, super-quick, super-cheap and super tasty!

Vietnamese Gac

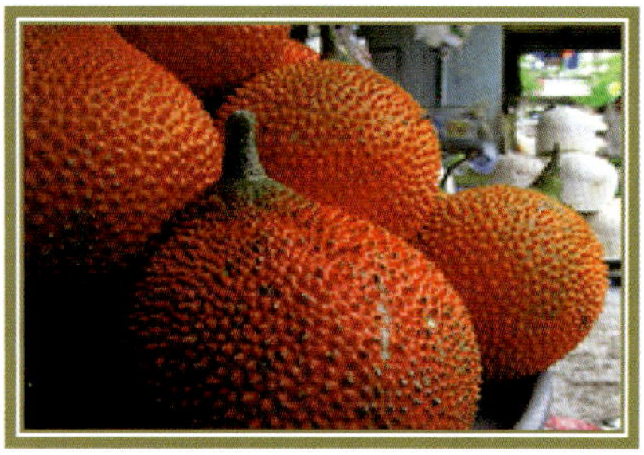

The exotic fruit is now emerging as the new "must have superfood", even threatening to tip goji off its perch particularly in the eyes of those convinced of the lycopene story and prostate cancer. Its other names include Baby Jackfruit, Spiny Bitter Gourd, Sweet Gourd, or Cochinchin Gourd in English. It is less abundant than other foods because it has a relatively short harvest season, which peaks in December and January. Gac is typically served at ceremonial or festive occasions in Vietnam, such as the Vietnamese New Year and weddings. It is most commonly prepared as a dish called xoi gac, in which the flesh and seeds of the fruit are cooked in a glutinous rice. More recently, the fruit has begun to be marketed outside of Asia in the form of dietary supplements.

Traditionally, gac fruit, seed and its leaves have also been used as a traditional medicine in the regions in which it grows. For example, the seed membranes are used to aid in the relief of dry eyes, as well as to promote healthy vision. Similarly, in China the seeds of gac, known in Mandarin Chinese, are employed for a variety of internal and external purposes. Recently attention is beginning to be attracted to it in The West, because chemical analysis of the fruit suggests it has high concentrations of several important phyto-nutrients, in addition to fibre and vitamins.

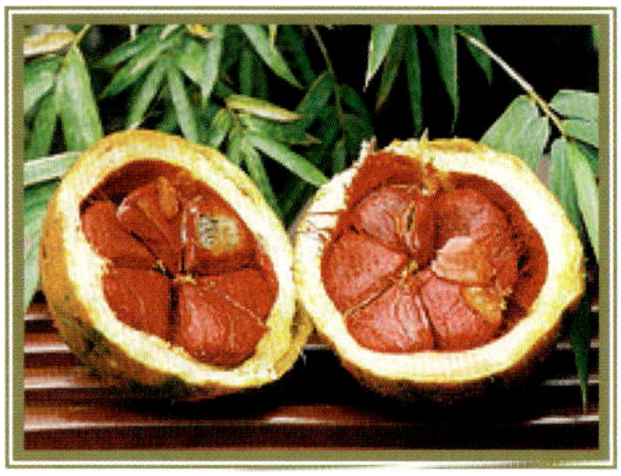

The fruit contains by far the highest content of beta carotene (Vitamin A) of any known fruit or vegetable – up to ten times more than carrots or sweet potatoes. More importantly, research has confirmed that the beta-carotene in the fruit is highly bio-available (easy absorbed into the blood stream). This was demonstrated in a double-blind study with 185 children, half of whom were given a dish containing 3.5 mg beta-carotene from gac, while others were given an identical-looking dish containing 5 mg of artificial beta-carotene powder. After 30 days, the former group eating natural beta-carotene had significantly greater plasma (blood) levels of beta-carotene than the latter with synthetic beta-carotene.

The oil of gac also contains high levels of vitamin E, essential long chain (healthy) fatty acids and lycopene. Relative to mass, it contains up to 70 times the amount of lycopene found in tomatoes. There has also been recent research that suggests that gac contains a protein that may inhibit the proliferation of cancer cells. It is important to eat the gac fruit when it is bright red otherwise is it not ripe enough to eat. They are at their peak when they turn a brighter red just before spoiling. Do not eat the sides, which are similar to the inner texture of a cantaloupe. This part of the fruit, as well as the exterior rind, are toxic and will make you feel ill if you attempt to eat it. The only parts that can be eaten are the inner soft, oily pulp surrounding the seeds and the seeds themselves.

Pomegranate (Punica granatum)

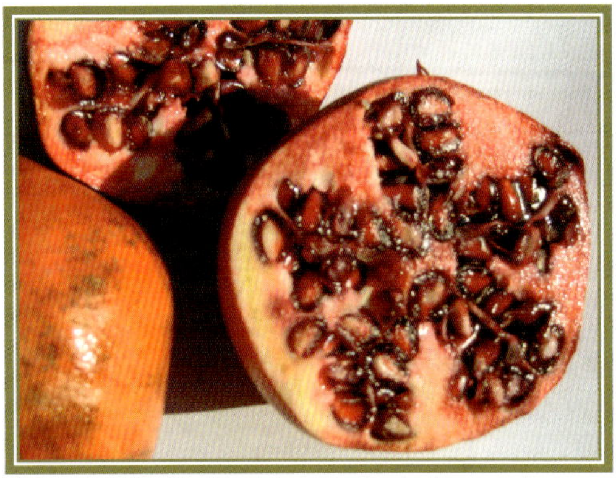

A fruit-barring shrub or small tree originally from the middle east but now grown across the world, particularly in warm climates. The pomegranate has been used extensively as a source of traditional remedies for thousands of years. The rind of the fruit and the bark of the pomegranate tree are used as a traditional remedy against diarrhoea, dysentery and intestinal parasites.

Pomegranate juice is a good source of vitamin C, B5 (pantothenic acid), potassium and antioxidant polyphenols. The most abundant polyphenols in pomegranate juice are the hydrolyzable tannins called punicalagins which have potentent free radical scavenging properties. The ORAC (antioxidant capacity) of pomegranate juice was measured at 2,860 units per 100 grams. In addition to this, there is also a tendency for their metabolites ellagitannins to accumulate in the prostate gland. As already described in the previous chapter, a North American study, sponsored by the Pomegranate Growers Association, gave pomegranate juice to 48 men with prostate cancer. All the patients had previously received radiotherapy or surgery but started showing evidence of their cancer returning in the form of a rising PSA blood test. There was a significant slowing in the rate of rise of the PSA after drinking the juice compared to before the study.

Berries

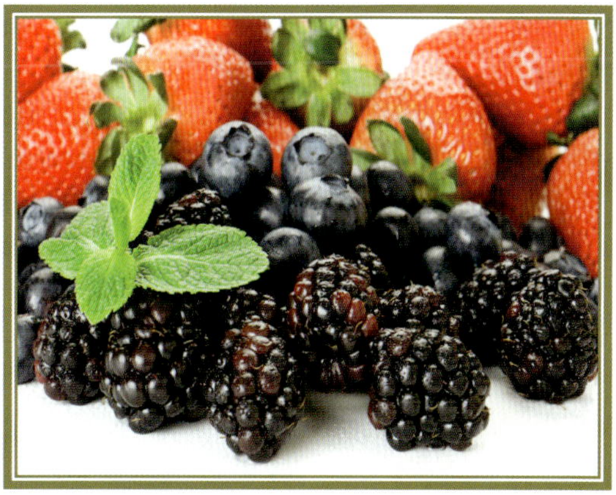

All edible berries are an excellent source of vitamins, fibre, minerals and the ORAC chart above shows how high they are in antioxidants, the dark and colourful varieties having the highest concentrations. The chart also shows that the wild varieties have higher levels than their cultivated cousins and have the additional advantage of not being sprayed with pesticides and herbicides. Blackberries have even higher ORAC rating than the much published blueberries and grow with abundance in the UK – a free, organic superfood virtually on the doorstep.

Make your own "Superfoods"

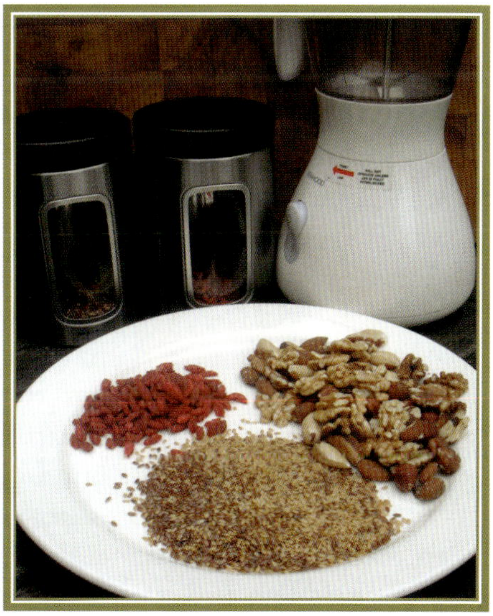

Although individual foods can be very healthy, mixing them together is a fantastic way to provide your body with a great variety of essential nutrients, with the reassurance that your diet is likely to be correcting potential deficiencies whilst avoiding excesses caused by one particular food type. Most health food shops, many cafes and supermarkets are now selling mixed foods, either ground in bags or in the form of health bars, cereals or drinks. They tend to be expensive and still have to be processed in some way. You can, however, make your own superfood mix very easily with the help of a liquidiser. It can be used to make a grain mix, fruit smoothies or soups all packed with goodness.

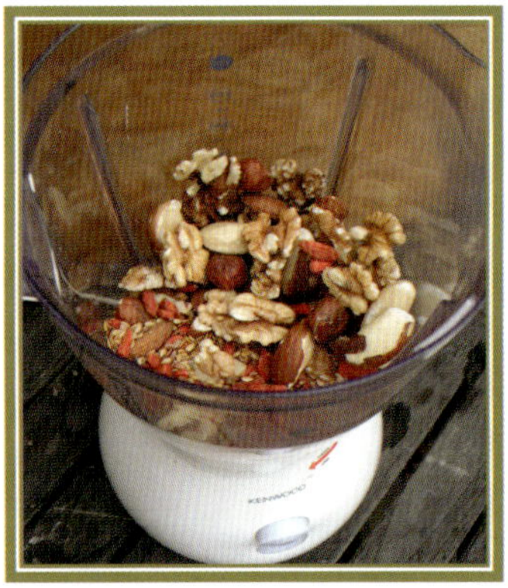

Grain mixes; These are great for increasing our intake of linseeds, which tend to pass through the system untouched unless ground. Ground they release their valuable omega 3 fatty acids, proteins and antioxidants. They can be mixed with seeds, nuts and goji berries for extra taste and nutrional value. Despite being ground, this is still an excellent source of fibre – a tablespoon of this mix a day will guarantee no further need for laxatives and will have a significant impact on bringing down the body's cholesterol. Once ground, a batch can be placed in an airtight container and used over several weeks. The mix can then be sprinkled on cereals or porridge, mixed with live yogurt or milk, added to smoothies or soups. Remember to clean out the container thoroughly before adding the next batch in order to avoid moulds. The mix can be altered each time depending on your nutritional needs. For example, if more omega is needed, add more walnuts, if more roughage more linseeds. If you are looking to add more vitamin E, add shelled pistachio nuts or if more antioxidants increase the goji berry content. The trick is to be organised to ensure your supplies do not run out. It would be better to invest in a rack of large storage tins or jars for the various ingredients and then buy the nuts and seeds in bulk to reduce the cost considerably.

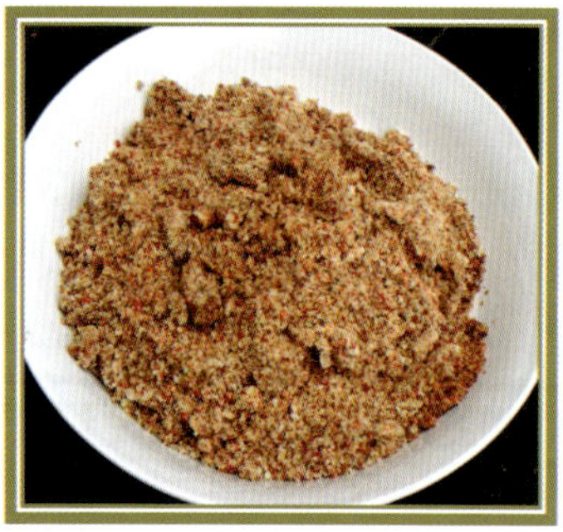

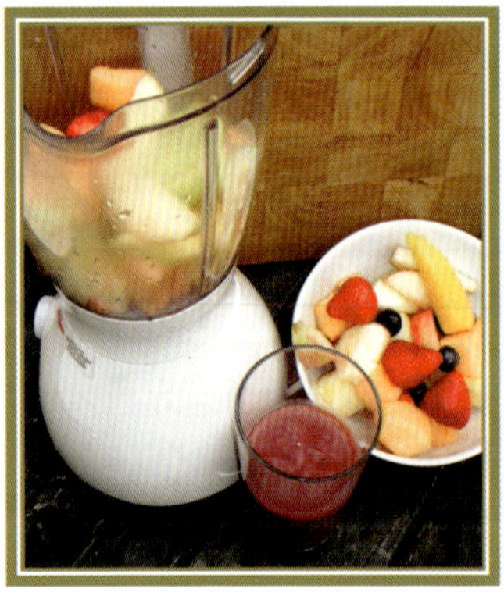

Fruit smoothies; Although these can be bought in cartons and bottles they tend to be expensive. Most have also usually have been pasteurised, understandably, to prolong the self life but this can alter the taste and may affect some of the healthy nutrients. They are still many times healthier than fizzy drinks and are very convenient when on the go, but if you have time, making you own is still a cheaper and better option. Use any fruit you fancy but a good tip is not to overdo the strawberries – it is not uncommon to get an allergic reaction to them when taken in large amounts and the seeds can give the drink a gritty texture. Otherwise, it's up to your individual taste and what fruits were on offer in the market that day.

Chapter Eight

Essential minerals
Evidence, benefits, advice

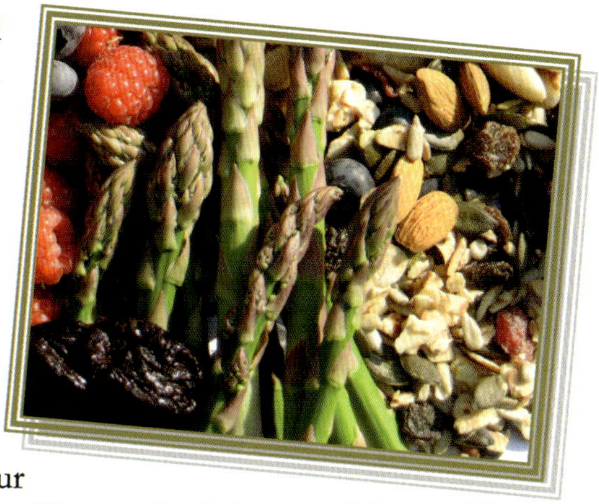

Intensive farming and sterile food processing are blamed for the reduced essential trace minerals and metals in the human diet, although reports of specific diseases caused by deficiencies are rare. Mineral deficiency syndromes have been recognised in remote areas of China, where the soil has extremely low selenium content. Population studies from Australia, the USA and Europe have shown that minor deficiencies of minerals commonly occur in western cultures and, while not causing illnesses in their own right, could contribute to others such as hypothyroidism (underactive thyroid gland) and cancer. In the west, as described later in this chapter, an increasingly important issue in humans is mineral excesses caused by over-enthusiastic consumption of dietary supplements. Studies are now emerging that excess blood levels of minerals are now contributing to an increased risk of cancer.

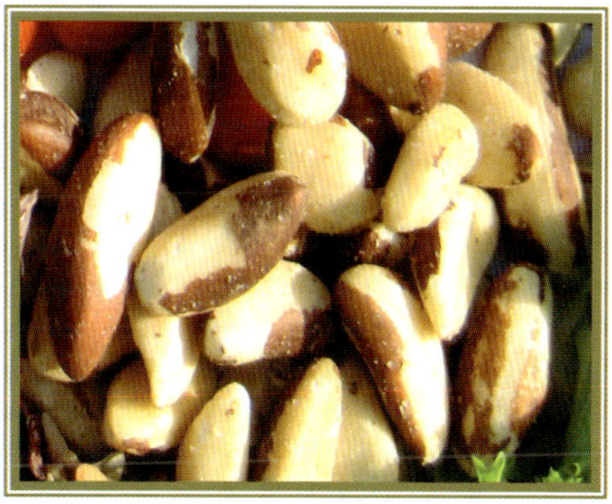

Selenium: The RDA for selenium is 60-75mcg/day and more than 200mcg/day is excessive. Selenium, in addition to helping flight cancer, also protects against mercury exposure such as that found in marine foods, by forming inert metal-selenium complexes. Brazil nuts are a reasonable source provided they are grown in South America and not China. Sardines, prawns, shellfish, eggs, crab and crab liver are also good sources. USA-grown wheat is relatively high in selenium, but the same cannot be said for European varieties because of the low levels in most European soils. Oily fish contains selenium, but this may well be bound to the mercury and made inert. Meat and other cereals contain small quantities.

In humans two major studies in 1980 and 1990 showed that a low selenium status was associated with an increased risk of developing cancer. They also indicated that in patients with selenium deficiency, the cancer they developed was more likely to be aggressive and fatal. The Harvard Health Professional Survey, for example, linked low selenium status (measured on toenail clippings!) with higher rates of aggressive prostate cancer. Both Finnish and Taiwanese studies have linked lower blood levels of selenium with higher rates of lung and a liver cancer called hepatocellular carcinoma (HCC). In China, where the incidence of HCC is high, the inhabitants of one village were supplemented with sodium selenite whilst another five villages were given simple salt. After six years, involving over 130,000 people, there was a 35 percent reduction in the HCC rate in the selenium-supplemented village, but no change in the others.

These data prompted the design and initiation of an excellent double-blind randomised trial in the USA called the Nutritional Prevention Study. It recruited 1312 individuals with a history of skin cancer and prescribed either a placebo or 220 micrograms of selenium a day. The primary aim (end point) was to see if dietary selenium supplementation could reduce the risk of recurrent skin cancer. There was no difference in the number of skin cancers between the selenium and placebo group. However, when the data was analysed in more detail, a significantly lower level of lung, bowel and prostate cancer was seen in the selenium group and this lived up to robust statistical evaluation. The largest study, published in 2009, was called the SELECT study. It gave either selenium and vitamin E or a placebo to a larger group of healthy men. After many years careful follow-up the rate of prostate cancer in the two groups was exactly the same. No measurements of underlying selenium or vitamin E levels were recorded in this study. Many suspect, however, that the people who would benefit from selenium supplements are those with a dietary deficiency in the first place, for example, those living in areas with low levels of selenium in the soil, although this needs to be confirmed in further research.

Good food sources of selenium include mixed nuts, particularly brazils – especially those grown in South America were there is plenty of selenium in the soil, raisins sardines, prawns, shellfish, eggs, crab and crab liver. Oily fish is also a good source selenium, but, as previously mentioned, this may well be bound to the mercury and rendered inert. Vegetables, salad, eggs, legumes and cereals contain small quantities. Barley and wheat can be good sources but levels very much depend on farming techniques and the levels in the soil. Meat can be a good source if the animal was reared free range and fed on grass which in turn contains selenium.

Calcium: The Australian and UK Medical Councils have recommended dietary calcium intakes of 1000mg/day for women and 800mg/day for men, and regard dietary calcium greater than 1500mg per day as excessive. Four prospective cohort studies, relating to calcium and prostate cancer, have been published. Two recommended a mean calcium intake of between 1330-1840 mg/day, which showed no benefit or risk, or associated risk. Two others, one involving 86,404 men in the CP II Nutrition cohort, with mean intake of >2000 mg/day from food and supplements, actually showed a significantly higher rate of prostate cancer. Five out of nine further questionnaire surveys associated high intake of dairy food with an increased risk of prostate and breast cancer, but interpretation of these was complicated by the fact that a diet high in dairy products was associated with high fat intake. The detrimental effect of excessive calcium is thought to lie in the finding that high dietary calcium can reduce blood and cellular vitamin D levels. This evidence shows that calcium supplements, on their own, may well have a detrimental effect on cancer but when combined with vitamin D are useful to treat and prevent bone loss. Foods high in calcium tend to be fatty foods such as milk and cheese. However, alternatives include skimmed milk, cheese, low fat and regular yoghurt, canned fish with bones (sardines, salmon) and spinach. Soya products often have calcium added. Low quantities are also present in salads, fruit and vegetables.

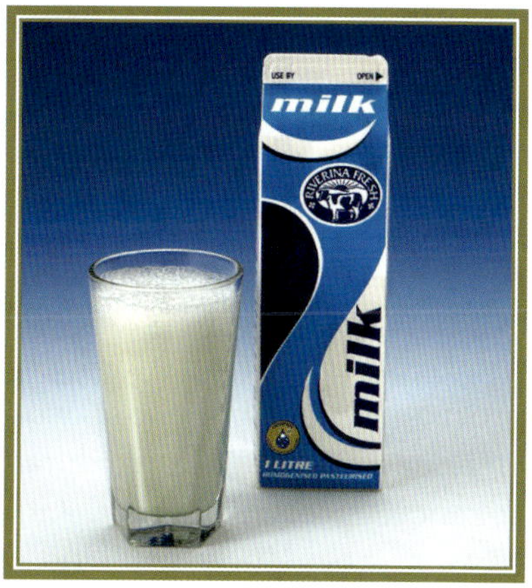

Zinc: This is required for the catalytic activity of approximately 100 enzymes and it plays a role in immune function, protein synthesis, wound healing, DNA synthesis, and cell division. Zinc also supports normal growth and development during pregnancy, childhood, and adolescence and is required for proper sense of taste and smell. A daily intake of zinc is required to maintain a steady state because the body has no specialized zinc storage system. RDA is 8mg/day (women) and 11mg/day (men, especially if sexually active as zinc is lost in the semen.) Research from animal studies has shown that there is an increased risk of cancer in the presence of copper, manganese, selenium or zinc deficiencies particularly under conditions of high carcinogenic attack where more SOD is needed. Zinc tends to accumulate more in the prostate, and one laboratory study suggested that this might offer some

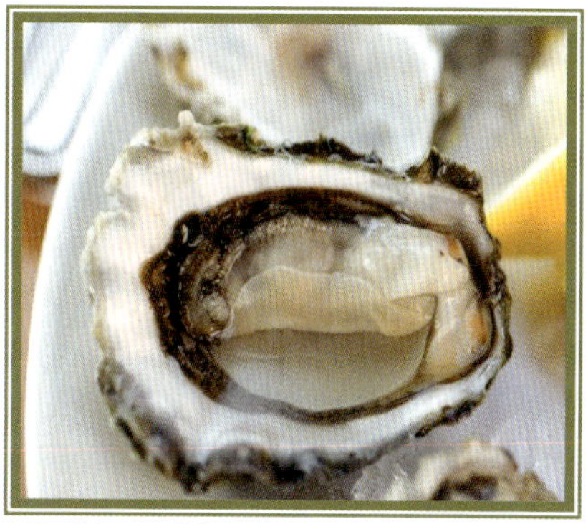

protection against prostate cancer cell growth. Zinc in excess, as you can image, is likely to be harmful. This was highlighted in the Health Professionals Follow-Up Study (HPFS). In this study, 50,000 health professionals were recruited between 1986 and 2002, from several medical fields. They were required to provide information on their eating, smoking and drinking habits, including the type of alcohol they preferred and supplements they took. During the study, 3,348 cases of prostate cancer were diagnosed. Further analysis of the diet and type of cancer showed that men who took normal amounts of zinc had the normal incidence of prostate cancer but those who took supplemental zinc at levels of more than 100mg/day, or for long durations, were more than twice as likely to develop advanced prostate cancer. Good dietary sources of zinc include oysters, crab, lobster other shell fish and seafood as well as fresh dark green salad and vegetables.

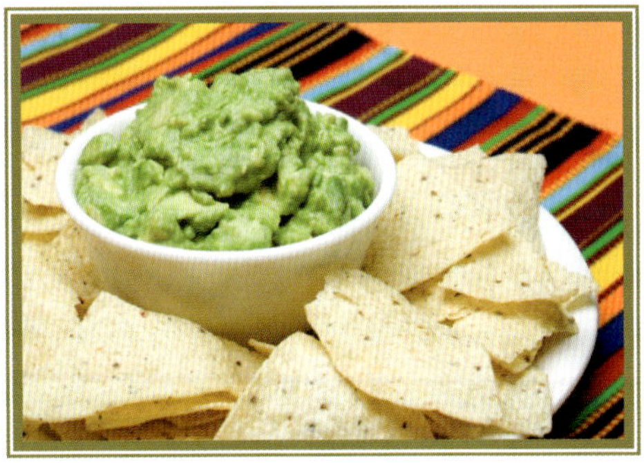

Copper: The estimated safe and adequate intake for copper is 1.5 – 3.0 mg/day. Many survey studies show that in the west we tend to consume 1.0 mg or less of copper per day. Copper is involved in the absorption, storage and metabolism of iron and the formation of red blood cells. It also helps supply oxygen to the body. The symptoms of a copper deficiency are similar to iron-deficiency anaemia. A study which removed copper from the feed of cows showed an excess of cancer and function of the enzyme SOD. Dietary sources of copper include avocado, bananas, brussels sprouts, butternut squashes, coconut and eggs.

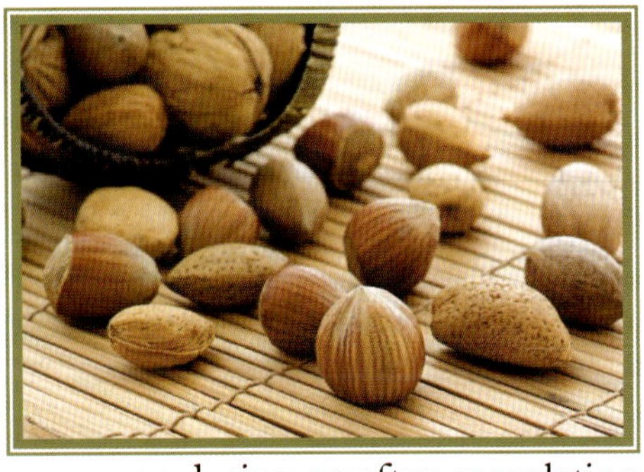

Manganese: The estimated safe and adequate intake for manganese is 2.0-5.0 mg/day for adults. The functions of this mineral are not specific since other minerals can perform in its place. Manganese does function in enzyme reactions concerning blood sugar, metabolism, and thyroid hormone function. It is worth measuring this metal along with urinary iodine if thyroid deficiency occurs during or after completion of cancer therapies such as chemotherapy or the biological agent sutent. Deficiency is rare in humans and good sources are nuts, Kiwi fruit, avocado, blackberries, lima beans, artichoke and nuts.

Magnesium: The fourth most abundant mineral in the body and essential to good health. Approximately 50 percent of total body magnesium is found in bone. Magnesium helps maintain normal muscle and nerve function, keeps heart rhythm steady, supports a healthy immune system, and keeps bones strong. A significant Japanese study in the Journal of Nutrition in 2010 showed a link with colon cancer. It followed 87,117 Japanese men and women, aged 45 to 74, for eight years to determine whether dietary magnesium could help prevent colon cancer. The analysis showed that men who consumed at least 327 milligrams of magnesium a day were 52 percent less likely to develop colon cancer, compared to those whose daily diets provided less than 238 milligrams. Although they did not see a similar association in women in this study, two other studies also saw a benefit of magnesium in women. The Iowa Women's Health Study, published in 2005 followed 41,386 postmenopausal women for 17 years. A daily magnesium intake greater than 351 milligrams – versus less than 245 milligrams – reduced the risk of colon cancer by 23 per cent. This was also supported by The Swedish Mammography Cohort, also conducted in 2005, which studied 61,433 women, aged 40 to 75 years, for nearly 15 years and found that women whose daily diets provided at least 255 milligrams of magnesium were 40 per cent less likely to be diagnosed with colorectal cancer compared to their peers who consumed less than 209 milligrams each day. Interestingly, those who took higher than necessary doses or nutritional supplements had no benefit, so the recommendation from all three was to gather magnesium from the diet.

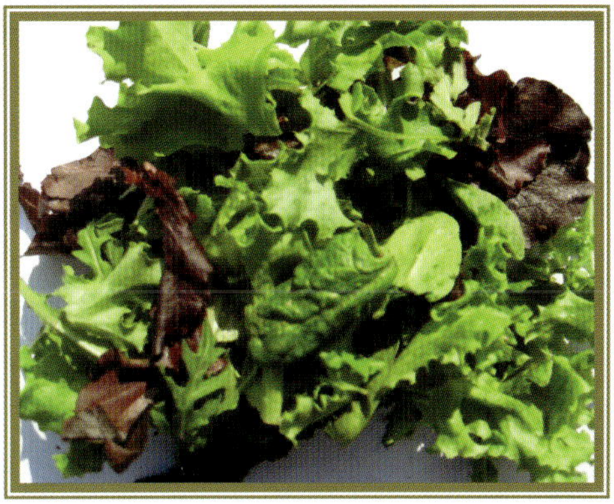

Green vegetables such as spinach are good sources of magnesium because the centre of the chlorophyll molecule (which gives green vegetables their colour) contains magnesium. Fish is also a good source as well as almonds, cashew nuts and soy beans. Some legumes (beans and peas), seeds, and whole, unrefined grains are also good sources of magnesium. Refined grains are generally low in magnesium. When white flour is refined and processed, the magnesium-rich germ and bran are removed. Bread made from whole grain wheat flour provides more magnesium than bread made from white refined flour. Tap water can be a source of magnesium, but the amount varies according to the water supply. Water that naturally contains more minerals is described as "hard". "Hard" water contains more magnesium than "soft" water.

Mechanisms of trace mineral benefits and risk.

These dietary trace metallic elements act as antioxidants because they are essential for the production of super oxide dismutase (SOD) and selenium is also essential for glutathione peroxidase. Together with catalase, these form the enzymatic defence against harmful carcinogenic chemicals. These three enzymes are responsible for the end stage of 'mopping-up' free radicals before they have time to damage the DNA. Research from animal studies has shown that there is an increased risk of cancer in the presence of copper, manganese, selenium or zinc deficiencies particularly under conditions of high carcinogenic attack where more anti-oxidant enzymes are needed. Selenium has also been shown to slow the progression of cancer cells when added to a culture medium in the laboratory. This effect was independent of the enzymatic SOD pathway, indicating that selenium on its own may have a direct anticancer effect.

If, however, trace minerals are taken in excess they start over loading biochemical pathways making the body's metabolism and immunity run less efficiently. High levels of one mineral may also interfere with the absorption of others leading to deficiencies. In short minerals in excess start acting as poisons.

Advice for optimal trace element intake

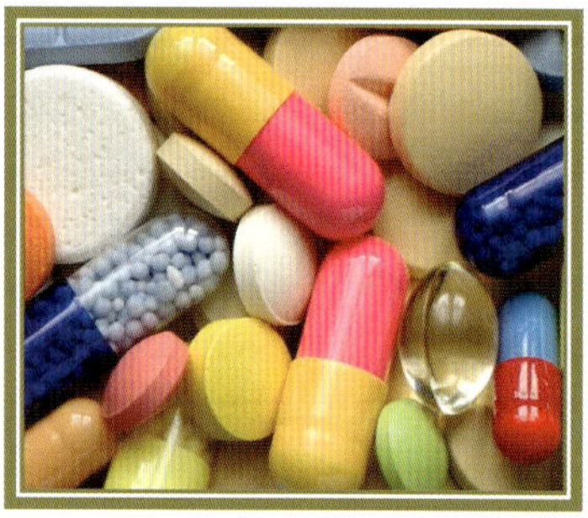

In additional to the minerals and salts mentioned above there are numerous other minerals and elements that we need to absorb from food and which are required in trace amounts. Fortunately the body is pretty efficient at extracting the ones we need, in the correct amounts, when we need it. Taking a "one fits all" supplement is not the answer to ensuring adequate intake. The section on supplements explains the dangers of having too much exposure to trace minerals and salts both in terms of general health and, indeed, cancer. The trick is therefore to diversify the foods sources and their country of origin and only rely on additives or supplements for short periods of nutrition deficiency such as after a spell of poor appetite or sickness. Not only will this ensure you will not be consistently eating a food deficient in a certain mineral or vitamin, it will also avoid overexposure to particular harmful chemicals.

If an individual has the time, motivation and money, the most reliable way to ensure adequate mineral intake is to measure the body's existing levels at regular intervals. There are now several tests which can be performed on a variety of body tissues from nail clippings, hair, saliva, red blood cells and urine. They can tell whether you are deficient or have an excess of a particular chemical.

Individuals then have the choice to modify the diet or take specific supplements. Regrettably, some of these tests can be expensive but they are not required very often and may provide considerable long-term health benefits if a deficiency or excess is found. Further information on bespoke testing can be found on the website cancernet.co.uk/nutritional-tests.htm

Summary – advice to ensure adequate trace mineral intake:

- Diversify your foods as much as possible
- Alternate your carbohydrates; consider
    - Different potato varieties
    - Brown or wild rice, as well as white
    - Couscous
    - Different types of pasta, especially wholemeal
    - Quinoa
- Alternate your daily fruits i.e. different varieties of apples, kiwi or bananas
- Snack on dried fruit, dates, pumpkin seeds and nuts including Brazil nuts
    - Alternate brands
    - Alternate mixes
    - Try to eat organic varieties if available
- Eat seafood such as crab and shellfish once or twice a fortnight
- Alternate fish between oily, freshwater and sea varieties
- Alternate water sources – tap, filtered and different mineral waters
- Alternate the countries of origin – different soils have different minerals
- Think about growing your own organic vegetables
- Avoid taking extra mineral supplements
- Consider measuring the body mineral levels to avoid deficiency or excess

Chapter Nine

Cancer-forming chemicals

Avoiding carcinogens

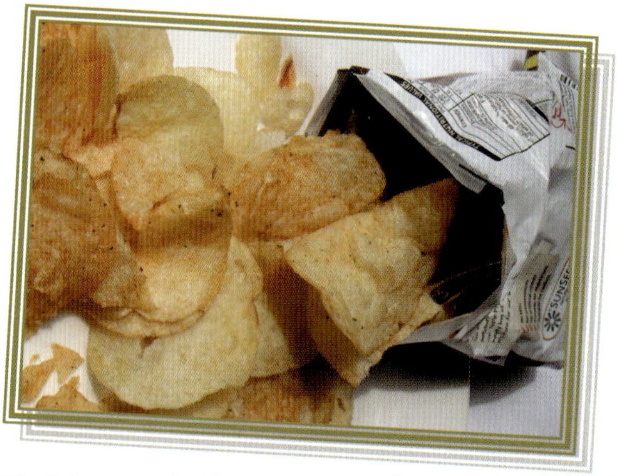

The section on antioxidants explained how certain chemicals (carcinogens) can generate super oxide free radicals which damage DNA and rearrange the genes within our cells, leading to the development of cancer. Although patients with established cancer have already sustained the initial DNA damage in order to mutate from benign to malignant cells, the cancer process can also be fuelled by continuing consumption of foods high in carcinogens. Further DNA damage can encourage the cancer to mutate into a more aggressive type or develop mechanisms to hide from the body's immunological defences. Avoiding carcinogens after cancer is also beneficial as it may reduce the risk of developing further cancers, which are also more likely in patients who may be susceptible from a pre-existing genetic vulnerability, or who have acquired vulnerability caused by chemotherapy or radiotherapy.

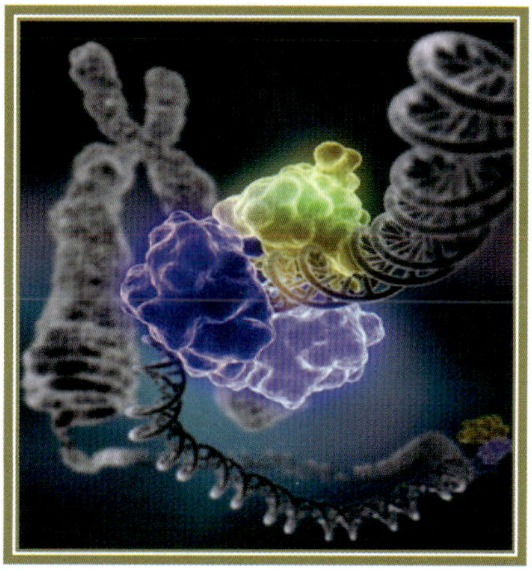

There is a wide array of known carcinogens in our diet and probably many others which are unknown. The American Food and Drug Administration (FDA) and similar organisations internationally are responsible for detecting and regulating carcinogens in our diet. They analyse chemicals using cultured cells in the laboratory and in animals. These carcinogenicity studies are subdivided into four broad categories of lesions – gene mutation, clastogenicity, DNA damage and cell transformation. They are legally bound to share their data with other countries via the Cooperative Research and Development Agreement (CRADA). Of this group of carcinogens the most commonly investigated and discussed are the acrylamides. The evidence for the risks of acrylamides stemmed from a report issued by researchers at the Swedish National Food Administration and Stockholm University in 2002. This reported finding that acrylamides associated with high temperature cooking of carbohydrate-rich foods were linked to cancer.

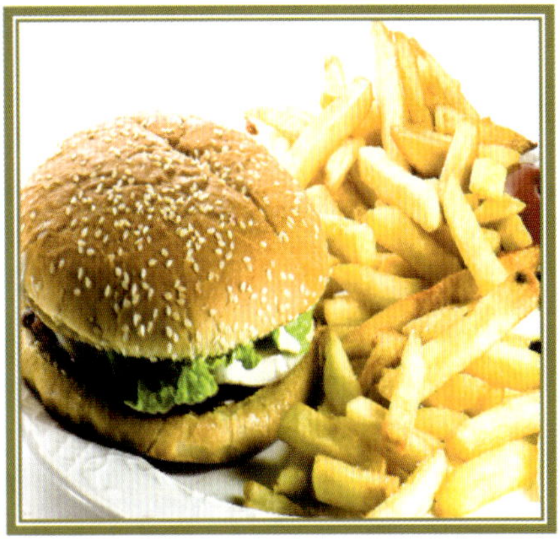

In animal studies many pesticides are carcinogenic, (e.g. organochlorines, creosote, and sulfallate) while others (notably, the organochlorines DDT, chlordane, and lindane) are tumour promoters. Some contaminants in commercial pesticide formulations may also pose a carcinogenic risk. In humans arsenic compounds and insecticides used occupationally have been classified as carcinogens by the International Agency for Research on Cancer. Human data, however, are limited by the small number of studies that evaluate individual pesticides. Epidemiologic studies, although sometimes contradictory, have linked phenoxy acid herbicides or contaminants in them, with soft tissue sarcoma (STS) and malignant lymphoma; organochlorine insecticides are linked with STS, non-Hodgkin's lymphoma (NHL), leukaemia, and, less consistently, with cancers of the lung and breast; organophosphorus compounds are linked with NHL and leukaemia and triazine herbicides with ovarian cancer. Few, if any, of these associations can be considered established and causal, although only a few hundred of the 20,000 chemicals in everyday use have been tested for their impact on health and the environment. Hence, further epidemiological studies are needed with detailed exposure assessment for individual pesticides, taking into consideration work practices, use of protective equipment, and other measures to reduce risk.

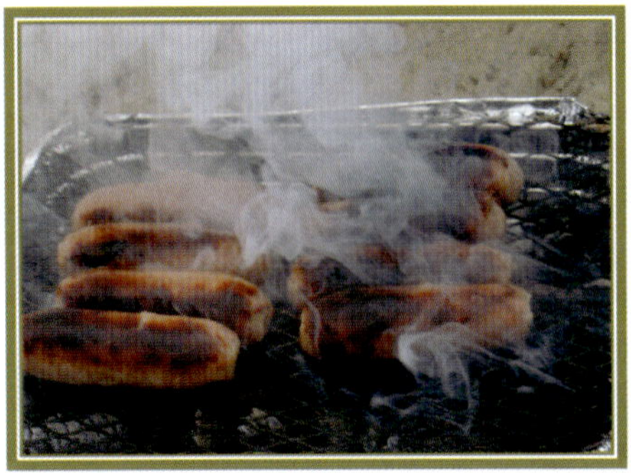

A direct link between environmental pollution and cancer in human beings was reported in the Lancet in 2005. Researchers have found that people with high levels of pesticides and chemicals known as organochlorines in their blood stream are far more likely to develop genetic mutations linked with cancer of the pancreas. The researchers studied 51 patients with pancreatic cancer and compared blood concentrations of the pollutants and the levels of mutation of a gene called K-Ras, believed to cause pancreatic cancer. K-Ras genes have been found to be targets for chemical carcinogens in laboratory studies of animals and this correlates with a more aggressive type of cancer.

A study published in the prestigious Journal of Clinical Oncology in 2010 looked at the blood levels and history of exposure to carcinogens of 623 men with prostate cancer and compared this to 671 similar men without cancer. The levels of carcinogens were significantly higher in the cancer group, indicating that they were a likely contributor to the illness. The risk was particularly high if men already had a genetic susceptibility to prostate cancer as measured by an analysis of their DNA. The carcinogen in question in this study was called Chlordecone (Kepone) a organochloride insecticide with carcinogenic and xeno-oestrogenic properties used extensively between 1973 and 1993 in the West Indies to control banana root disease.

Similar stories from across the world are now emerging and, with expansion of industrial farming methods especially in the Far East and as farmers have to supply food for a rapidly growing world population; the issue is not getting better. A classic example is the production of goji berries, which originally were gathered naturally in the wild by Tibetan monks – organic by default. Now following world demand vast farms have been established in China, many heavily sprayed with pesticides and herbicides and fertilizers to keep up production. It is impossible to avoid carcinogens but here are some examples of the most types commonly present in the west:

- Acrylamides – high temperature cooking of carbohydrates
- Acetaldehyde – manufacturer of acetic acid, flavourings and plastics
- N-nitroso compounds – particularly bloody red meat
- Hydroperoxide, alkoxy and epoxides – heated proteins
- Polycyclic or aromatic hydrocarbons – smoked foods, burnt,barbecued foods
- Allylaldehyde (acrolein), butyric acid and other nitrosamines – heated fats
- Nitropyrene, benzpyrene and nitrobenzene – heated oils and smoke
- Methylglyoxal and chlorogenic atractyosides in over roasted coffee
- Pesticides, fertilizers, herbicides – water, crops and vegetables
- Benzene, formaldehyde, ammonia, acetone – alcohol, smoke
- Hydrogen cyanide, and arsenic – smoke
- Lead – exposure industrial batteries
- Diesel exhaust – occupational exposure to commercial vehicles
- Atrazine - widely used as a herbicide

Acrylamides

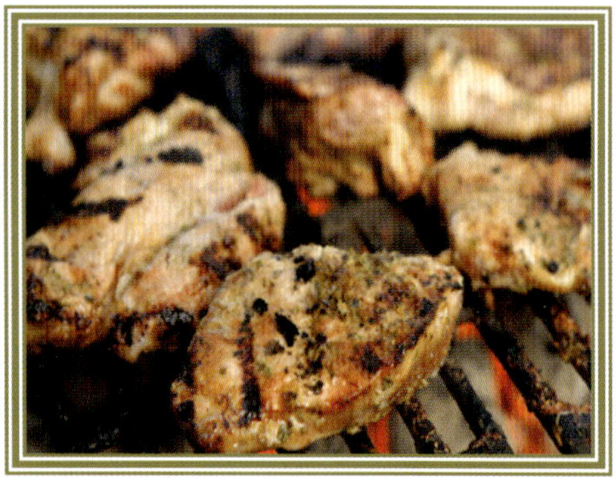

The most familiar group of carcinogens are the acrylamides, usually generated by cooking or processing, particularly when food is cooked at 117°F (47°C) for three minutes or longer. For example grilling, high temperature oven baking or frying of meat, fats, and starchy carbohydrates such as potatoes (making crisps), chips and baked snacks. The Food and Drug Administration (FDA) regularly analyse a variety of U.S. foods for acrylamide concentrations and publish league tables such as these examples below.

Summary – acrylamide concentrations in common foods (FDA 2010):

Often greater than 1000 ug/kg

- Burnt barbequed meat or fat
- Burnt toast, pizzas
- Veggie chips, potato snacks or potato crisps
- Dry roasted oat or wheat bran crackers

Usually between 500-1000 ug/kg

- French fries / chips
- Processed baked potatoes or hash browns
- Ginger snap cookies, pretzels or sesame/nut snacks or tortillas
- Cream crackers and dried biscuits
- Low fat bruschetta / vegetable crackers
- Dried soup powder

Usually between 200-500 ug/kg

- Butter flavoured popcorn
- Frozen potato skins, corn flaked cereals or corn chips
- Processed prune juice
- Toast not burnt

This table can only be used as a rough guide because the levels of acrylamide (AA) depend not only on the foods we buy and eat, but the individual cooking processes. Boiling meat would have significantly lower levels than frying it for example. The levels of AA may also significantly alter between different brands of the same product by the way it has been processed. To make it clearer, there are now moves to legislate for the introduction of AA labelling on food products.

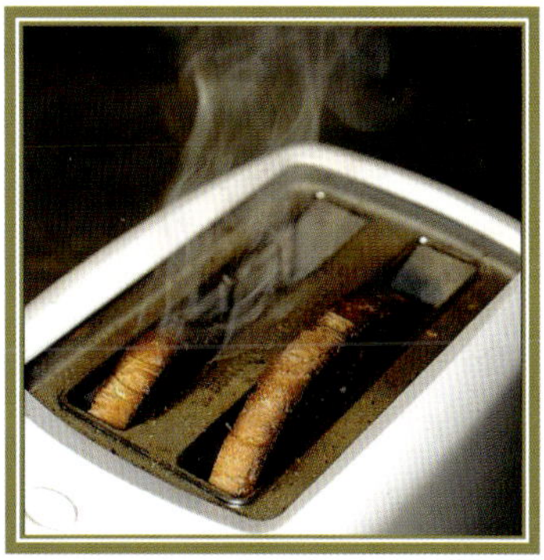

It must also be remembered that total ingested AA is more important than the concentration within each foods. For example, a small quantity of a food with high levels of AA such as a cream cracker is still safer than a large quantity of food with lower levels such as baked potatoes. Furthermore, the level of antioxidants in the same food or meal can also counterbalance the negative affects of the AA. A study from Philadelphia, USA showed that marinating meat in spices such as turmeric and sage before frying can significantly help, as can eating fresh salad and vegetables at the same time.

Xenoestrogens, environmental chemicals

Some chemicals can increase the risk of breast cancer not by directly damaging the DNA, like the acrylamides above, but by having a chemical structure similar to oestrogen. This stimulates breast tissues to grow rapidly and often in an uncontrolled way. These are termed xenoestrogens and are usually environmental pollutants or man-made chemicals. The most common group of chemicals are the polychlorinated biphenyls (PCB) and organochlorines found in sources which include car pollution, fuels, drugs and polycarbonate plastic baby bottles and food containers. It is difficult to avoid these chemicals in a modern environment as they are ingested in small quantities over long periods of time.

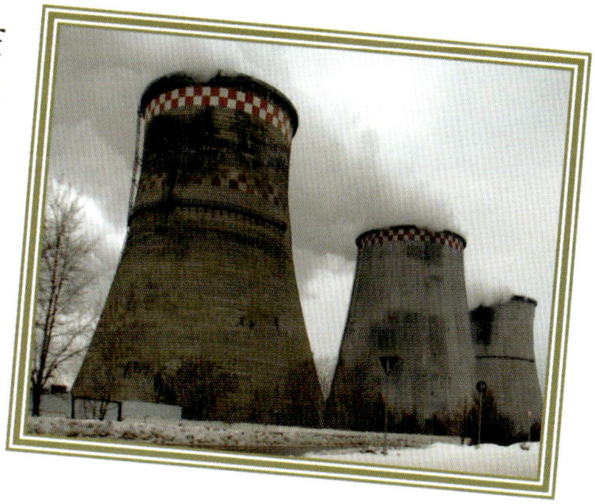

Researchers from five USA academic centres demonstrated that if the same oestrogenic pollutants in our environment are given to laboratory mice, they induce and promote mammary cancers. A further study in 1993 showed that rhesus monkeys developed a thickened uterus (the first stage to develop cancer) and endometriosis after being fed food that contained dioxin, a xenoestrogen,

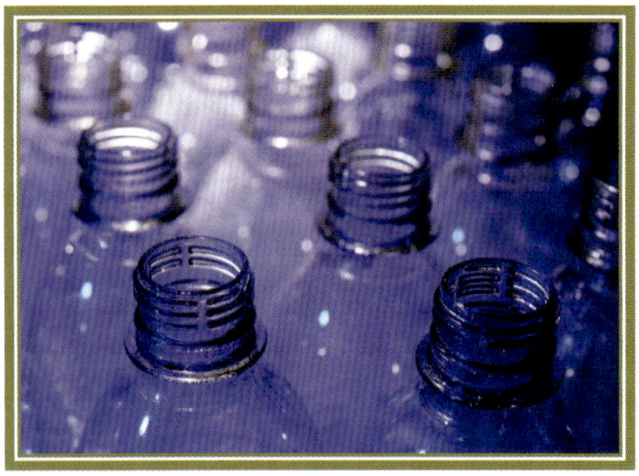

over a four-year period. Both endocrinologists (specialists in disorders of endocrine glands such as ovaries and testes) and reproductive biologists have suggested that long-term exposure to xenoestrogens might underlie the rise in endometriosis, fibroids, infertility and breast cancer in women. In men, many scientists believe that oestrogenic pollutants are responsible for some disturbing trends such as decreasing sperm count and function and decreasing testosterone production. In the animal kingdom, plastic infiltrating the water supply may explain the shrinking sizes of alligator penises!

Pesticides, fertilizers and herbicides

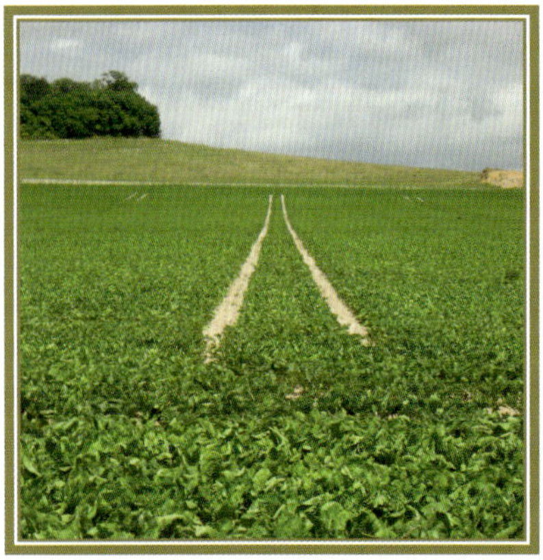

There are over 350 permitted pesticides allowed in western farming but researches have estimated that more than 70,000 other chemicals have been detected in our food chain, and most of these have not formally been tested for health risks. These pesticides, herbicides, fungicides, fertilizers and industrial pollutants are in our water because of rain erosion runoff from landfills and agricultural lands. Obviously, without them it would have been hard to feed the world, and many are safe, but their use is now geared to over commercialisation. Some of these, as well as being carcinogenic have also been found to be oestrogenic.

A report published in the International Journal of Andrology has linked pollutant oestrogenic chemicals in mothers' breast milk with an increased rate of testicular cancer in their male children. More specifically, researchers found that Danish men were up to four times more likely to have testicular cancer as men in neighbouring Finland. Investigators measured levels of 121 chemicals in 68 samples of breast milk from women in Denmark and Finland. They found a dramatic difference between the two countries, as Danish breast milk had significantly higher levels of some chemicals, including dioxins, polychlorinated biphenyls (PCBs) and pesticides, than Finnish breast milk. Why women in Denmark should have more of the chemicals in their breast milk than their Finnish neighbours remains unclear. Nevertheless, this study reinforces the view that environmental exposure to oestrogenic pollutants increases the risk of cancer and also in this case high rates of other male reproductive disorders, including poor semen quality and genital abnormalities.

In addition to hormone related conditions and cancers, such as testicular and breast cancer, animal studies have shown that polychlorinated biphenyls increase the risk of liver cancer and lymphoma by up to 65 percent compared to animals fed a chemical free diet. These chemicals are in our food supply – in plants, animals, fish and grains. They cannot be avoided and of an even greater concern is that switching to a diet with more fruit, salad and vegetables may paradoxically mean higher exposure to pesticides and herbicides unless extra precautions are taken to avoid them.

Smoke from lamps and candles

Burning everyday paraffin-wax candles can emit a multitude of toxic chemicals, including toluene and benzene. While it is nowhere near as harmful to light an occasional candle as it would be, for example, to smoke a pack of cigarettes a day, researchers at South Carolina State University suggest that frequent candle burning in tight, unventilated areas has been implicated in lung cancer, asthma, and skin rash.

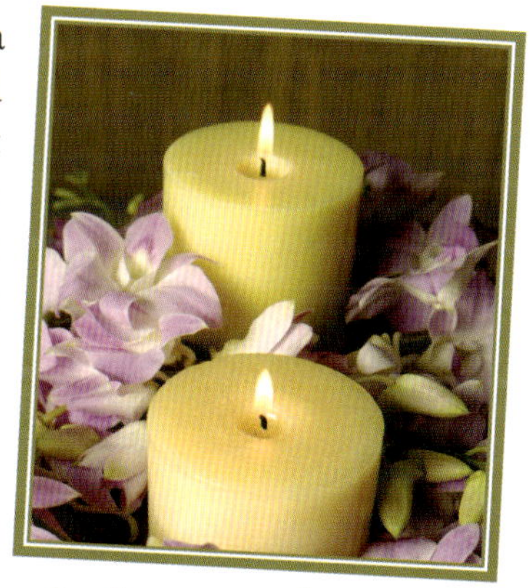

Speaking before a chemical society meeting, the researchers explained that the candles, which are made from petroleum, are a source of known human carcinogens and indoor pollution. However, candles made from beeswax or soy, although more expensive, are apparently safer, because they do not release potentially harmful pollutants.

Cosmetics, parabens and aluminium

A class of preservatives found in some deodorants and cosmetics are called parabens which, in the laboratory, have also been found to have harmful xenoestrogenic properties.

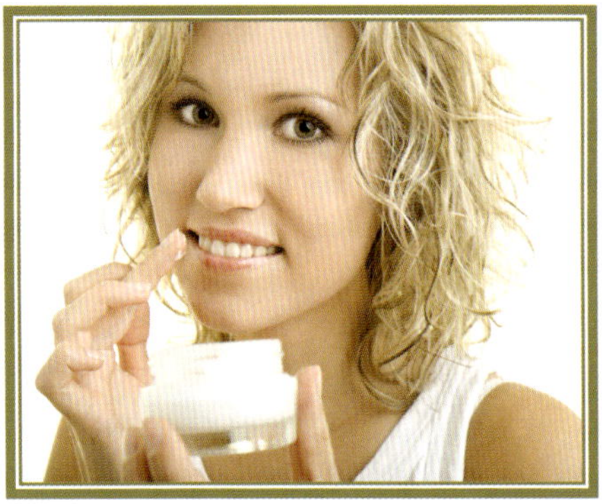

An initial concern in humans was raised following a study in 2004 from Reading University, UK, which demonstrated higher quantities of parabens in the outer part of the breast and within breast cancer cells themselves. Although a direct link with cancer is not proven it did encourage some manufacturers to remove parabens from their products, but in many items such as shower gels and shampoo they can still be seen on the label.

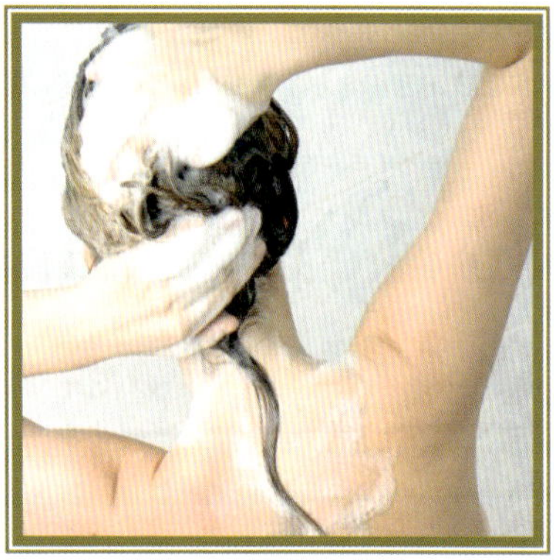

Aluminium salts are responsible for the anti-sweating affect of antiperspirants. A study in 2007 from Keel University created a lot of media activity when it showed higher quantities of aluminium in the upper outer area of the breast in those who used antiperspirants regularly. Aluminium has also been shown to have harmful oestrogenic properties when tested in the laboratory and consequently comes under the classification of metaloestrogens. Users of Aluminium based antiperspirants are understandably concerned that the higher levels in the breast may increase the risk of cancer, although this has not been proven in a study, which would be very difficult to design. Nevertheless, breast cancer specialists also have concerns over oestrogenic chemicals within cosmetics.

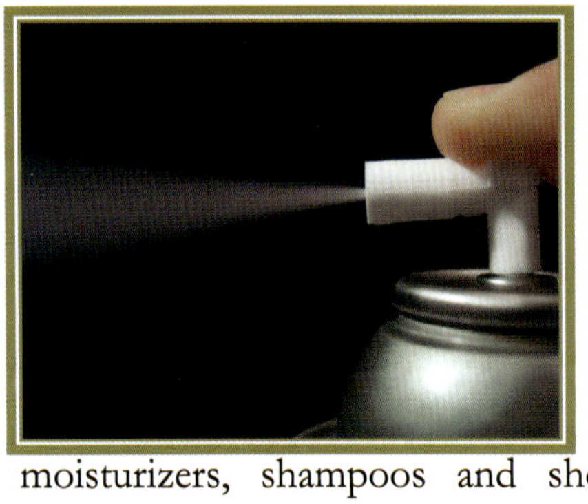

In the prestigious San Antonio Breast Cancer Symposium a presentation reported the finding that widely available moisturizers contain parabens and other chemicals which mimic oestriol or estrone, two powerful oestrogen-like compounds that could increase breast cancer risk if absorbed through the skin. They concluded that women with breast cancer should forgo using topical moisturizers, shampoos and shower gels that contain parabens or other oestrogenic preservative, as there is a chance that they may interfere with their treatment and increase the long term risk of relapse.

Non-chemical carcinogens and lifestyle factors

Not all carcinogens are in the form of chemicals yet some of these can be just as harmfull to our DNA. Sunlight is a carcinogen, if taken in excess and this has already been discussed on page 92. Other factors are described below:

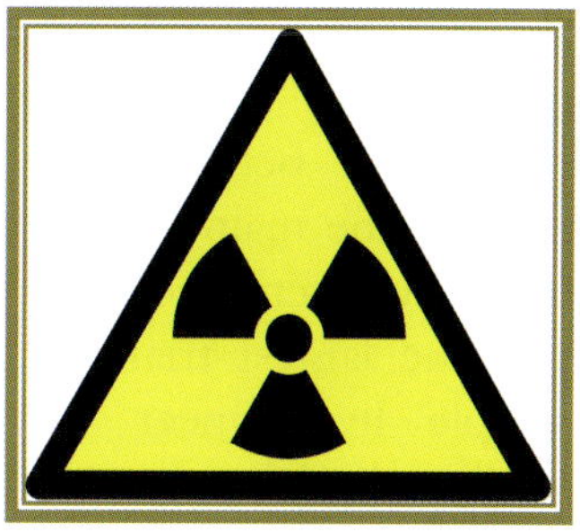

Radioactivity can arise from a number of sources. Survivors of the Second World War atomic bombs had an increased risk of cancer. However, a study which assessed survivors lifestyle over the period of many years showed that those who had a high intake of antioxidants and avoided other carcinogens successfully reduced their risk. This was an important study because it showed that the risk of cancer following exposure to one carcinogen can be made worse by exposure to a completely different type (an additive effect). Medical x-rays are also a significant source of radioactivity and although this is small, there should be a good reason to have an X-ray. Another source is radon gas which is naturally released from stones, particularly granite and concerning levels have been found in stone cottages especially in Cornwall. A recent study also recorded increased levels of radon gas in kitchens with granite work surface and advised keeping these rooms well ventilated. If you are worried about radon gas levels in your house there are various agencies which will measure them for you. Acceptable levels are less than 2pCi /L of air, if levels are above this, and certainly above 4 pCi/L adaptions to the house may be advised.

Electricity pylons, power lines and aerials. An Italian court has been investigating the 60 huge steel aerials erected on farmland by the Vatican during the last century to transmit Vatican Radio programs around the World. The courts commissioned a team from the National Tumour Institute and did conclude that there was a connection between the towers and cancer incidents. This included 19 child deaths from leukemia or lymphoma between 1980 and 2003. The risk appeared to be higher in children under 14 who lived less than 7.5 miles from the masts. They also found evidence of a link between the radiation and adult cancers but only among those who lived much closer to the antennae. Consequently, six officials of Vatican Radio have been placed under investigation for manslaughter. This Italian study does not, however, match the finding from other scientists across the world. The University of California, Los Angeles investigated link between electrical fields from improperly laid power lines or kitchen appliances exacerbated children's cancer risk. Although prior studies had suggested a flimsy association between extremely low-frequency magnetic fields (ELF-MFs) and leukaemia, their review of 10 studies, showed no proven link.

A study of 1,397 cancer cases in the UK, published in British Medical Journal, reported that children whose mothers lived close to a mobile phone tower while pregnant did not appear to be at any higher risk of cancer than children whose mothers lived farther away. The team also gathered detailed data about all 81,781 mobile phone towers that were operational during that time. The researchers found that, in virtually every permutation of their calculations, there was no correlation between the towers and the cancer cases. The main author of the paper, John Bithell of the University of Oxford, commented that this was the largest trial in the world of its kind and people living near cell phone towers can be reassured. Other international studies analysied by the World Health Organization (WHO) have found no link between electricity pylons and cancer.

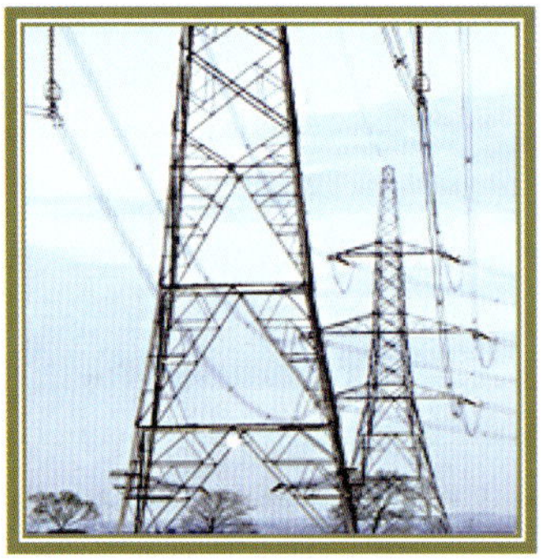

Mobile phones. There have been a number anecdotal reports that heavy users of cell phones have an increased risk of brain tumours caused by the electromagnetic fields and radiation. The WHO, therefore, decided to review the world evidence to find out whether this was true. The decade-long investigation was conducted in 13 countries involving 12,800 people. Researchers interviewed tumour sufferers and people in good health to see whether their mobile phone use differed. They found that six of eight studies found some rise in the risk of glioma (a common brain tumour) and two of seven showed an increase in benign tumours (neurinoma). Despite this, following a combined analysis, the overall conclusion was that the weight of scientific evidence has not linked cell phones with any health problems. The American FDA also reported that "The best science doesn't show a link between cell phone use and cancer of any kind. No link whatsoever."

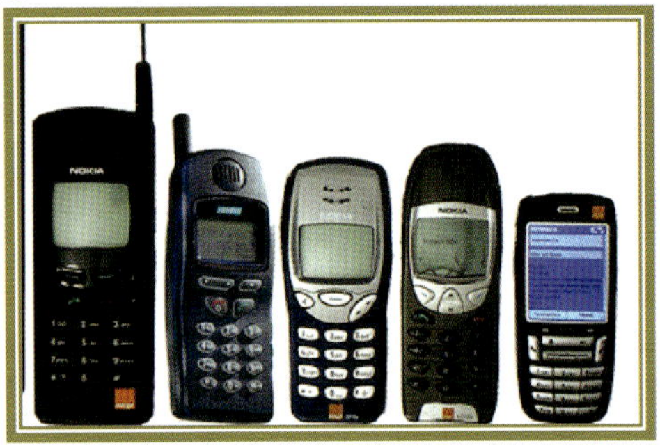

Marriage A study published "Cancer" showed that married cancer patients lived longer than single ones. Data indicated that 65% of married patients survived at least five years after diagnosis, compared with 57% of those who had never been married, 52% of the divorced patients and 47% of widowed. The researcher did not claim that being single was carcinogen but postulated that married patients have a built-in support system and are more likely to stick to their treatment regimens. It is also likely that they may even be in better health to begin with.

Having a desk job. An analysis of 45,000 men aged 45 to 79 appearing in the British Journal of Cancer found that those who had highly physical jobs were 28% less likely to develop prostate cancer than those who spent most of their working lives sitting.. The researchers, from the Karolinska Institute in Sweden, concluded, "Findings from this study show that not sitting for most of the time during work or occupational activity and more active living (walking or cycling) is associated with reduced prostate cancer incidence.

Watching TV A study published in "Circulation" described a link between the time an individual spends watching television and his or her risk of death.. They tracked the TV-viewing habits of 8,800 adults and followed them for six years. Every hour of daily TV watching increased the risk of dying from any cause by 11% percent. for cardiovascular diseases the increased risk was 18 percent, and for cancer it was 9 percent. The research point out that this effect probably correlated with lack of exercise rather than a direct negative effect of the TV's rays – although more research is needed

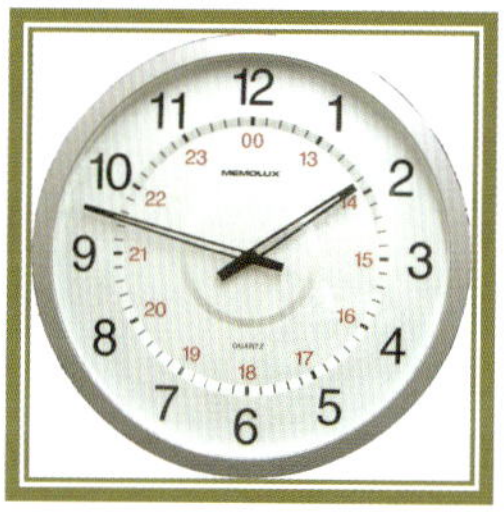

Night shift workers Emerging evidence is suggesting that individuals who have an exposure to light at night have a higher incidence of cancer. This largely applies to night shift workers in factories, hospitals and restaurants. The cause is thought to be a disruption of normal circadian rhythm which in turn upsets the excretion of melatonin. The hormone produced by the pituitary gland in the head has an influence on oestrogens and growth hormones.

In conclusion

There are thousands of potential cancer-forming chemicals (carcinogens) in our environment. Some are man-made and others occur naturally. It is impossible to eliminate contact with all environmental carcinogens, even if we recognised all of them. Fortunately, the body is generally pretty good at dealing with small quantities from time to time. The type of risk also varies between individuals depending on their genetic susceptibility and combination with other carcinogen and antioxidants. What is particularly dangerous is either a large quantity over a short period of time – although this is more likely to act as a poison and make you ill – or, more relevant to cancer, regular amounts over a long period of time. The evidence for the harmful effect of anti-perspirants and other oestrogenic cosmetics is anecdotal and indirect but remember many people apply these to their bodies very day from a young age, meaning that their lifetime exposure is considerable. This may not be harmful for most people but women with a family history of breast cancer, for example, may well have greater concerns. A comprehensive list of carcinogens is outside the scope of this book as they would fill a book on their own! Those with a morbid curiosity can download a list of over a thousand from cancernet.co.uk/carcinogens.htm.

Summary – general advice to avoid carcinogens:

- Steer clear of heavily processed foods
- Avoid foods high in additives, unhealthy fats, salt and sugars
- Avoid reheating fats and oils
- Avoid super-heated snacks such crisps, chips and cheap breakfast cereals
- Reduce the intake of smoked, barbequed or burnt foods
- Reduce red meat intake
- Limit foods with high AA concentrations from the list above
- Try eating as much raw (healthy) food as feasible
- Stop smoking
- Avoid passive smoke
- Avoid burning paraffin candles

Tips to avoid pesticides, herbicides and fertilizers:

- Buy a good salad spinner
- Soak lettuce leaves and herbs in water thoroughly, then dry before eating
- Wash fruit before putting them into the fruit bowl
- Wash vegetables first and change the water before cooking
- Buy organic foods if possible

Tips to avoid other xenoestrogens and metaloestrogens:

- Avoid petrol and diesel fumes
- Avoid excessive amounts of deodorants and antiperspirants
- Use soap instead of shower gels which contain parabens
- Use glass rather than polycarbonate plastic bottles where possible
- Try not to reuse plastic water bottles
- Rinse soap and detergents thoroughly from cups and dishes after washing
- Avoid storing food in plastic food containers including plastic film

Chapter Ten

Alcohol, coffee, sugar Evidence, benefits, advice

Alcohol, resveratrol and sulphites

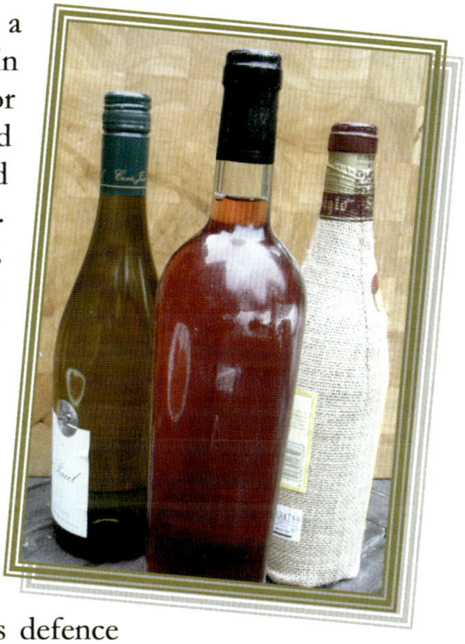

The majority of us would like to think that a few glasses of red wine are good for you. In terms of heart disease this may be correct. For example, red wine made from grapes has good levels of natural phytochemicals and antioxidants which have anti cancer effects. The most significant of these are resveratrol, catechins and tannins, which red wine contains more of than white wine because the making of white wine requires the removal of the skins after the grapes are crushed.

A lot of attention has recently been given to the benefits of resveratrol, a type of polyphenol called a phytoalexin, a class of compounds produced as part of a plant's defence system against disease. It is produced in the plant in response to an invading fungus or ultraviolet irradiation. Resveratrol has been shown to reduce tumour incidence in animals by affecting one or more stages of cancer development. It is known to inhibit growth of many types of cancer cells in culture. Evidence also exists that it can reduce inflammation, inhibit the COX-2 pathway and boost the immunity. Further laboratory studies of prostate, breast and bowel cells have shown that resveratrol can act on initiation, promotion, and progression of cancer cells.

In humans, research studies published in the International Journal of Cancer show that drinking a glass of red wine a day may cut a man's risk of prostate cancer in half and that the protective effect appears to be strongest against the most aggressive forms of the disease. It was also observed that men who consumed four or more glasses of red wine per week have a 60% lower incidence of the more aggressive types of prostate cancer.

Sources of resveratrol: Spanish wines have the highest levels among the red wine variety, followed by the pinot noir varieties. As well as in red wine high levels of resveratrol are also found in grapes, blueberrys raspberries, peanuts and peanut butter. More exotic sources include white hellobore and Japanese knotweed.

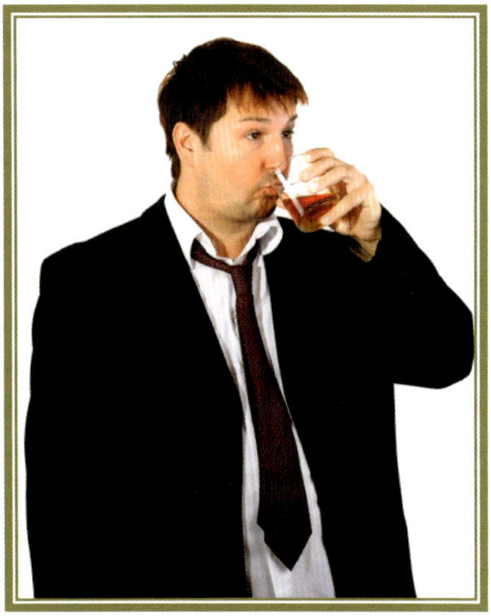

Before you rush out and start guzzling red wine for breakfast there is a sting to this seemingly positive tail. Unfortunately, the antioxidant in red wine overall does not seem to counterbalance the harmful affects. International health organizations such as the World Health Organisation now agree that alcoholic drinks can increase the risk of breast cancer as well as others such as mouth, oesophagus, bowel and liver. This can be accepted as a real independent risk, although the evidence for an increased association between alcohol and cancer is compromised by the knowledge that heavy drinkers also tend to smoke, eat poorly and lack exercise. The most convincing evidence for this comes from the Million Women Study published in 2009. Since 1996 this study has been gathering detailed information from 1.28 million women ages 50 to 64 years. Amongst other lifestyle factors, they examined how much alcohol women reported consuming when they volunteered for the study and again three years later, examining whether there was any link with the 68,775 cancers they subsequently, as a group, they developed over the next seven years. There were statistically significant increased risks of cancer in those who regularly consumed alcohol. Another study by Thun and his colleagues indicated that more than one drink a day increased the risk of breast cancer, but up to one drink was not associated with an increased risk. A further study from the University of California (2009) showed that men who drank heavily (>50g of alcohol or four drinks daily) doubled their risk of prostate cancers compared to other men. What's more, the cancers they developed tended to be more advanced and have a higher grade, implying that drinkers have a poorer prognosis.

A study in 2006 evaluated a group of survivors following head and neck cancer, recording alcohol intake for a median follow-up of one year. There was a significant difference in the rate of relapse, which in these cases almost entirely led to death. Survival in those who continued to drink excessively was less than 10 percent whereas in those who gave up or drank in moderation was four times higher.

The evidence of alcohol and risk of relapse after breast and other cancers is less convincing. In fact, one study from the Catholic University and the National Research Council in Italy showed that a glass of wine a day may cut the risk of treatment-linked skin toxicity by two-thirds in women undergoing radiation therapy for breast cancer. They evaluated the drinking habits of 348 women with breast cancer and found that patients who drank wine on the days they had their treatment had lower rates of acute toxicity than those who did not.

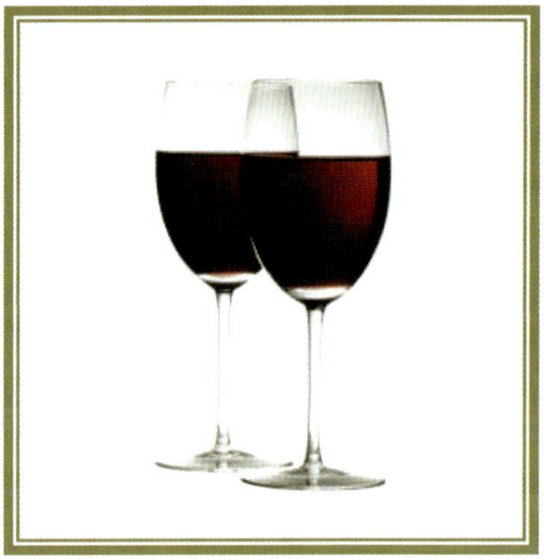

This observation did beg the question that wine may also reduce the effectiveness of radiotherapy, but relapse rate was not measured in this study. A further study in 2009 examined a group of 365 women with ER+ve breast cancer who had later developed cancer in the other breast. He compared their lifestyles with 726 matched controls. Consumption of more than 7 alcoholic beverages a week, obesity and smoking were all associated with the risk of cancer in the other breast.

Why could alcohol be harmful?

Some researchers feel the independent alcohol risk lies in the understanding that alcohol is converted into a chemical called acetaldehyde. Acetaldehyde is carcinogenic, damaging DNA and preventing it from being repaired. People who smoke and drink heavily have very high levels of acetaldehyde in their saliva. Alcohol is also fattening, and this leads to a higher cancer risk. Alcohol excess over long periods of time can lead to liver cirrhosis, which greatly increases the risk of liver cancer. Recent studies have specifically linked breast cancer and one study published by Cancer Research UK calculated that a woman's risk of breast cancer rises by 6 percent for each extra alcoholic drink she consumes on an average daily basis (7 percent on international measures). This is thought to be caused by alcohol's ability to increase your own body's oestrogen levels.

Advice to drink alcohol sensibly

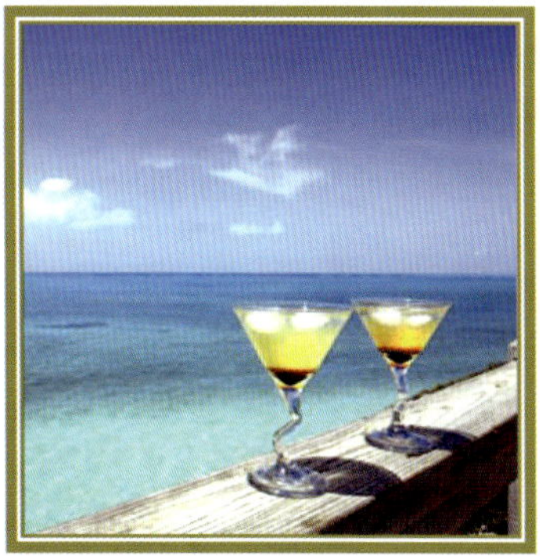

How much alcohol is harmful? This depends on other lifestyle factors such as smoking and diet. Even small amounts of alcohol can increase the risk of breast cancer and correlates with a higher risk of relapse. A group of scientists who analysed almost 100 previous studies found no safe lower limit for alcohol intake. Another study from the USA showed that mortality from breast cancer was 30 percent higher among women reporting at least one drink daily than amongst non-drinkers. Another American study found that one drink a day increased the risk of bowel cancer by 70 percent. A Japanese study found that people triple their risk if they drink three to five units a day, and quadruple their risk if they drink five units or more. As the safe limit is difficult to determine, the DoH have issued sensible guidelines based on available evidence – although these are largely related to the heart, brain and liver-related damage – which currently stands at 14 units per week for women, 21 units per week for men. (A premium pint of lager, beer or cider (5% vol) contains 3 units, a standard 175ml glass of wine (11-12% vol) contains 2 units. A double (35ml) shot of spirits (40% vol) contains 3 units.)

From a symptomatic point of view many alcoholic drinks use sulphites to preserve the fruits. As well as contribution to the all too familiar hangover, sulphites have been associated with an exacerbation of hay fever or asthma in vulnerable individuals and an increase in joint pains, a problem which is already common enough among women taking hormone therapies for breast cancer. Individuals taking biological drugs such as herceptin often complain of a blocked nose and this can be made worse by sulphites.

Although their inclusion is regarded as safe, the EU have designated an "acceptable daily intake" of 0.7mg per kg. That's 42mg a day if you are a 60kg female. A medium glass of white wine contains about 26mg; five dried apricots have 80mg. Last year the EU also introduced new rules that foods containing more than 10mg of sulphites per kg or litre must now be labelled. There is also a maximum permitted level: for dried fruit, cured meats, processed food and concentrated cordials this is 600-2,000mg per kg. For wine it's 200mg per litre. The trouble is that the quantity over this threshold is not declared so the levels of sulphites in wine will vary a good deal and can vary from label to label, or even from year to year. Good wines will generally be lower in sulphites, as are most organic brands, and Champagne has lower amounts because it's fermented in the bottle, although this does not apply to most sparkling wines which are the worst of the lot. Cider is generally high in sulphites because apples oxidise readily, but due to strict brewing laws German beers are also very low in sulphites. Beware of mixers and squashes – particularly lime cordial – which are usually very high in sulphites, as are juices made from concentrate.

After chemotherapy some patients complain of a bloating and gassy feeling in their abdomen. This may be due to an upset in the normal gut bacteria. Taking probiotics can help but until the natural balance is returned there may be a temporary wheat or barley intolerance which may have not been present previously. In this setting it is worth avoiding beer and lager or, if not, certainly check these symptoms do not get worse after drinking a beer – which may be several hours later or even the next day.

Summary – tips for cutting down alcohol intake:

- Keep an alcohol diary and set yourself an alcohol limit and stick to it
- Pace your drinks by sipping them slowly
- Try not to choose export beers which have high percentage alcohol
- Red wine contains more antioxidants than white so may be less harmful
- Premium German beers have less sulphites
- Organic UK beers have less chemicals and sulphites
- Try to choose wines with lower alcohol content
- Alternate alcoholic drinks with soft drinks
- Remember alcohol is fattening
- Try not to drink at home unless socialising
- Try to find something else to do instead e.g. a hobby or exercise class
- Have alcohol-free days to remind yourself
- Remember you don’t always have to drink to have fun

Coffee – pros and cons

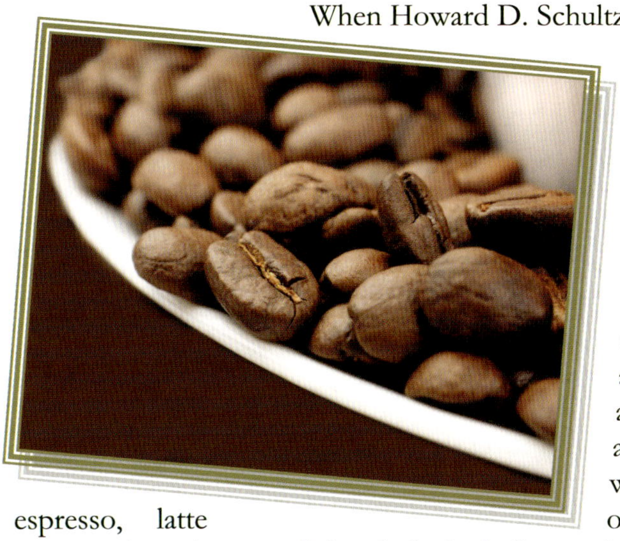

When Howard D. Schultz founded the company in 1985 that would become the wildely successful Starbucks chain, no one had to tell him that coffee was becoming the world's leading beverage and caffeine its most widely used drug. But, as with any product used to excess, producers and consumers often wonder about the health consequences, as even small amounts would affect millions of customers who daily order a double espresso, latte or cappuccino. Coffee drinks are complex mixtures of chemicals, including antioxidants and caffeine, several of which may independently affect health.

Cancer: Panic swept this coffee-dependent nation in 1981 when a Harvard study published in the British Medical Journal tied the drink to a higher risk of pancreatic cancer. The researchers later concluded that perhaps the association with smoking, not coffee, was the culprit. Later in an international review of 66 studies last year scientists found coffee drinking had little if any effect on the risk of developing cancer. In fact, another review in 2008 suggested that compared with people who do not drink coffee, those who do have half the risk of developing liver cancer. Finally, an observational study reported in 2010 suggested that regular coffee consumers have a lower incidence of prostate cancer. This benefit probably comes from coffee's antioxidants and chlorogenic acid.

Heart disease: The Centre for Science in the Public Interest in the USA published a comprehensive appraisal of scientific reports in its Nutrition Action Health letter. They analysed 10 studies of more than 400,000 people and found no increase in heart disease among daily coffee drinkers, whether their coffee came with caffeine or not. Another consensus report from cardiologists at the University of California, San Francisco, in 2000 concluded that there was little evidence that coffee and/or caffeine, in typical dosages, increases the risk of heart attacks. In a study from Johns Hopkins Hospital of 155,000 nurses, women who drank coffee with or without caffeine for a decade were no more likely to develop high blood pressure than non-coffee drinkers.

Bone loss: Some observational studies have linked caffeinated beverages to bone loss and fractures. This was confirmed by human physiological studies which found a slight reduction in calcium absorption had no effect on calcium excretion. The effect on bone is therefore mild and worse in consumers of caffeinated sugary drinks rather than coffee, which is often taken with milk. Dr. Robert Heaney, a bone density expert of Creighton University, quoted that caffeine's negative effect on calcium can be offset by as little as one or two tablespoons of milk. He advised that coffee and tea drinkers who consume the currently recommended amount of calcium need not worry about caffeine's effect on their bones.

Weight gain: Although caffeine speeds up metabolism, no long-term benefit to weight control has been demonstrated. In fact, in a study which followed more than 58,000 health professionals for 12 years, both men and women who increased their caffeine consumption gained more weight than those who didn't.

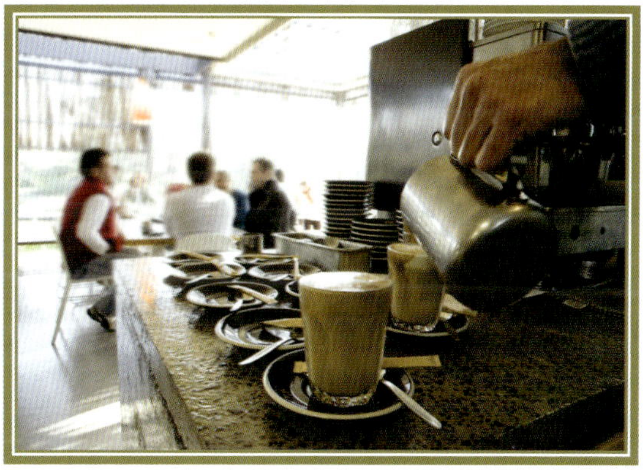

Mental ability and fatigue: Coffee drinkers are all too aware of the immediate "lift" after their morning brew. Researchers have confirmed this with studies that show that coffee has an immediate ability to enhance mood, mental and physical performance, and to improve a sense of well-being, happiness, energy, alertness and sociability. The trouble is that like all additive drugs there is a upside and a downside. In excess it can cause anxiety and the "shakes". Furthermore, when the positive "lift effect" wears off there may be a drop in "energy levels" caused by the withdrawal of caffeine from the blood stream, leading to fatigue. Individuals suffering from fatigue after cancer may be advised not to drink strong coffee as this withdrawal may cause more problems over the course of the day. Finally, for those who have trouble sleeping, remember that the caffeine in coffee can stay in the blood stream for 6-7 hours. Even having a coffee late afternoon can affect the ability to fall asleep at night.

Sugar and salt

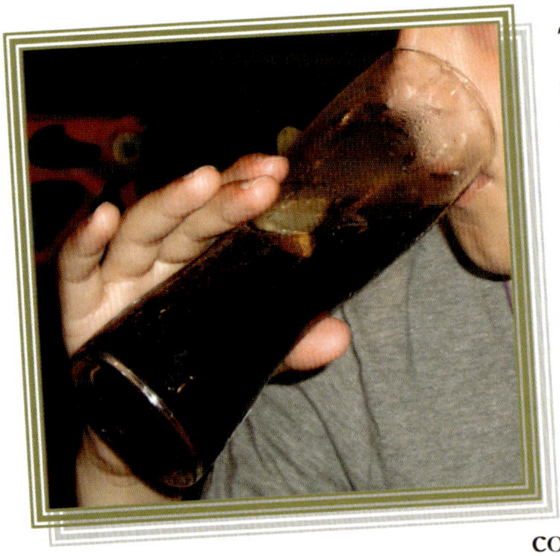

The link between processed sugar and cancer has been under appreciated in the passed although the scientific community is beginning to turn its attention towards its harm. Many nutuitionalists have always had their deep suspicions that "sugar feeds tumours" and many oncologist now believe the magnitude of the carcinogenic effects of sugar are Certainly, as foods packed with added sugars, and for that matter salt, are also likely to be heavily processed and contain more fats and carcinogens and increase the risk of obesity and high blood pressure. Chronic excessive sugar intake is associated with an increase risk of type II diabetes which is associated with an increased risk of cancer and increased risk of the cancers they develop being more aggressive and being. Even before diabetes is established chronic refined sugar intake leads to insulin resistance. In this scenario, the pancreas has to work harder to regular or bring down blood sugar levels. This is one of the features of a condition called "The metabolic syndrome". The precise definition varies but is usually defined as increased abdominal fat disposition, high blood pressure, insulin resistance and high blood sugars.

Evidence for a risk of sugar intake and cancer comes from a study published in the Public Library of Science Journal. They measured blood sugar levels in 274,126 men and 275,818 women from Norway, Austria, and Sweden and found that those individuals with excess blood sugar were more likely both to develop a range of cancers and also to die from it. Researchers found that women were more vulnerable than men and the risk was worst in those who were also overweight.

A study from University of Minnesota suggests that drinking two sugary soft drinks a week nearly doubles the risk of developing cancer. The study, funded by the National Cancer Institute looked at the dietary habits of more than 60,000 adults in Singapore for 14 years. More specifically the researchers found that two or more those who drank sugar-sweetened carbonated beverages were 87 percent more likely to develop pancreatic cancer than those who did not.

Why could salt and sugar be harmful?

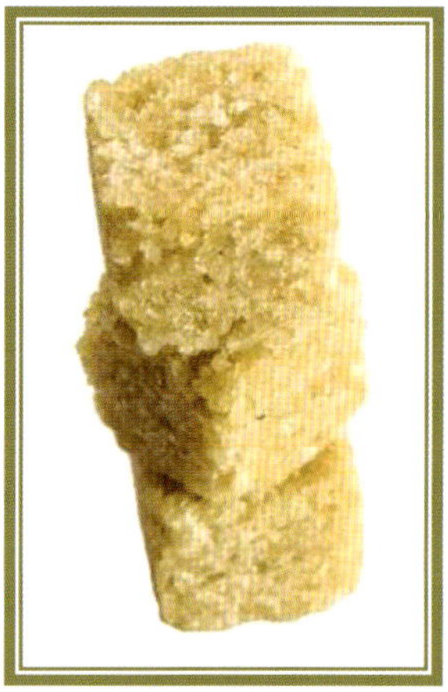

Refined sugars lead to higher insulin levels that have been shown to encourage cancer progression. High sugar and insulin levels also lead to over production of Insulin like Growth Factor (IGF) which as described above is implicated in carcinogenesis (the formation of cancer), cancer progression and metastasis. They also lead to increased food intake and obesity, which is also harmful. Studies have also found that sucrose cannot metabolise completely in our bodies, resulting in the formation of metabolites, such as pyruvic acid, and unstable sugars containing harmful five carbon atoms. These toxic by-products have been linked to lowering vitamin E levels and the formation of free radicals or oxidative metabolites. There have also been reports that sugar excess results in damage to the non-insulin secreting part of the pancreas. This can impair the production of enzymes such as trypsin and chymotrypsin, linked to a weakening of the healing processes and immune attack against cancer.

Advice to reduce table salt and sugar intake

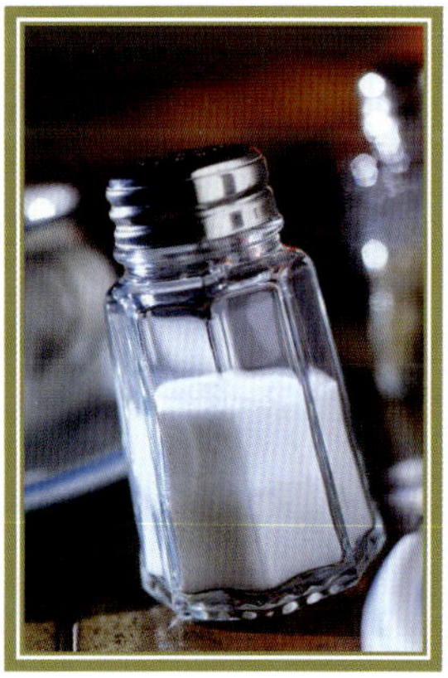

Refined sugars have had their fibre, proteins, vitamins and minerals removed so that they are rapidly absorbed into the body producing a 'sugar rush'. The pancreas interprets this as a big meal and responds by pumping insulin into the blood stream. Very shortly, the sugar levels drop drastically leading to hypoglycemia (low blood sugar) causing dizziness, hunger and tiredness that is only satisfied by eating more sugar, repeating the vicious cycle. On the other hand, sugars contained in natural whole foods are absorbed slower and are metabolised better, and do not produce this roller-coaster high and low sugar ride. It is clear that sugar is added to fizzy drinks, candy, sweets and cakes so it is worth reading the label of other processed foods such as "ready meals" where sugar is also added to supposedly enhance the favour. Some Indian restaurants add sugar to their curries – you can instruct the waiter to ask the chef to omit the sugar.

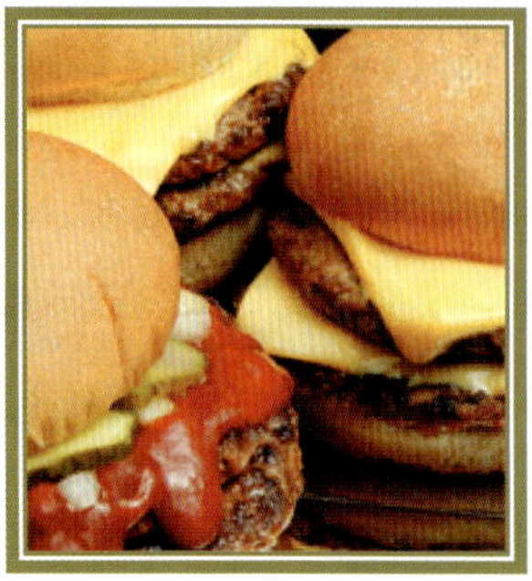

Salt protagonists argue that reducing the salt content of food may appear to reduce their flavour but, in fact, the opposite is true. After only one week of reduced salt intake the chemical structure of your taste buds changes so that sensitivity to salt increases. In reality food tastes just as salty with less salt in it. Furthermore, with salt not drowning out other flavours, the finer subtleties of taste can be appreciated. About 75 percent of the salt we eat comes from the food products we buy. There are obviously sources such as crisps, savoury snacks, pastries, burgers and pies but there may be high salt content of less obvious foods such as breakfast cereals, biscuits, bacon, ham, soups, sauces, ready-prepared meals. So it's important to shop carefully. If you can, try to choose products that say 'no added salt' and compare the nutritional information on different products. Try to avoid 'diet' foods – These are very salty and have artificial sweeteners to enhance taste. Although there is no evidence that artificial sweeteners are linked to cancer, they perpetuate the sweet-tooth phenomenon.

Summary – tips to reduce salt and refined sugar intake:

Reduce or avoid:

- Processed foods
- Pre-packed ready meals or those labelled as 'diet'
- Sweet snacks: cakes, sweets, biscuits and chocolate bars
- Sweet drinks: such as cola or other fizzy drinks
- Salty snacks: crisp, highly flavoured corn or potato snacks
- Salty food: such as cheese, bacon, pickles and anchovies
- Adding sugar to tea or coffee or salt to food during cooking
- Restaurants which add sugar to their meals

Alternatively:

- Taste food first, rather than initially adding salt or sugar
  — For snacks, consider raisins, crunchy vegetables, dried fruit
  — Easy-to-eat fruit such as grapes, bananas and Satsumas
  — Unsalted nuts (not for under-5s due to a risk of choking)
- Drink water or juices instead of fizzy drinks

Artificial sweeteners

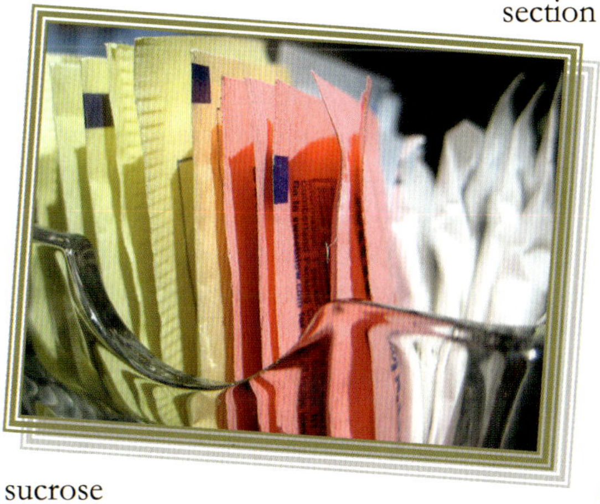

It is a little unfair to include artificial sweeteners in the "what to do less of" section of this book when the evidence for any harm is very poor despite the previous newspaper headlines. Nevertheless, they are present in prolific quantities in our diets so they are worth discussion, especially as their influence on cancer has been the subject of much debate.

These sugar substitutes are substances that are used instead of sucrose (table sugar) to sweeten foods and beverages. Questions about artificial sweeteners and cancer arose when early studies showed that a particular brand called Cyclamate (no longer used) in combination with saccharin, caused bladder cancer in laboratory animals. However, results from subsequent carcinogenic studies on these sweeteners and other approved sweeteners (i.e. studies that examine whether a substance can cause cancer) have not provided clear evidence of an association between artificial sweeteners and cancer in humans. Subsequent studies in rats showed an increased incidence of bladder cancer with high doses of saccharin consumption, especially in male rats. However, mechanistic studies (studies that examine how a substance works in the body) have shown that these results apply only to rats. Human studies have shown no consistent evidence that saccharin is associated with bladder cancer incidence.

Aspartame, distributed under several trade names (e.g. Nutrasweet® and Equal®), was approved in 1981 by the US Food and Drug Association after numerous tests showed that it did not cause cancer or other adverse effects in laboratory animals. Questions regarding the safety of aspartame were renewed by a 1996 report suggesting that an increase in the number of people with brain tumours between 1975 and 1992 might be associated with the introduction and use of this sweetener in the United States. However, analysis of current statistics showed that the overall incidence of brain tumours began to rise in 1973, eight years prior to the approval of aspartame, and continued to rise

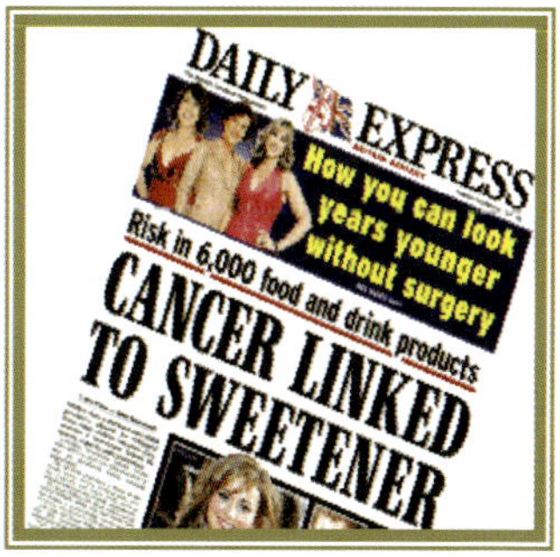
DAILY EXPRESS

How you can look years younger without surgery

Risk in 6,000 food and drink products

CANCER LINKED TO SWEETENER

until 1985. Moreover, increases in overall brain cancer incidence occurred primarily in people aged 70 and older, a group that was not exposed to the highest doses of aspartame since its introduction. These data suggest there is no link between the consumption of aspartame and the development of brain tumours.

Likewise, an early laboratory experiment found more lymphoma and leukaemia in rats fed very high doses of aspartame (equivalent to drinking 2,083 cans of diet soda daily). However, there were some inconsistencies in the findings. Subsequently, the National Cancer Institute of the USA examined human data from the largest Dietary and Health Study involving over half a million retirees. Increased consumption of aspartame-containing beverages was not associated with the development of lymphoma, leukaemia or brain cancer.

In addition to saccharin and aspartame, there are three other artificial sweeteners currently permitted for use in food in the United States. Acesulfame potassium (also known as ACK, Sweet One®, and Sunett®) was approved by the Food and Drug Administration in 1988 for use in specific food and beverage categories. It was later approved as a general-purpose sweetener (except in meat and poultry) in 2002. Sucralose (also known as Splenda®) was approved by the FDA as a tabletop sweetener in 1998, followed by approval as a general-purpose sweetener in 1999. Neotame, which is similar to aspartame, was approved by the FDA as a general-purpose sweetener (except in meat and poultry) in 2002. Before approving these sweeteners, the FDA reviewed more than 100 safety studies that were conducted on each sweetener, including studies to assess cancer risk. The results of these studies showed no evidence that these sweeteners caused cancer or posed any other threat to human health.

In conclusion, there is little good evidence that sweeteners cause cancer in humans but they do not reduce the cravings for sugar and remember, they are a man-made chemical – it may be wise not to take them in excess

Chapter Eleven

Other lifestyle issues
Evidence, benefits, advice

Aspirin, salicylates cancer and diet

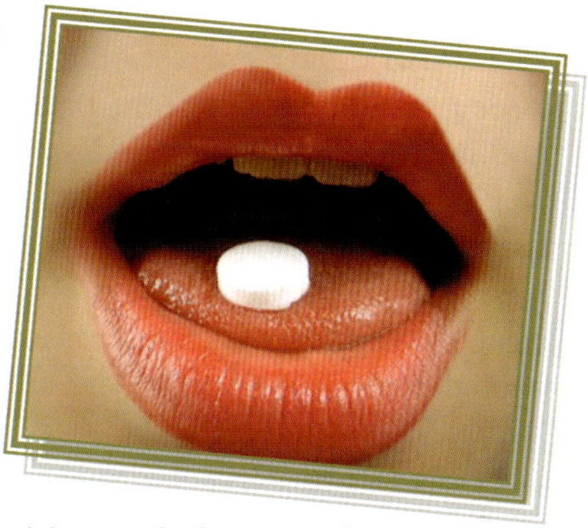

Over the last few years there has been great excitement and interest shown in an enzyme called cycloxidase (COX), which is modified by the salicylate chemical found in aspirin-like drugs or some foods, and has been strongly implicated in the cancer pathway.

Interest in the anti-cancer properties of salicylates or the most widely available type, aspirin (acetyl-salicylate), has emerged following a discovery, via questionnaire survey, that people who took aspirin regularly seemed to have a lower incidence of cancer. The most notable of these was the Health Professionals Follow-up Study (HPFS) cohort at Harvard University, USA, which reported a decreased risk of advanced prostate cancer among men with regular aspirin use.

In an observational study published in the very reputable Journal of Clinical Oncology in 2010, researchers evaluated 4,164 women who had been diagnosed with early breast cancer. They found that those women who just happened to be taking aspirin somewhere between two and five days a week, there was a reduction in the risk of dying of the breast cancer. More specifically, although in women who took aspirin just once a week there was no benefit, those who took aspirin two to five times a week experienced a 71 percent reduction in the risk of dying from a return of the cancer.

Two prospective randomised trials involving individuals with polyps and bowel cancer evaluated the benefits of aspirin. The first involved participants who had polyps removed from their large bowel – half were given aspirin and the other half placebo. At two years there was a significantly lower number of polyps in the aspirin group compared to the placebo group. The same benefit was found in a second study involving patients who had actually had bowel cancer. Not only did aspirin reduce the incidence of subsequent polyps, it reduced the incidence of new secondary cancers in the bowel.

Mechanism of action of salicylates.

Many cancer cells have been shown to over-express a type of cycloxidase protein called COX-2 in laboratory studies. This protein has been found to be integrally involved in the fundamentals of cancer progression, namely: reduced apoptosis (***immortality***), spreading to adjacent organs (***invasion)***, development of new blood vessel formation (***angiogenesis***) and spreading to other areas of the body (***metastasis***). Over-expression of COX-2 has not been found in normal cells, but is seen in those taken from patients with bowel, prostate and ovarian cancers. Anti-inflammatory drugs and salicylates found in painkillers can block COX-2 over expression and hence they may have an important role in blocking the malignant process. More importantly, fresh vegetables also contain natural salicylates so the mechanisms of their health benefits are likely to include an influence on the malignant process through the COX pathway, and not just through their vitamin, fibre and antioxidant mechanisms.

A scientist recently found that the expression of COX-2 increased when a slow growing (indolent) tumour mutates into a more aggressive type. Salicylates inhibit the function of the COX-2 protein, thereby potentially preventing early cancers from growing, becoming more aggressive, invading or spreading to other organs.

Not surprisingly, in view of this theoretical and laboratory background, numerous studies were conducted and published using salicylates, or non steroidal anti-inflammatory drugs (NSAID's), in patients with cancer. These, however, have mainly been designed to determine if they helped prevent cancer coming back after initial treatment, rather than a direct treatment in itself. Researchers have also tended to use the newer, highly selected NSAID's known as pure COX-2 inhibitors, which are thought to avoid the unwanted gastro-intestinal side effects, whilst amplifying the anti-cancer COX-2 effects.

The benefits of these pure COX-2 inhibitors over natural salicylates (those in tablet form or those found naturally within the diet) have not however been established. Concerns have also arisen about the safety of some pure COX-2 inhibitors. Firstly, the reduction in gastrointestinal side effects of pure COX-2 inhibitors has not been as strong as expected when tested clinically, and indigestion and gastric damage remains high. Secondly, pure COX-2's adversely affect blood pressure and, following long-term use, can affect the kidneys. Thirdly, most of the prospective studies so far have actually shown a reduced incidence of malignancy associated with aspirin rather than other more pure NSAID's. Fourthly, the only prospective randomised clinical studies in oncology published to date used ***aspirin***, showing a protective benefit against recurrent bowel cancer. Finally, the cardiac safety of some third generation NSAID's has more recently been put in doubt with some trials actually showing an increased death rate caused by heart attacks. The answer, as is often the case, may lie in nature. People with diets rich in fruit and vegetables, particularly vegetarians, have serum salicylate equivalent to a dose of up to 80mg a day – usually more than enough to initiate COX-2's likely biochemical anti-cancer process (the conversion of arachidonic acid to prostaglandins). A higher intake of fruit and vegetables, as well as delivering numerous other health benefits, actually protects the stomach and digestive pathway, reducing the risk of adverse gastrointestinal symptoms such as indigestion.

There is much we still do not know about the full benefits of COX-2 inhibition and a number of interesting trials are ongoing amongst patients with established cancer. One study, described in a previous chapter, has shown that up to 40 percent of men with progressive prostate cancer had a temporary stabilisation in their PSA following a program of diet and salicylates. A measure of COX-2 over-expression in cancer cells and its inhibition within further dietary intervention studies would be useful. It would be particularly interesting to compare improved diet with salicylate supplementation but as this would be difficult to design and has no commercial interest, it would be unlikely to attract funding.

Grapefruit and breast cancer

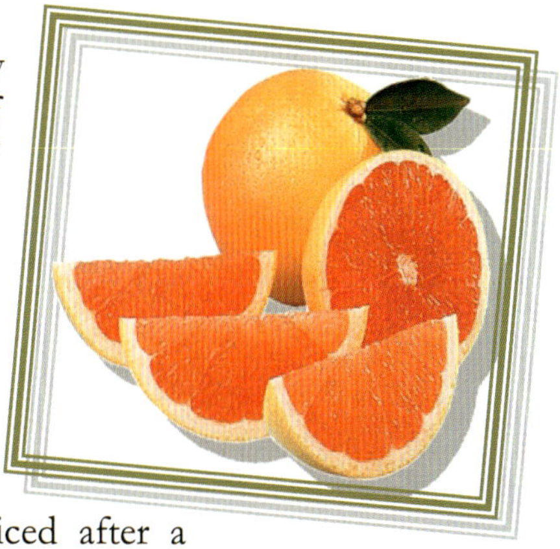

It seems incredible that a nice-tasting healthy looking fruit can actually increase the risk of cancer, but there have been a number of studies confirming this. The culprit is thought to be its inhibition of an enzyme in the gut called cytochrome P450 or CYP3A4. Studies have shown that by tampering with this enzyme it interferes with more than 60 percent of orally administered drugs, including alcohol, which then results in increased blood levels. This effect was noticed after a single glass of grapefruit juice, with the peak effect about 24 hours after consumption. It was later found that this enzyme is also involved in the metabolism of oestrogens. This was confirmed in a study of post-menopausal women who were found to have 30 percent higher oestrogen levels if they consumed the equivalent of ¼ of a grapefruit a day.

As the risk of breast cancer is increased with higher oestrogen levels, further studies were conducted. One notable study did confirm that grapefruit consumption increased risk of developing breast cancer. A study published in 2007 equated a population of 50,000 post menopausal women between 1993 and 1996. There was a significantly higher risk of breast cancer in grapefruit eaters. There was approximately a 21 percent increased risk if women consumed more than ¼ of a grapefruit a day on average. This went up to 36 percent in high grapefruit consumers (>60g/day). Lean women (BMI< 25) had a slightly higher risk than their more full-bodied counterparts. This was because oestrogen levels are already higher in overweight women, so a further increase has less of an effect on the risk of breast cancer. For the same reason pre-menopausal women (with naturally high oestrogen levels) had no increased risk with grapefruit consumption.

So, unlike phytoestrogens such as soya, which lower your own body's oestrogen levels through a process call negative feedback, grapefruit actually increases your own oestrogen levels. Although no direct link with breast cancer relapse has been found in view of the increased risk of developing breast cancer in the first place, it is best avoided if post-menopausal naturally, or if you have been rendered post-menopausal after cancer therapies. As grapefruits also contain many healthy substances such as vitamins, antioxidants and fibre, they would be a useful regular addition to the diet in pre-menopausal women and men, provided they were not taken with prescribed medication.

In conclusion, if you have had breast cancer, have an extra risk of developing it or simply want to reduce your risks, it would be wise to avoid grapefruit juice, especially if you are post-menopausal and normal to thinly built.

Chapter Twelve

Dietary supplements
Nutritional testing

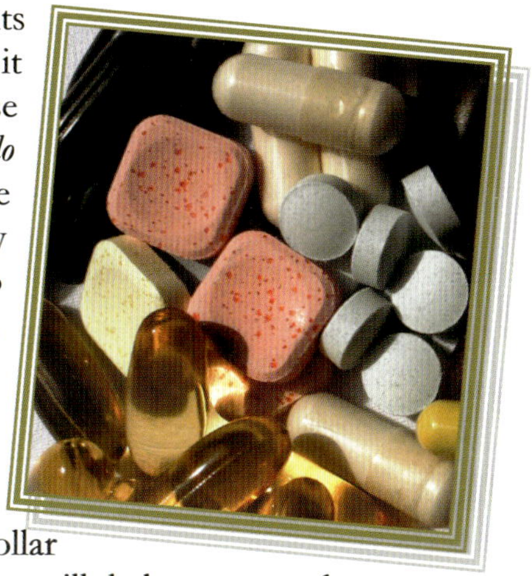

The decision to take dietary supplements requires a chapter of its own, not just because it is a complex and confusing subject, but because the issue does not fit neatly into the '*What to do more of*' **or** '*What to do less of*' sections. There may be situations where a supplement may help and others where the same one could do harm. Some individuals may benefit and yet, for others, the same substance could be harmful. This section considers the evidence for the pros and cons of supplements not influenced by the enormous pressures on you to pop a pill from the multimillion dollar supplement industry. Hopefully this evidence will help you reach your own decisions and look objectively at supplements, even when you are bamboozled with advertisements every time you open a magazine, walk into a chemist or supermarket or even glance at the side of a bus.

Advertising campaigns concentrate on the concept of a quick fix, simple pill which is a very attractive option, if true. They often show bored children munching through piles of unappetising looking vegetables alongside smiling attractive muscle men savouring the beauty and splendour of a single wonder pill. Unfortunately life is not that simple, especially when considering integrating genetics with the constantly changing biochemical cancer pathways. Supplements attempt to concentrate separate anti-cancer constituents of food and process them into convenient tablets or potions. Cancer is, however, a devious creature, evolving and interacting with mankind's genes and environment for millions of years, capable of changing it's makeup in order to avoid attack from the body's internal immunology. It is naive or indeed arrogant to assume that we fully understand the interaction of diet with the cancer process, or indeed our body's genetic makeup. The idea of pulling out one or two aspects of the dietary jigsaw and putting them into a simple pill is therefore inherently flawed. Cancer will form new pathways to avoid environmental or chemical attack. If diet or other lifestyle factors are to have any impact on established cancers, especially in the long term, they need to influence as many stages in the cancer pathway, and as many biological and immunological processes, as possible. Eating whole foods, with as much diversity as possible, is more likely to avoid deficiencies in these vital defence pathways, and to fuel the body's anti-cancer armamentarium.

This chapter provides a brief overview of the most commonly taken supplements, and offers a broad explanation of some of the advantages and disadvantages of taking them. Although much of the evidence has already been described in the evidence section of this book, as the topic is so relevant to many individuals it is worth summarising the issues again here. It must be emphasised that a complete overview for the evidence for supplements is outside the scope of this book, particularly as evidence for and against supplements being published week after week. For specific information regarding individual supplements it is probably best to refer to designated government websites such as www.nci.org. For ease of explanation the issue of taking supplements has been split into the pros and cons:

Pros and concerns with supplements

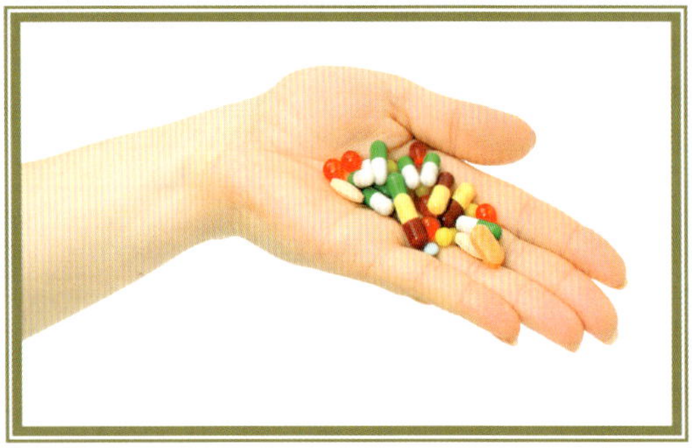

Apart from the expense, most supplements in moderation are probably harmless. Taking excess supplements, however, especially when they are not needed may have dangerous adverse risks. Some studies have clearly demonstrated that prolonged and excessive supplement intake actually increased the risks of developing a number of illnesses including cancer. Previous chapters have already described in detail these international studies, but in view of their importance, and in case you skipped them, this chapter will summarise the salient points again:

Carotenoid and vitamin A supplements

Prostate cancer cells and mice in the laboratory demonstrated an anti-cancer effect after being fed with vitamin A. However, in a study involving 10,472 U.S. men with an adequate diet, no reduction in prostate cancer incidence was demonstrated in those given vitamin A supplements. In this regard they may well be a waste of money and effort but the studies in which they are combined with beta-carotene show they may have more sinister consequences such as stroke and heart disease. These natural pigments have an anti-oxidant effect and people with higher dietary intake tend to have a lower rate of cancer. A substantial European study gave alpha-tocopherol (vitamin E) and carotenoid supplements in the form of beta-carotene to individuals who were either heavy smokers, or who had previously had cancer of the throat. The trial showed an elevated risk of lung and prostate cancer!

Vitamin E supplements

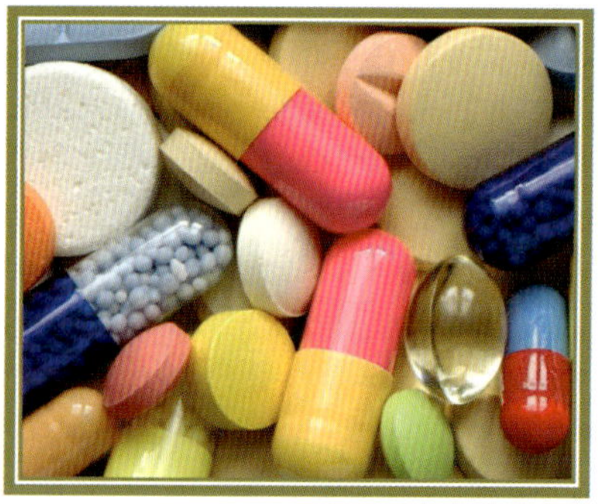

The tocopherol forms have also been shown to prevent less aggressive tumours changing to a more aggressive type. However, a study of vitamin A involving 30,000 male smokers, found that there was a reduction in the incidence of prostate cancer, but the incidence of lung cancer was actually higher. Other studies showed that smokers had lower vitamin E levels, but that this correlation was particularly high with the isoform of vitamin E called gamma-tocopherol which is the main vitamin E found in healthy foods, as opposed to the alpha-tocopherol found in man-made supplements. A further study which supplemented women with alpha-tocopherol, demonstrated no reduction in cancer, but the incidence of heart disease was slightly worse. Finally, another study of male smokers demonstrated a higher rate of cerebral haemorrhage if they also had high blood pressure.

Vitamin C

Vitamin C helps DNA sense and repair the damage caused by free radicals, such as hydrogen peroxide. Convincing experiments in humans in relation to cancer have either not been conducted or are inconclusive. Studies using high dose vitamin C, particularly if given via a vein (intravenous), caused kidney damage in some individuals.

Zinc

This essential metal is one of the elements needed to produce the superoxide dimutase (SOD) enzyme important to defend the body against the attack of dangerous free radicals. Laboratory experiments have shown that cells deficient in zinc are more likely to become cancerous. The role of zinc supplements in humans was highlighted in a study of 50,000 health professionals, 3348 of which developed prostate cancer. Detailed analysis showed that men who took normal amounts of zinc had the normal incidence of prostate cancer, but those who took supplemental zinc at levels of more than 100mg/day, or for long durations, were more than twice as likely to develop advanced prostate cancer.

Selenium supplements

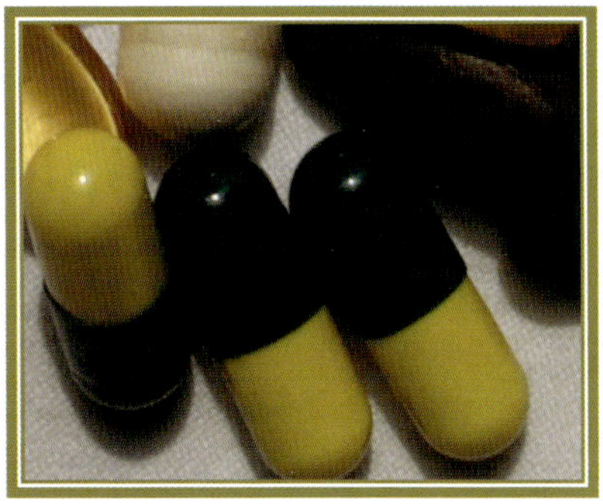

An eloquent trial, described above, gave 200 micrograms of dietary selenium or placebo to a large group of Americans. After several years there appeared to be a significantly lower level of lung, bowel and prostate cancer in the selenium group. Several large ongoing prevention studies are now underway across the world to try to confirm these findings and fine-tune the optimal selenium dose required. However, few have confirmed this finding including the large SELECT study of selenium and Vitamin E published in 2009 which showed no difference in the number of prostate cancers compared to the placebo. There was a suggestion that men who took supplements had a higher incidence of more aggressive tumours. Many suspect that the people who would benefit from selenium supplements are those with a dietary deficiency in the first place and taking selenium when the levels are normal actually increases the risk. There is evidence from studies involving blood / hair samples and toenail clippings that many areas of the world have populations deficient in selenium, including the UK, Central Europe and China, and this is thought to arise from low indigenous soil levels. The problem for an individual is knowing what the body's underlying levels of selenium are. As a consequence, the safest route is to ensure an adequate diet of selenium-containing foods, as this is unlikely to lead to excess absorption of minerals or metals which can occur with supplement intake. The most reliable, but more expensive, route is to measure the body's selenium levels from time to time and take supplements only if the levels are low (see nutritional testing below).

Phytoestrogens as supplements

Natural plant foods containing phytoestrogens generally contain other healthy substances such as fibre, vitamins, trace elements and antioxidants. The mild oestrogenic qualities are likely to reduce the body's own oestrogens via a process called negative feedback and have a beneficial effect. What's more, although they bind to the oestrogen receptor in the tumours they only very weakly stimulate them. Effectively, therefore, they block the binding of the more powerful oestrogen of the body itself. However, concentrating oestrogenic elements of food into a pill may alter the natural structure of the oestrogen which, by isolating it and enhancing its oestrogenic properties. It may then start acting as a stimulant to hormone sensitive cancer cells after they have bound to them. In clinical trials, phytoestrogen pills have not been shown to be harmful or beneficial but despite this lack of evidence in view of their potentially hazardous properties, most cancer doctors would discourage their patients from taking them. This is especially true for individuals with tumours originating from the breast which can be stimulated to grow by oestrogens.

Supplement / chemotherapy interactions

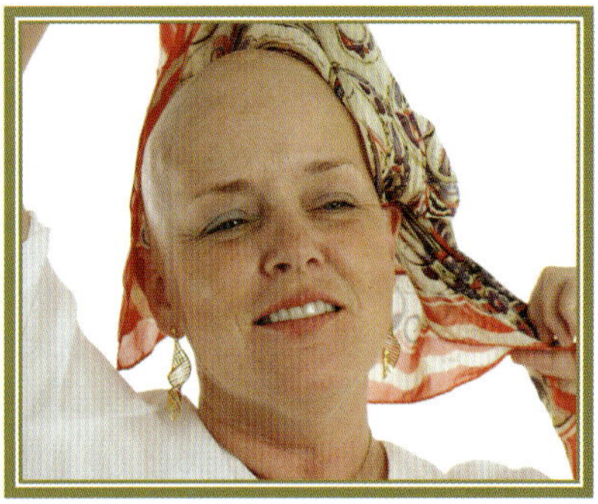

In recent years it has become evident that some over- the-counter remedies can influence chemotherapy drug metabolism, leading to reduced effectiveness or increased toxicity. Unfortunately, patients often do not realise that these products may interfere with their treatment as their use is mostly not discussed with their cancer team. Furthermore, as they are usually branded as natural, a possible harmful interaction is usually not considered. This should be regarded as an oversight as other research has shown that up to 84 percent of patients dabble or regularly take complementary medicines after their diagnosis of cancer.

Among the most widely used herbal supplement is St John's wort (Hypericum perforatum), thought to have anti-depressant properties. Like smoking, mentioned above, this interacts with one of the liver enzymes (CYP3A4) decreasing the concentration of the chemotherapy drugs irinotecan, docetaxol and the biological agent imatinib.

Although the evidence for a number of other complementary therapies is less compelling, potential interactions have been reported with echinacea, grape seed and gingko (caution with most chemotherapy drugs), ephedra (increases blood pressure during cancer therapies, particularly with sutent and nexevar) and kava-kava (increases the risk of liver damage). In short, supplements are chemicals and need the body's metabolic processes to excrete them. As the body is already under a lot of pressure and there is some evidence that antioxidant, herbal or vitamin supplements may interfere with the effectiveness of conventional therapies, on balance it is best not to take them as they make matters worse.

Summary – concerns of dietary supplements:

- They offer an attractive quick fix to health
- They may distract people from the real need for a diverse healthy diet
- Nutritional deficiencies are best corrected with a balanced diet
- Very few trials have shown a cancer benefit
- Correcting an underlying deficiency has been shown to be most beneficial
- For people with adequate levels, supplementary vitamins are particularly harmful
    - Some trials show an increased risk of cancer
    - Others show an increased risk of heart disease
    - Others show an increased risk of cerebral haemorrhage
- Phytoestrogen supplements may stimulate breast cancer cells
- The long-term risks remain uncertain until more data is available
- Supplements are expensive and add to the cost of living
- Herbal supplements can interfere with chemotherapy agents and risk liver disease

Potential benefits of supplements

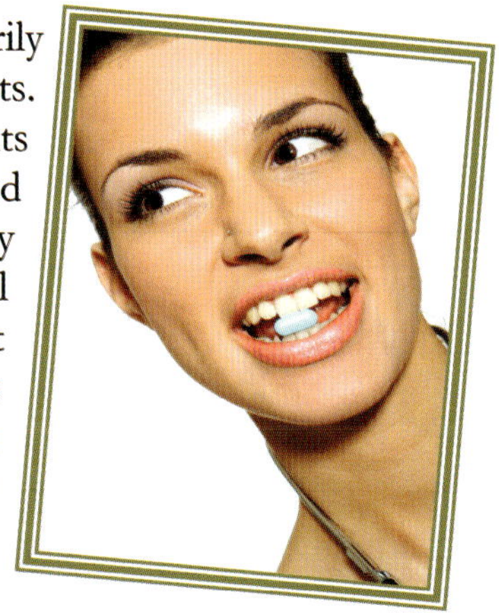

The concerns outlined above do not necessarily imply that there is no place at all for supplements. On the contrary, short-term use of supplements after a period of illness, particularly if associated with a poor appetite or weight loss, may be very useful. A good quality vitamin and mineral supplement may help restore dietary balance, but only until the person is back to a normal diet. It is the habit of taking long-term supplements which can expose the individual to the risks of chemical excess, but there may still be a place for them, especially if caution and monitoring are observed. In general, further evidence from ongoing clinical trials is required, although there are some categories of supplements which are worthy of a mention.

Fish oils

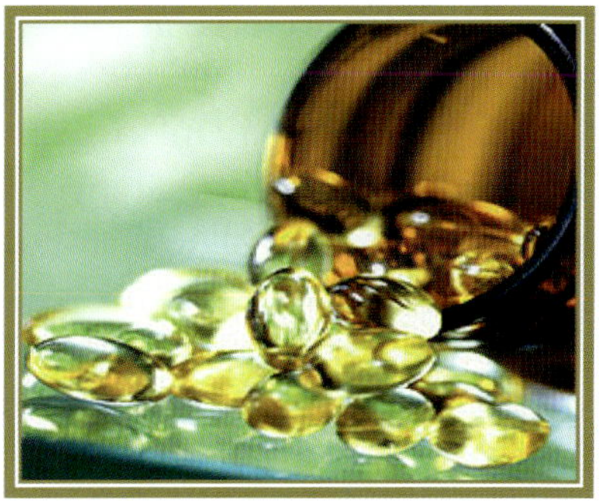

The main components of these are long chain omega-3 fatty acids but they are also high in vitamins A, E and D. Cod liver oil is particularly high in Vitamin A which, if you are deficient in it, would be beneficial. The problem for most of us with normal levels is that taking excessive vitamin A actually increased the levels of lung cancer, especially in ex-smokers. Unless we measure our baseline Vitamin A levels (see nutritional tests below) it is safer to take fish oil rather than the traditional cod liver oil, because it has lower vitamin A levels.

There is genuine trial evidence for the benefits of fish oil for joint point pain and arthritis. Not only have well conducted trials shown a reduction in joint discomfort, but they have demonstrated a reduction in the underlying damage to the joint. A trial involving patients with rheumatoid arthritis took 1 g of cod liver oil (one capsule) daily for 3 months. Half reported a reduction in stiffness, and 40 percent a reduction in pain and swelling. An extremely eloquent study from Cardiff University in 2004 examined the discarded arthritic knees of people who had undergone knee replacement surgery. Some were treated with Omega-3 fatty acids for 24 hours in a laboratory, others were not. A chemical was added to mimic an inflammatory response, and the samples examined four days later. When researchers looked at the cartilage pieces, they found enzymes which are responsible for destroying cartilage in arthritis present in the untreated group. But they were 'turned off' in those treated with Omega-3 fatty acids, as were the enzymes which cause inflammation and pain in joints. This research, therefore, showed that not only does fish oil reduce pain and inflammation in the joints of people with osteoarthritis, but it also turns off the enzymes responsible for destroying cartilage. If you have joint stiffness and pain, it is certainly worth taking fish oil.

There are other benefits of fish oils. Regular intake has been shown to reduce cholesterol and help reduce the risks of heart attacks, dementia and strokes. Fish oil is also high in vitamin D which is difficult to take in recommended amounts, particularly in the northern hemisphere. As deficiencies in vitamin D have been linked to a wide range of cancers, for this reason alone there may be a place for daily fish oil supplements, at least in the winter months.

Probiotics and prebiotics (healthy bacteria)

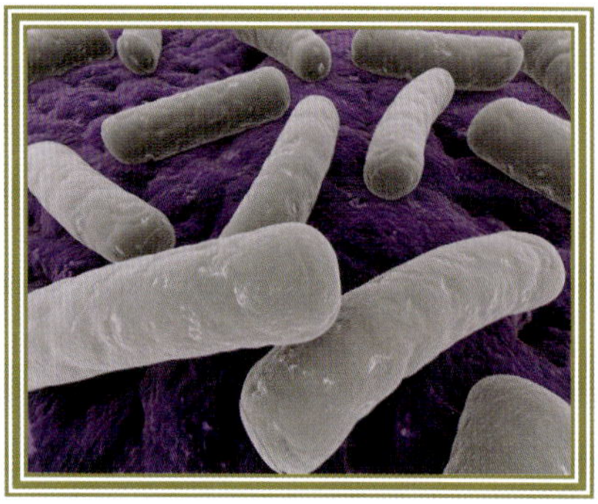

The healthy bacteria in our gut have lived with mankind for millions of years. We have learnt to rely on them to help us digest our food. During chemotherapy or radiotherapy, after a prolonged illness, following a course of antibiotics, or for no apparent reason, these healthy bacteria can be damaged, and there is now very good evidence that taking an extra amount in the form of a dietary supplement may be helpful.

The most numerous probiotic bacteria normally inhabiting the small intestine are a species of lactobacilli. In the colon, the majority are mainly bifidobacteria. Most probiotic products consist of one or more species of bacteria from one or both of these types.

Lactobacillus acidophilus is by far the most well known species of probiotic, which has led many people to refer to probiotics simply as "acidophilus". This strain, amongst other benefits, has been shown to increase levels of interleukin and tumour necrosis factor, which suppress cancerous tumour growth. Other research has shown that L.acidophilus alleviates lactose intolerance by producing significant amounts of the lactose-digesting enzyme, and inhibits gastrointestinal pathogens by producing antimicrobial substances such as acidophilin. It has also been shown to help conditions outside the gut such as eczema and other inflammatory skin conditions. Chemotherapy agents such as fluorouracil can cause diarrhoea, which can not only be uncomfortable, but can also lead to dehydration, concentration of the drug in the blood stream and generally greater side effects and risks. A study in 2007 randomly allocated 100 patients, receiving fluorouracil, either Lactobacillus acidophilus, or supplements. There were no adverse effects in the probiotic group, but the rate of moderate to severe diarrhoea was significantly better in the lactobacillus group.

Lactobacillus rhamnosus combined with acidophilus, has also been shown to reduce or prevent radiotherapy-induced diarrhoea in three separate clinical studies. There is a growing amount of evidence that L.rhamnosus can help treat and prevent gut infections. Valuable controlled trials performed on hospitalised children who had acute diarrhoea showed that L. rhamnosus reduced the duration of diarrhoea. Some placebo controlled studies also suggest that probiotics are of benefit in the treatment of antibiotics-associated diarrhoea, and in the prevention of viral diarrhoea. There have also been a number of studies which suggest a protection against the 'superbug' clostridium difficile plaguing hospitals around the world, so a course of probiotics before coming into hospital for an operation would be wise.

Lactobacillus bulgaricus. This organism usually passes through the digestive system and leaves the body in the stool, untouched. It has been shown to enhance the digestibility of milk products and other proteins, and to produce natural antibiotic substances that specifically target pathogenic bacteria, whilst sparing friendly species. In another study it was shown to stimulate activity in part of the gut immune system called the Peyer's patches.

Lactobacillus salivarius has been shown to inhibit the bacteria Helicobacter pylori (H.pylori) which are responsible for the creation of peptic ulcers. It has been discovered that L.salivarius produces large amounts of lactic acid acting as an antibiotic, inhibiting the growth of H.pylori and reducing the associated inflammatory response. The first bacteriocin (natural antibiotic substance) to be isolated and studied at the genetic level was taken from a strain of L.salivarius.

Lactobacillus probiotics have also been shown to help alleviate food intolerance and allergic conditions. Food intolerance leads to uncommon periods of bloating, wind and colicky indigestion – this is often labelled irritable bowel syndrome. This can develop for no apparent reason at any stage of life but it is even more likely if you have had a prolonged illness, taken antibiotics or received chemotherapy. Often this is related to the development of a mild intolerance to wheat or yeast, but it may also be caused by other foods. Although this does not usually lead to full-blown bowel damage or malabsorption seen with conditions such as *Coeliac Disease*, it can be uncomfortable and distressing. As well as bloating, you can be prone to alternating diarrhoea and constipation, passing offensive wind and an overall sensation of not having a satisfactory bowel movement. As well as identifying the foods which upset you – e.g. bread, beer or wheat pasta – a course of probiotics for a week or so every month, may help to restore the natural balance.

Prebiotics are indigestible carbohydrates known as oligosaccharides, and feed probiotic bacteria and encourage their growth. Oligosaccharides are found naturally in certain fruit and vegetables, including bananas, asparagus, garlic, wheat, tomatoes, artichoke, onions and chicory. Prebiotics can be taken on their own or with a probiotic supplement. The most common types of prebiotics available in supplements are fructooligosaccharides, inulin and galactooligosaccharides.

Calcium and vitamin D supplements

Vitamin D in the form of calciferol fed to cancer cells and rats in the laboratory reduced cancer growth and progression and inhibited the formation of new blood vessels. Humans with sub-optimal levels of vitamin D have been linked with a high risk of cancer. Clinical studies of high dose calciferol, however, had to be abandoned because it dangerously increased serum calcium.

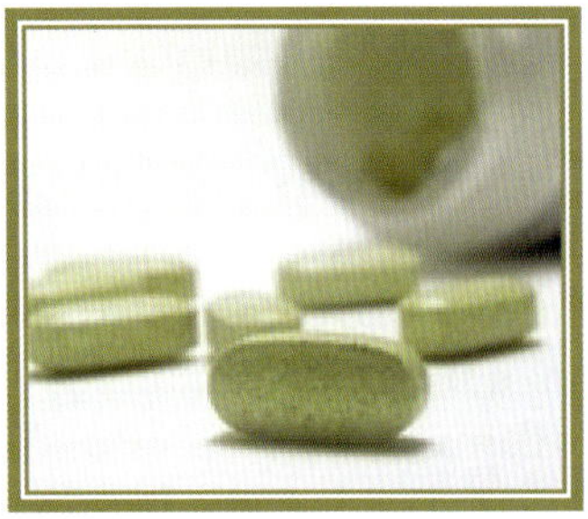

Calcium supplements taken without vitamin D have been evaluated in two human studies at doses of between 1330-1840 mg/day, and showed no benefit or risk of cancer. Two other large studies at doses >2000 mg/day from food and supplements, actually showed a significantly higher rate of prostate cancer. Five of nine further questionnaire surveys associated high intake of dairy food with an increased risk of prostate and breast cancer, but interpretation of these was complicated by the fact that high dairy consumption was associated with high fat intake. The detrimental effect of excessive calcium is thought to lie in the finding that high dietary calcium can reduce blood and cellular vitamin D levels. Nevertheless, calcium and vitamin D supplements taken together in moderation are very useful in the maintenance of bone density and preventing osteoporosis. Bones are at risk following a number of cancer therapies. The paragraph in the 'cons' section above, however, summarises the concerns with a high calcium intake on its own. The reasons for the negative effects of calcium are likely to be its association with food of high fat content and its tendency to lower vitamin D levels. Combining calcium with vitamin D in a supplement will avoid these factors and, in theory, may be safe. Although confirmation of this theory in a clinical trial is required, it provides some reassurance that it is likely to be safe and can be taken if bone loss is a concern.

Antioxidant food supplements

In general the best advice is to eat a variety of foods with naturally high levels of anti-oxidants. These food categories are also usually high in fibre, mineral, vitamins and other healthy substances, some of which are yet to be discovered. These foods, as well as being healthy, are often tasty – remembering the famous quote from Oscar Wilde "We don't eat to live, we live to eat". Removing a single chemical from a particular food risks losing the benefits of the whole food. A good example of this is the lycopene versus tomato powder experiment mentioned above. The physician, Howard Cao, who developed the antioxidant scale (ORAC), put this succinctly by quoting, "The combinations of nutrients found in foods have greater protective effects than each nutrient taken alone."

Although individual extracted antioxidant chemicals are not advised there may a place for taking an extra boost of the whole *superfood* in a more convenient dried form which would have a high and varied antioxidant content. This would help to ensure enough antioxidants are on board to combat the carcinogens which are perpetually being bombarded upon us daily in what we breathe, eat, drink, wash with, or put on our skin. The busier an individual the less time he or she has to concentrate on their lifestyle and all too often tend to drift into bad habits – fast foods for example, although convenient, tend to contain more carcinogens and less antioxidants. These food supplements should be differentiated from anti-oxidant chemical supplements which have had the chemical stripped out and separated from the food. Good examples of a *superfood* supplements would be those which have dried whole foods e.g. pomegranate, green tea, broccoli and curcumin. As the antioxidants within them are heat resistant, they remain intact and functional. Combining different *superfoods* further ensures an even wider variety of different antioxidants. Although not a substitute for a healthy diet, taken in moderation an antioxidant food supplement such as this would ensure adequate intake of a wide variety of antioxidants and ensure individuals are continually armed against daily carcinogenic attack. Several such products are available from health food stores or via the internet, most made in a variety of countries under varying quality standards. The problem for a consumer is – who to trust and what to take?. If you are considering taking an antioxidant rich food supplement, it would be a good idea to check that the company has been accredited with UK GMP (Good Manufacturing Practice).

Our recommendation: If you feel you may wish to boost your diet with an extra anti-oxidant rich food supplement, the UK based supplement manufacture *natureMedical*, has a high standards of hygiene and food preparation. They have designed a supplement which contains Pomegranate, Green tea, Broccoli and Turmeric. By having four different whole food constituents originating from different sources (fruit, vegetable and spices) a wide range of antioxidants are included avoiding excess of one particular variety. More information can be found on the website www.keep-health.com

Chondroitin and Glucosamine tablets

These are complex sugars that are present in the cartilage of joints. They are used widely to treat arthritis, and are often taken in large quantities by body builders who are convinced that they would not be able to lift the weights without extra protection for their joints. Their springy chemical structure provides much of the resistance to compression of cartilage on weight bearing, and its loss is a major cause of joint pain and osteoarthritis.

Chondroitin appears to be made from extracts of cartilaginous cow and pig tissues, particularly trachea, ear and nose, although alternative sources include bird and shark cartilage. The dosage of oral chondroitin used in human clinical trials is usually 800–1,200 mg per day. Since chondroitin is not a uniform substance, and is naturally present in a wide variety of forms, the precise composition of each supplement will vary. As a result Chondroitin is under the jurisdiction of the FDA in the U.S. as a dietary supplement and as there are no mandatory standards for formulation, there is no guarantee that the product is correctly labelled. One report, in the year 2000, analysed 32 chondroitin supplements. Only 5 were labelled correctly and more than half contained less than 40 percent of the labelled amount. Fortunately, at least in the US, testing standards now exist for the identification and quantification of chondroitin.

Glucosamine is a monosaccharide amino sugar found as a major component of the exoskeletons of crustaceans, but is also found abundantly in fungi and higher organisms. It is produced commercially by crushing crustacean exoskeletons. Like chondroitin, glucosamine is commonly used as a treatment for joint pains, although its acceptance as a medical therapy varies.

Multiple clinical trials in the 1980s and 1990s, all sponsored by the European patent-holder, Rottapharm, were conducted on patients with a wide variety of arthritic problems. Although these trials were small and not particularly well designed, they did show a clear benefit for glucosamine treatment. There was not only an improvement in symptoms, but also an improvement in a feature of arthritis seen on an x-rays – joint space narrowing. This suggested that glucosamine can actually help prevent the destruction of cartilage as well as reduce pain. On the other hand, several subsequent studies, independent of Rottapharm, but again small and poorly designed, did not detect any benefit from glucosamine. As a result of the conflicting evidence both for and against glucosamine's efficacy, there remained a debate amongst physicians about whether to recommend glucosamine treatment to their patients.

This situation led the prestigious National Institute of Health in the USA to fund a large multi-centre study of people with pain and osteoarthritis of the knee, evaluating both agents. It compared groups treated with glucosamine, chondroitin or a combination of both, to both placebo and a standard anti-inflammatory pain killer. The results of this 6-month trial found that patients taking glucosamine HCl, chondroitin sulphate, or a combination of the two had no improvement in their symptoms compared to patients taking a placebo. The group of patients who took the standard pain killer, not surprisingly, did have a statistically significant improvement in their symptoms. These results suggest that glucosamine and chondroitin did not effectively relieve pain in the overall group of osteoarthritis patients, although no significant side effects were reported. There still remains, however, some hope for the fate of this supplement. A subgroup analysis suggested that the supplements may have been effective in patients with pain classified as moderate to severe. Also the main commercial manufacturers of glucosamine claimed that glucosamine sulphate should have been used in the study instead of HCL, as this is more effective. Although this concern is not shared by pharmacologists, many conclude that the question of these agents' efficacy will not be resolved without further updates or trials.

Summary – potential benefits of dietary supplements:

- Empirical unmonitored ***short term*** supplementation may be helpful, e.g.:
  - — a multi vitamin and mineral to cover a period of poor nutrition
  - — vitamin B following a period of heavy alcohol intake
  - — oral iron following a heavy menstrual period or other bleeding
- Correcting a known deficiency has been shown to be most beneficial
  - — initial assessment of a deficiency is required
  - — monitoring is required to ensure over-correction does not occur
- Selenium deficiency is relatively common and may need supplementation if diet fails to provide adequate quantities
- Fish oils are a good source of long chain omega-3
- Glucosamine & chondroitin may help arthritis, (more evidence is needed)
- Probiotics help with:
  - — chemotherapy induced diarrhoea
  - — radiotherapy induced diarrhoea
  - — abdominal bloating caused by lactose and wheat intolerance
  - — protection from infective diarrhoea including C. difficle
  - — protecting the stomach from infective indigestion (H.pylori)
- Calcium and vitamin D help with bone density, but should be monitored.
- Whole dried food capsules may be a useful way to boost antioxidant intake

In the meantime, as the evidence remains inconclusive, in addition to the lifestyle measures it would not be unreasonable to try a short course of these supplements to see if they have any beneficial effect on your joint pains. Although expensive, at least they are well tolerated and, unlike vitamins and minerals, are unlikely to lead to accumulative toxicity. If they help you, you may avoid the toxicity and risks of standard painkillers.

Micro-Nutrient testing – Pros and cons

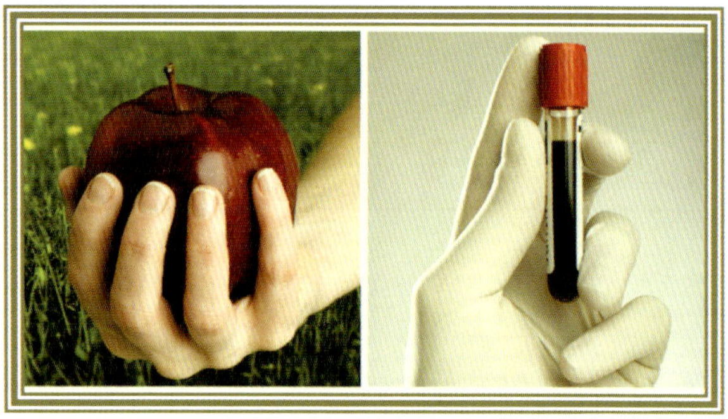

Many cancer survivors are turning to nutritional testing in order to empower themselves with the optimal lifestyle choices. Very few of the clinical trials described above measured participants' baseline nutritional status, but those which did showed a benefit to correcting a deficiency. They also showed a risk to health if the intervention resulted in an over correction a normal level of vitamin or mineral. Not surprisingly, therefore, the results of most of the large supplement studies showed no benefit as the population examined would have included those benefiting from the intervention and those being made worse by it. The studies which did measure the levels of nutrients at the start, however, have clearly shown that:

- Deficiencies in vitamins, minerals and trace metals can lead to a reduced chance of fighting cancer, and the cancers developed in individuals with deficiencies have a tendency to be more aggressive.

- Correcting deficiencies has been shown to improve the ability to fight cancer, but over-correcting a normal level is harmful and could increase the risks of cancer and other illnesses.

It is becoming clear that just simply popping a general dietary supplement, without a recognised need, is not the answer as amongst those with a generally good diet this behaviour may cause more harm than good. Furthermore, there is little consensus on the dose and type of dietary supplement required or for how long it should be taken. Moreover, nutritional needs are likely to differ over time for each individual and vary considerably between different people depending on their dietary history, country of origin and genetic susceptibility.

Ideally, all future dietary trial designs should include a baseline micro-nutritional assessment to identify those individuals with sub-clinical imbalances. Sensitivity can be helped by more complex tests, which match the blood levels of the micro-nutrients, with specific biochemical, molecular and genetic pathways. In the meantime a good start would be to measure blood for the levels of micro-nutrients which the clinical trials, summarised above, have shown to be implicated in the cancer process either in excess or deficiency. These should include the vitamins, antioxidant levels, function of the antioxidant enzymes (catalase, glutathione S-transferase glutathione, superoxide dimutase), levels of essential minerals, salts and fatty acid including omega 3, 6, 9 and the ratios between them.

Empowered with this knowledge individuals can modify their lifestyle to correct their specific nutritional profile and optimise their cancer risk. This could either be by eating more of the foods they need and less of those they do not need, or the intake of selective food supplements. Ideally, the impact of integrating these complex tests into a bespoke nutritional or supplement management would have to be tested in well-designed studies, whose results would take many years to mature. In the meantime, there are some bespoke tests which are accessible commercially. These are currently not available in routine oncology or community doctor practices but are available directly online privately. There are several companies in the UK which offer this service but it is important to ensure they are reliable, accurate and cost effective:

The Cancer Risk Nutritional Profile.

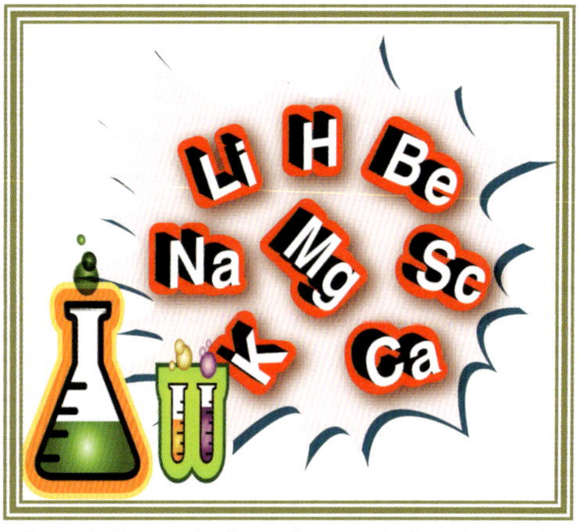

This test uses the largest and most established micro-nutritional testing laboratory in the UK and provides a comprehensive report relevant to each individual's profile. The test can be ordered online from the website (cancernet.co.uk/nutrional-tests.htm) anywhere in the UK. A blood sample kit is sent directly to the address given. The client then goes to their local blood taking facility (usually the GP's practice or hospital phlebotomy room) and after the blood has been put into the specific bottles, it is sealed and sent it back to the laboratory in the designated packaging provided.

Following analysis, the results are sent to the consultant oncologist for interpretation and writing of the specific lifestyle and dietary report. The report then will highlight specific levels of essential nutrients and provide relevant lifestyle recommendations together with easy to follow advice sheets. These sheets may advise more in take of some foods or certain activities and less of others in order to restore the body's nutritional balance. If the blood test shows particularly low levels of one or more essential nutrients, certain dietary supplements may also be advised for a specified length of time.

Although not cheap and further research in cancer prevention is needed, based on available evidence, micro-nutrient analysis is money well spent as an imbalance in the body's essential chemicals can exist for many years before an illness develops.

Chapter Thirteen

Exercise and cancer
Evidence, benefits, advice

Evidence that exercise helps fights cancer

It is well known that people who exercise regularly have a reduced risk of developing cancer. In terms of prevention, it has been shown that being sedentary and overweight could account for 14 percent of male and 20 percent of female cancer deaths in the UK. With bowel cancer, for example, most environmental studies have demonstrated a reduction in the order of 40–50 percent for those at the highest levels of physical activity. Further studies, from the Harvard Centre for Cancer Control, estimate that at least 15 percent of colon cancers could have been prevented by 30 minutes of daily exercise. These data suggest that increasing physical activity is one of the major factors that are amenable to modification by individuals wishing to reduce their risks of cancer.

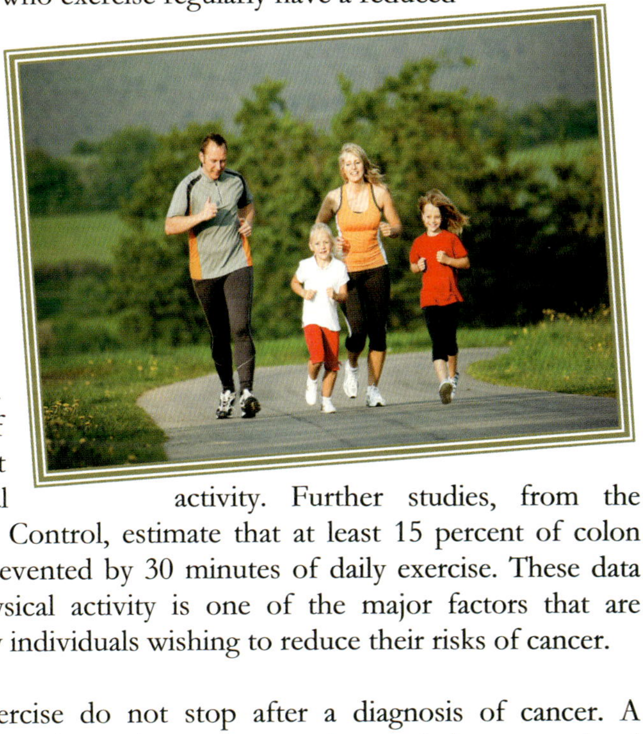

The benefits of exercise do not stop after a diagnosis of cancer. A number of studies have proven that patients who exercise regularly are associated with a lower risk of their cancer returning and generally surviving longer. The two most convincing studies involved men and women with bowel cancer. The first involved 526 patients, recruited between 1990 and 1994, with either cancer of the rectum or colon carcinoma (CRC) from the Melbourne Collaborative Cohort Study, Australia. At trial entry, shortly after their diagnosis, body fat measurements were taken and patients were interviewed about their physical activity over the prior six months. Information about the established risk factors was also recorded, such as tumour size, grade and treatments given. The body mass index was calculated from the weight, height, and waist to hip ratio measurement. Patients were defined as 'exercisers' or 'non-exercisers'. Exercisers were defined as those taking recreational activities or sports one or more times per week that made them perspire or feel out of breath. Body composition was also measured by bioelectrical impedance using a single frequency electrical current. The numbers of patients in the two groups who relapsed or died over the next five years were compared. The results showed that, taking into account the standard risk factors, 57 percent of patients were alive at five years in the non-exerciser group, and 71 percent in the exerciser group. This 14 percent difference was statistically highly significant. As regards death, specifically from bowel cancer, there was a 12 percent difference (61 percent v 73 percent), again very significant. This benefit was seen across all stages of cancer but was even greater for patients with higher risks of relapse (stage II – large cancers and stage III – spread to local nodes).

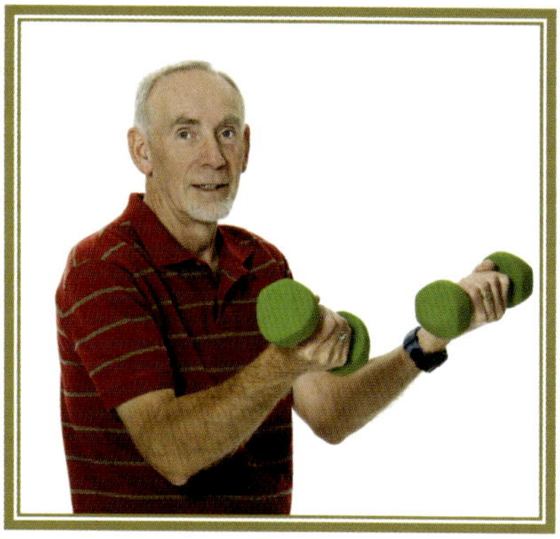

A similar finding was demonstrated in an American study involving 816 patients with cancer of the colon. All patients had a disease that was completely removed but also had evidence of it spreading to the local lymph nodes (stage III). They completed detailed lifestyle questionnaires during and after additional chemotherapy that generally lasted for six months. Increased physical activity was associated with a lower chance of the disease relapsing and an improved overall rate of survival. In practical terms this equated to a 35 percent difference in relapse rate for individuals in the highest quintile of regular physical activity, compared with the lowest quintile. This study also evaluated blood samples from the patients who exercised and those who did not. They found differences that are helping to explain the underlying mechanisms of how exercise helps to fight cancer.

A presentation made at the Frontiers in Cancer Prevention Research conference in 2010 described the role that exercise could play in the fight against prostate cancer. An analysis of activity levels among 2,686 prostate cancer patients showed that men who jogged, played tennis, or participated in other comparable exercise for an average of three or more hours per week had 35 percent lower mortality rates than those who exercised less frequently or not at all. As for walking, those who did so for four or more hours per week had overall mortality rates that were 23 percent lower than those of men who walked for fewer than 20 minutes per week.

In conclusion, despite the limitations in distinguishing the benefits of exercise from other lifestyle factors, there is now persuasive evidence that exercise improves the physical and psychological function of patients with cancer, reduces the risk of recurrence, and possibly improves survival. There are, however, other benefits of exercise after a diagnosis of cancer. In particular, it has been shown to increase the degree of empowerment for both the patients and carers, who can also join in with the activity. It creates an overall sense of well-being, improves mood, lowers anxiety and risk of depression, and improves social integration and self-esteem.

How exercise influences cancer?

There are five accepted underlying mechanisms of how exercise could potentially fight cancer:

Body fat levels – obesity: Although seemingly obvious, the observation that exercise helps to reduce weight among patients with cancer is supported by a large prospective study which reported a significant decrease in body fat after physical exercise intervention. Exercise also decreased the fat to muscle ratio, which helps the metabolism of some drugs. The mechanisms of harm of being overweight are described earlier.

Oestrogen levels: A trial from Alberta randomised 320 sedentary postmenopausal women for moderate to vigorous exercise over the course a year or not. They found reduced levels of oestradiol in the exercise group compared with those achieved by controls. There were no significant differences the levels of the male hormones androstenedione and testosterone.

Decreasing bowel transit time: Exercise decreases the time it takes for a waste to pass through the bowel. Stagnant stools in the colon are thought to increase the risk of cancer by exposing the carcinogens that have not been absorbed in our diet to the mucous membrane of the bowel lining for longer. Exercise is particularly helpful after surgery to the abdomen, which has a tendency to cause fibrous tissue to form between the loops of the bowel, slowing the normal flow of motion. Likewise, some chemotherapy drugs and painkillers can do the same thing. Patients who have developed one bowel cancer are more likely to develop a second. Reducing the carcinogen exposure time to the gut is likely, therefore, to be even more helpful in this higher risk group.

Prostaglandin and immune pathway: Prostaglandins are essentially involved in the healing process of the body. They are biologically active, healthy lipids, generated from arachidonic acid via the enzyme cycloxidase (COX). The COX-1 subtype is activated in response to trauma, infective or chemical injury, producing prostaglandins that contribute to the inflammatory response we are all familiar with, for example, following a wasp sting or healing from a skin cut leading to redness, swelling and pain. Prostaglandins created by activation of COX-1 are also involved in several important physiological processes including protection of the lining of the stomach and stickiness of blood platelets that ensure we stop bleeding when cut. The COX-2 subtype has very interesting implications in the cancer process, which have been described in detail in the dietary section of this chapter. Exercise inhibits COX-2 production and may therefore have a direct anti-cancer affect via the same pathway as aspirin-like drugs, fruit or vegetables.

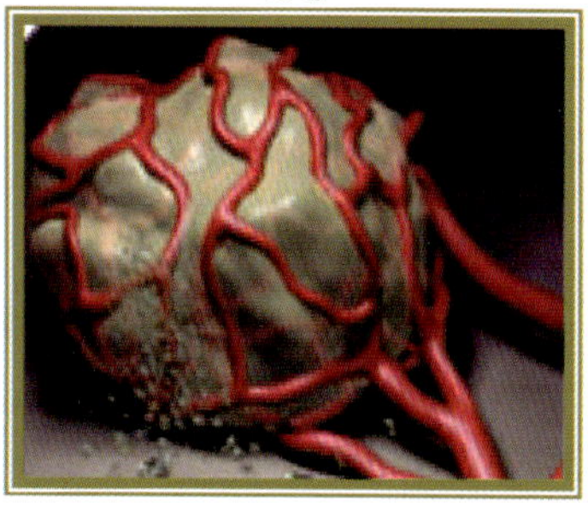

Altering insulin-like growth factor axis: The most compelling emerging evidence so far supports the idea that physical activity might exert its beneficial effect on cancer via a protein called insulin-like growth factor (IGF) axis. A number of large studies involving patients with established cancer (particularly those with bowel cancer) have shown higher blood levels of insulin-like growth factor 1 (IGF-1) and another protein called C peptide. The benefits of lowering IGF-1 may be linked to its central role in the growth regulation processes. The main stimulus for IGF-1 production comes from growth hormone. The stimulatory effect of growth hormone is modulated by insulin, which increases growth hormone receptor levels and in turn IGF-1. Early studies have shown that after binding to its receptors, which are found on normal colonic mucosal cells as well as colon cancer cells, IGF-1 can stimulate cells to grow faster and in an uncontrolled way (**proliferation**), inhibiting the normal life cycle i.e. stopping cells from dying of old age when they ought to (**apoptosis**). Other studies have also shown that IGF-1 binding triggers the formation of new blood vessels essential for tumours to grow rapidly (**angiogenesis**). In the circulation, as over 90 percent of IGF-1 is bound to a protein called IGFRBP-3 (Insulin-like Growth Factor Binding Protein-3), binding inhibits the action of IGF-1 by limiting the availability of free hormone. This explains the finding that higher blood levels of IGFBP-3 are associated with lower levels of IGFR-1. Conversely, patients with lower levels of IGFBP-3 are associated with a worse outcome and higher free levels of IGFR-1. People who exercise regularly have been convincingly shown to have lower IGF-1 and higher IGFBP-3 levels.

The most compelling evidence that this correlates with cancer outcomes comes from a study of 41,528 people aged between 27 and 75 years with colorectal cancer. Patients recruited between 1990 and 1994 had their exercise activity recorded along with regular blood tests. Confirming previous studies, lower IGF-1 and higher IGFBP-3 levels significantly correlated with higher exercise activity. More excitingly, these factors, at diagnosis, were associated with a lower chance of the cancer returning and a higher chance of being alive after five years. A similar study conducted by the Melbourne Collaborative Cohort Study Group looked at exercise patterns after diagnosis and found the same relationship – confirming the intriguing role exercise and IGF-1 have in the cancer recurrence mechanism.

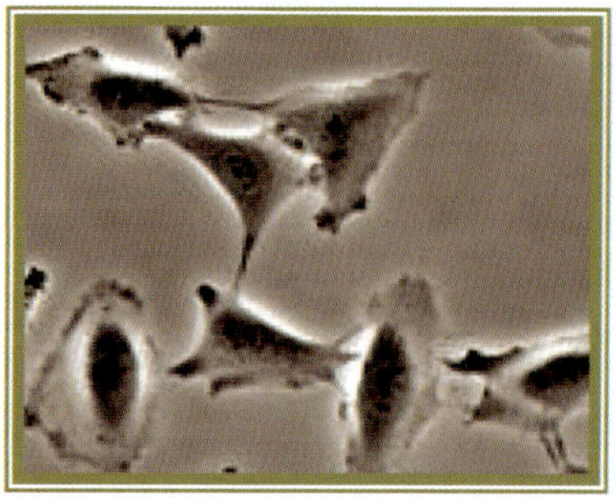

Blood fat levels: Regular exercise has been shown to help control the body's levels of serum lipids and cholesterol. High serum fat levels have been particularly associated with a greater risk of a more advanced and aggressive type of cancer, with a higher risk of relapse after initial therapy. Men with prostate cancer, with lower serum lipids, have better prognostic features including lower PSA, lower aggressiveness of cells (grade) and less advanced stage of the cancer. These factors correlate with better outcomes. A clue to the mechanism of fat levels, at least in prostate cancer, comes from the finding that lower serum fat levels correlated with lower testosterone. Exercise also helps repair infection-fighting T-cells, restoring the immune system after it has been damaged by chemotherapy.

A note on Heat shock Proteins and exercise before chemotherapy A report in September 2011 from Ohio suggested that exercising before chemotherapy can counterbalance the cancer killing effect of the drugs. The press obviously overemphasised the conclusions mostly failing to mention the overwhelming body of evidence that continuing to exercise during chemotherapy reduces risks, improves well-being and may well add to the killing effect via IGF described above. The study from Ohio reported that adding a chemical called heat shock protein (HSP) to cancer cells growing in a petri dish increase their resistance to chemotherapy by allowing he cells to heal themselves more efficiently. The author and many newspapers went on to suggest that exercise before chemotherapy should be avoided. Although an interesting academic experiment, this was based on the assumption that HSP can increase in humans after exercise.

HSP are activated by the body in response to cellular stress such as attack from chemicals, high temperature, infection or lack of oxygen (hypoxia). The main stimulus for the body to produce HSP is a raised temperature (associated with infection), lack of oxygen (such as a heart attack). People who exercise regularly tend to have higher baseline HSP levels, and is one of the explanations why they tend to look younger. There is some clinical evidence that vigorous exercise can increase levels HSP especially if associated with a lack of oxygen, although not all experiments agree with how much it would rise and what level of exercise is required. For example, a study from Toronto measured HSP in muscle in mice while they were exercising. They found that there was no increase in levels when mice where exercising normally on a wheel. Only those exercising anaerobically (sprinting) and simultaneously heated to 40 degrees had any increase in their HSP – condition which would be hard to emulate in humans. Tests in humans show that regular exercisers do not tend to have a sudden rise in HSP when they then exercise more vigorously but blood levels can rise if strenuous exercise is taken in a previously sedentary individuals.

Even if the authors are correct and HSP are raised to a significant amount in human after vigorous exercise there is little information on whether increased blood and tissue levels of HSP would actually increase levels within cancer masses themselves. Furthermore, the report failed to mention the beneficial effect of HSP on normal cells. If indeed HSP were increased in the body, it also would also diminish the harmful damage on the normal tissues from chemotherapy including the heart. Although this has not been proven, I suspect the benefit in terms tissue protection would out way the cancer sparing effect - thus actually increasing the therapeutic ratio of chemotherapy. So, exercising vigorously could just as easily be beneficial. Certainly a therapeutic procedure called hyperthermia (used with chemotherapy and radiotherapy) suggests that heating the tissue actually kills more cancer cells without killing the normal cells. In other words, there is no evidence, at all, that in humans exercise diminishes the chemotherapy effect. There are several benefits of exercising during chemotherapy. However, in view of this new Ohio experimental data more research is necessary to see if exercise may be a way to further increase the therapeutic ratio. In the mean time, continue regular exercise during chemotherapy and afterward but to be on the safe side, although the evidence is poor for any risk, avoid extreme aerobic exercise (sprinting) 48 hours before chemotherapy especially in very hot climates/ rooms especially if you do not exercise regularly.

Advice to improve your daily exercise

Just do it – a familiar sports brand slogan may have relevance to the fitter members of the general public, but for those recovering from the battering of cancer and its therapies, it is not as simple as that. A more realistic motto should be – "How can I do it?" This chapter aims to provide an insight into the answer.

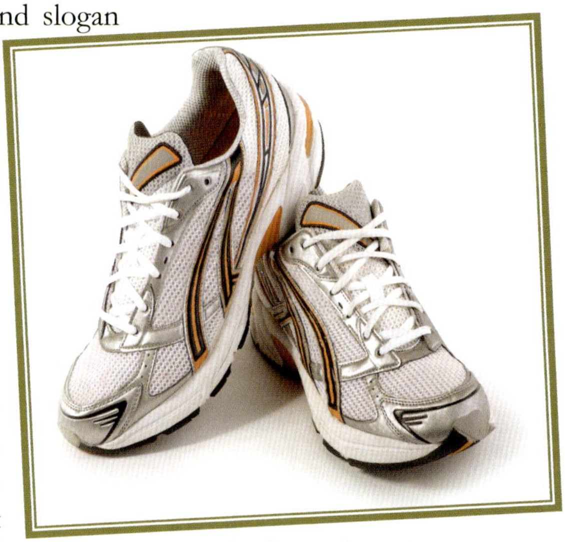

Following cancer therapies, a more flexible and innovative approach to exercise strategies is required as most patients, even those who had exercised regularly before their diagnosis, may not have the same motivation or abilities afterwards. The cancer itself, surgery or the anticancer treatments, may have caused physical disability, fatigue, weight gain, reduced self-esteem and body-image concerns. Many people, when contemplating exercise, see it as an insurmountable hurdle and require significant encouragement. Although individual patient motivation remains the strongest determinant to the intensity of exercise, support and encouragement from friends, relatives and physicians plays a fundamental role in promoting exercise. One study, for example, found that patients who were encouraged by their oncologist exercised significantly more than patients who were not. Individuals who recognise the barriers to starting regular exercise and are able to ask for help are much more likely to succeed. With help, tasks can be re-learnt or new exercise patterns initiated, often with a broader range of activities which may not previously have been contemplated.

Within the normal activities of daily living: Throughout the day we have several choices which require different levels of exertion – you should try to take the more active option. For example, walking instead of using the car for short journeys; getting off the bus or underground at one stop earlier; using the stairs instead of the lift and walking rather than standing on the escalator. When watching TV or sitting at a desk, you could try to get up and walk around for a few minutes, at regular intervals. A comfortable pair of training shoes for walking around the block for ten minutes every evening before the evening meal is a good idea. This is great for your circulation and digestion, and will help with weight reduction. Although this is a relatively low level of exercise, the trick is to perform it regularly. If an evening's exercise is missed out you could consider an additional lunchtime walk instead. If a day's exercise is missed, you could consider going for a walk twice the following day to catch up. All too often people who, when asked closely, say that they exercise regularly have excuses, often legitimate, for missing most of the days of the week. It may be worth keeping a wall chart or an exercise diary as an *aide memoir*. Basic, gentle stretching is as important as exercise, so you should try to set aside five minutes every day for a gentle session. Just before getting into bed is a good time.

At home: The advantage of exercising at home is that it is time efficient and convenient. It doesn't, however, have the social interaction of group activities unless a friend is invited round for a joint exercise session. Exercising with someone else is always more fun and usually ensures a higher level of activity. Furthermore, most people are keen to help after a diagnosis of cancer – and what better way to do so? If you have decided to start exercising at home it is worth having a semi-formal program to follow. There are many useful gadgets available to make it more feasible (exercise bikes, treadmills, rowing machines, etc). Alternatively, you could follow an exercise video – there are literally thousands to choose from, but it is necessary to set aside a good hour, preferably when an interruption is unlikely. Always remember to perform some gentle stretches before and after exercise, and trying to get a little breathless and sweaty during exercise. If you can afford an exercise professional to come to your home this could be a good investment. Most would be sympathetic to your abilities and needs and would keep you focused and motivated. A nice shower or bath afterwards is a good reward and massaging yourself on the previously treated or sun-exposed areas, with olive oils, before getting into the shower is a plus.

At the office or workplace: After a cancer diagnosis it is important not to remain sedentary for long periods of time. This can happen in the work place, particularly during long meetings or sitting at a desk. Commuting to work by car or train, especially in a confined space, can also be disadvantageous. Walking as much as possible, maybe to the bus, train or underground station, should be encouraged. Also use the stairs instead of the lift and walk on escalators. It may be better to commute wearing training shoes and change to more professional attire on arrival. Getting up from your desk every 30 minutes or so and walking for two minutes could be considered. Walking or some other exercise at lunchtime will be beneficial. If walking is not feasible, desk exercises could keep you alert, especially when getting tired or sleepy. Ignore any negative comments – people will secretly admire your enthusiasm.

Within your social life: There is an alternative to the pub or watching TV. Exercise can and should be sociable and enjoyable – finding something that is fun and which can be integrated into your social life can be a great benefit. Dance, aqua aerobics and fitness classes are very cordial places and, particularly if you go regularly, are somewhere to form new friendships and make new acquaintances. A good example of this was demonstrated by a male patient who decided to give up alcohol and, as a distraction, took up ceroc dancing. Within a month or so of attending twice a week, he could dance five or six moves with ease – certainly enough to participate in a class. His job also required travelling from time to time around the country. Previously he would go to the pub, drink and then walk back to his hotel with a greasy kebab. He has now discovered that there are ceroc classes in most major towns (most of these can be found on the Internet). With a little planning, he now confidently attends classes elsewhere in the UK, exercising and meeting new friends and avoiding the temptation of alcohol in the pub. His business is booming because he is waking up refreshed, invigorated and able to work more efficiently.

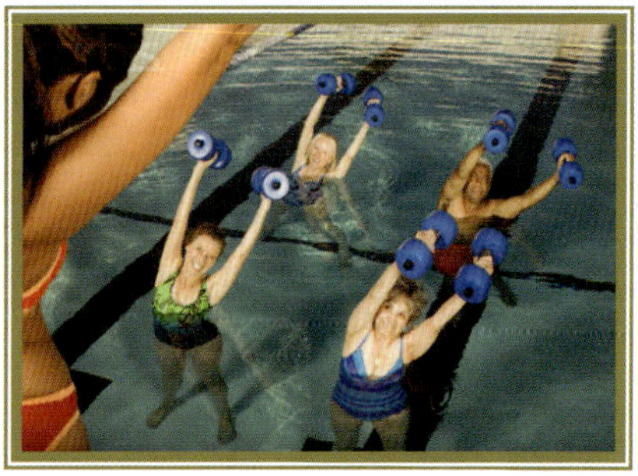

Another patient, treated for bowel cancer, found that his love of watching sport on TV encouraged him either to sit at home or go to a pub and inevitably eat salty, unhealthy snacks whilst there. One of his friends, eager to help, suggested meeting to watch a game in the local gym. They ran on a treadmill and cycled, albeit fairly slowly, for most of the game wearing headphones. During moments of excitement, the surge of adrenaline, instead of putting up their blood pressure, encouraged them to run momentarily faster – exactly what nature intended. They now meet in the gym with a group of friends regularly once a week to exercise and watch the game. What's more, the patient, who also had high blood pressure and cholesterol for five years before his diagnosis, managed to stop all his medication as well.

It's a question of changing your frame of mind and adopting a fresh approach to socialising. The majority of recreational and sports activities have a strong social aspect to them. There are a lot of choices, perhaps arranging a gathering with family and friends, looking at the availability of activities in the area, and then deciding which one would be best for the group. The following section provides some ideas, but the choice most often depends on the quality and availability of local recreational activities.

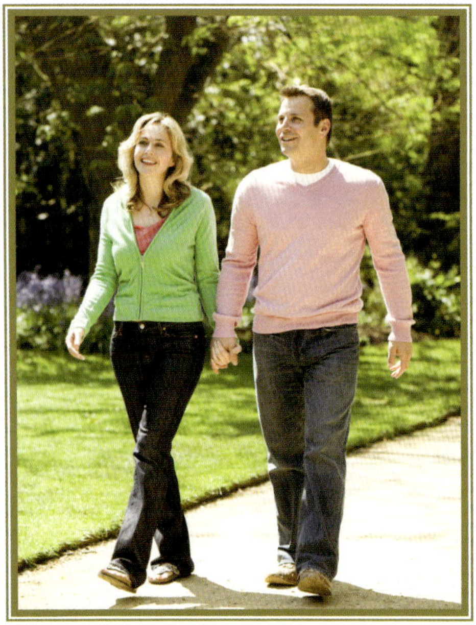

Walking and jogging: In addition to integrating walking into our daily lives, social walking groups are available in many areas and are a good way to meet new people, view interesting scenery and exercise to a variety of ability levels. Numerous walking groups exist around the country often meeting once or twice a week. There are numerous other ideas for exercise groups, but if these are not convenient the fall back of buying a good pair of training shoes and jogging or briskly walking around the block or local park is always available.

Golf is a good encouragement to walk and clubs are available throughout the world for all levels of play. The handicap system allows for people of all abilities to take part and enjoy themselves. To get started driving ranges and coaching are easily accessible.

Cycling socially with the family or as part of a daily commute, even if only once or twice a week, can be fun and even save money. You could consider buying a bicycle with a basket or panniers for the shopping.

Other sports: Traditional sports are often overshadowed by the hype surrounding the trendy genre of 'inner strength, street dancing, and meditation classes' but they remain excellent outlets for stress and exercise. They often require more organisation than simply turning up for a class, as they usually involve a group. The local sports centre, however, sometimes brings groups together without anyone else having to organise it – for a range of activities from five-aside football, squash, tennis, badminton, basketball, volleyball and netball. Not all tennis clubs are expensive and they do not require their customers to be experts. Most have group lessons for all abilities and social communal days when individuals can join in. Athletics clubs, although generally aimed at the young, often have different age categories and run groups for different abilities.

Exercise classes: There are numerous enjoyable ways to exercise in groups at a variety of levels. Many of these are available at the local gym or sports hall. The most common classes include aerobics, water aerobics (a good one to start with), spinning (cycling in a group), body pump and circuit training. Once a level of fitness has been achieved, higher and often more diverse forms of exercise unfold, from boxing and kick-boxing classes, jazz funk aerobics, rock climbing and core stability classes.

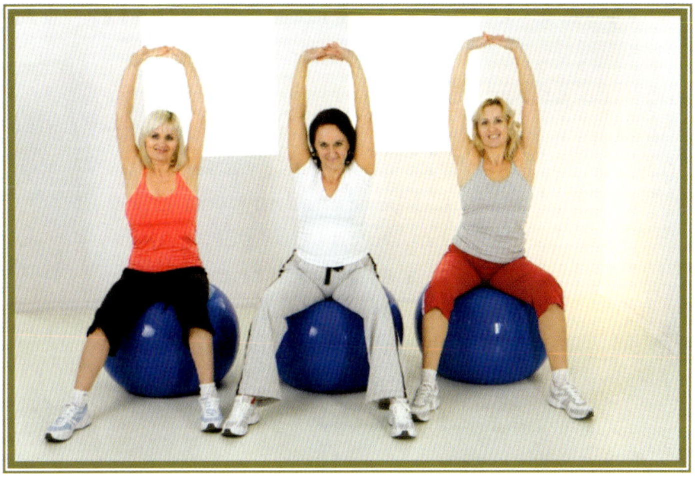

Stretching classes: Gentle stretching is advisable before and after any exercises. Yoga and Pilates are recommended for balance and core strength, both of which are often impaired by cancer treatments, especially if steroids have been given during chemotherapy. They are also recommended for joint and muscle suppleness and posture. Don't worry if even touching your toes is impossible – yoga and Pilates are not about the lotus position anymore. Individuals with any level of flexibility can gain major benefits if the stretches are conducted regularly.

Swimming: Many pools offer classes to learn to swim, classes for disabled, single sex or water aerobics. Swimming is particularly good for building up stamina whilst protecting most of the weight-bearing joints. On a word of caution, however, breaststroke is not so good for the knees and crawl can aggravate shoulder and neck problems.

Dancing; There are numerous dance classes available in most towns, either in private or municipal gyms or dance studios. The most common choices include conventional ballroom, line dancing, rock and roll, Latin American, ceroc and salsa. Some traditional studios offer ballet and the trendier ones, jazz, funk, and even street dance.

Advice for formal training programmes

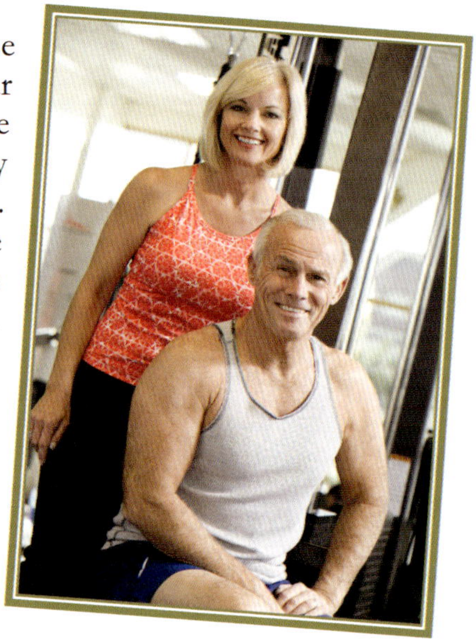

The type of regular or more vigorous exercise programme you choose to do depends on your preferences and abilities as well as available time and facilities. It should be something you enjoy otherwise it will be given up very soon. Whether exercising at a gym or at home, alone or supervised within each session the emphasis should be on whole body conditioning. A typical session should therefore ideally include:

- A warm up
- Aerobic exercises and conditioning
- Resistance training,
- Balance
- Flexibility
- A warm down, general and specific stretching.

In terms of order, resistance training should generally be performed after the aerobic exercise. Balance training may be integrated into the resistance training portion of the session or specific balance exercises can be integrated into the program. Within the warm-down session, as well as general stretches, those relevant to their previous treatments can be emphasized. For example, if an individual client has had a surgery or radiotherapy to the breast, abdominal or pelvis (see specific exercises and stretches sections of this book).

Aerobic exercises; Aerobic conditioning should be taken at a moderate level in both intensity and duration. In a gym, tread mills, cross trainers, arm cycling, and rowing machines are all suitable as is outside jogging or strides in the local park or if fortunate enough, a beach. Aerobic exercise can improve heart and lung fitness fitness, reduce fatigue and improve psychological distress. The Karvonen formula can be used to calculate target heart rate (THR) based on estimated maximal heart rate (MHR), resting heart rate (RHR), and the desired exercise intensity (%HRR):

THR = (MHR – RHR) x %HRR recommended + RHR
[Maximal heart rate (MHR) can be estimated using the following equation:
MHR = 207 – (0.7 x age)]

The %HRR depends on the condition of the individual. Those who have been sedentary, are in poor health, or have a low fitness level should begin exercising at an intensity of 30–45% of HRR. Active cancer survivors who are in good health may begin an individualized exercise intervention at 50–60% of HRR

The duration of a single bout of specific aerobic exercise depends on the emphasis of the session for that particular day and how much aerobic exercise has been performed by themselves during their activities of daily living. On training days that include resistance training, 20–30 minutes of aerobic exercise is ideal. On non resistance training days, 30–60 minutes of aerobic exercise is appropriate, as recommended by the American Cancer Society. Aerobic exercise duration may also be limited by the presents of fatigue. In this case, it may be necessary to recommend shorter bouts of exercise throughout the day as this has been shown to obtain similar improvements as one longer gym session without the associated fatigue. For example, three 10min sessions jogging or walking briskly morning, afternoon and evening. This of course is more time consuming and requires more self motivation.

Resistance training; Light regular resistance training is an ideal way to increase strength, improve fatigue and can be combined with core and balance exercises. Although many factors lead to the development of cancer-related fatigue, skeletal muscle wasting resulting from cancer wasting is a contributing factor. An exercise intervention that focuses on resistance training to stimulate protein synthesis is especially valuable for individuals experiencing cancer muscle wasting. Resistance training also attenuates the common age-related decrease in muscle protein synthesis. It is important to incorporate balance and core training with resistance training by using apparatus such as physioballs. As there may be deficiencies in balance and positional awareness (proprioception) it is vital to get supervision for in gym terminology to be "spotted" closely. Improving strength and endurance of all of the major muscle groups should be the focus of resistance training. Personal trainers will help determine the areas that need additional attention and provide specific advice.

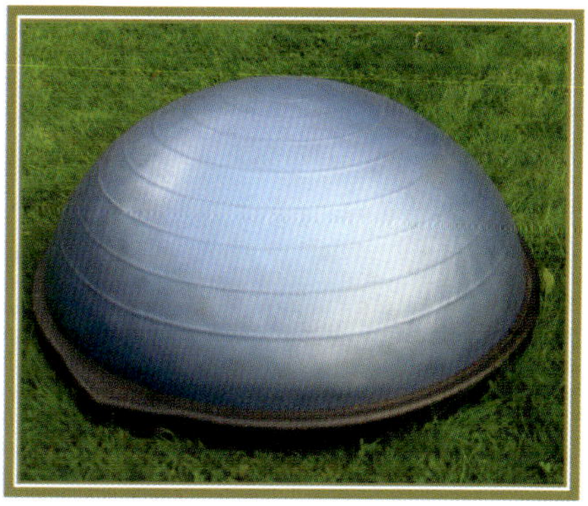

Balance training: Cancer treatments may lead to deficiencies in and balance, this may be caused by weakness in core strength, damage to the nerves which sense the position of the limbs (proprioreception) or damage to the sensory nerves in the arms and feet (peripheral neuropathy). These can also be exacerbated by a general lack of confidence in physical ability. Balance training exercise requires the use of the core muscles for balance as well as the large muscles of the lower body. Initially, balance training can be the primary

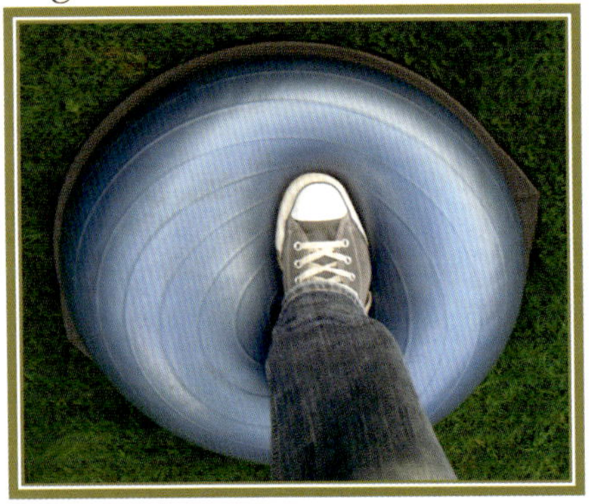

focus of a work out but should eventually be integrated into other resistance training exercises to shift the focus to functional, dynamic balance. There are a wide variety of balance and core devises available in most gym ranging from balance balls to specific floor exercises with the half balance ball being particularly useful. In the first instance, however, simply standing on one leg may suffice, later combining this with light biceps curls with dumbbells. The use of walking poles (e.g. Nordic-walking.co.uk) will decrease the difficulty of this exercise and may be a good way to begin balance training. Once balance disc walking with walking poles becomes relatively easy try without the assistance of walking poles. As you get more advanced try a half ball balance trainer (e.g. Bosu.com). It can be used in two ways. Stand on two feet with the flat surface uppermost then squat slowly up and down. This can be made harder by carrying some dumbbells. Alternatively, put the flat surface on the ground and stand with one leg in the centre, then step on a off repeatedly. Another advanced exercise

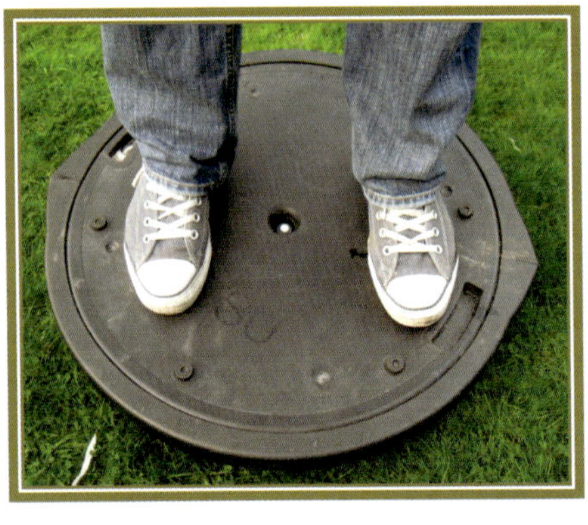

consists of throwing and catching a light medicine ball while seated on a stability ball. Adopted a stable position while sitting on a stability ball, begin tossing a light medicine ball from a close distance. Moving farther apart will make this exercise more difficult. To integrate balance training into resistance training exercises that require standing on the floor, the exercises can be performed on a balance pad, balance discs, or a balance trainer. Performing biceps curls on the balance trainer not only targets the biceps muscles but also improves balance and body position awareness. Progression from a balance pad, to balance discs, to the balance trainer will increase the difficulty of the exercise.

Flexibility, warm down and specific stretches; Training sessions should end with a low intensity warm-down and stretching. The aim is to try and stretch the entire body with different emphasis on different areas in different sessions depending on the resistance training schedule. Try to introduce an order as an aide memoir and ensure areas are not missed. For example, start with the right hand, wrist, arm elbow, shoulder, then repeat left side. More to the neck, thoracic spine, then feet and knees, hips and lower back. In addition to generally increasing your flexibility, there are some situations where specific exercises and stretches will aid recovery, improve local symptoms and help prevent long term complications such as neck or shoulder stiffness. It is important that these exercises and stretches are performed regularly and correctly. If not sure ask the medical team or physiotherapist or well qualified exercise professional in the local gym. The frequency depends on the severity of the condition but they should be performed two to three times a day at first, until the problem resolves, and then once a day there after. It is also important to continue the exercises long term, even if the apparent need has resolved, as continuing them will ensure that the symptoms are less likely to return. Two to three times a week may be enough in the long term, but you should set a realistic target and try and stick to it. If, for example, you miss one day, consider doing two the next to make up for it.

Exercise regularly and aim for the long-term

Whichever exercise you decide on, the essential point is that it should not just be a passing fad, but a regular way of life. The ultimate choice depends on numerous practical factors such as local availability, ability, previous experience, preferences, cost, time pressures and what friends and family also like to do as well. If an activity is to be sustained it should be enjoyable and convenient. There is little point putting yourself through torture, as even the most motivated person will give this up fairly quickly. Hopefully, after overcoming the initial barriers, exercise should be the norm, and not exercising will feel unusual.

Depending on your condition and ability, try two to three times a day at first, until the problem resolves, and then once a day. It is also important to continue the exercises long term, even if the apparent need has resolved, as continuing them will ensure that the symptoms are less likely to return. Two to three times a week may be enough in the long term, but set yourself a realistic target and try and stick to it. If, for example, you miss one day, do two the next to make up for it. Although the activities are relatively straightforward, you may not be particularly confident in the first instance. In this case, it may be appropriate to ask for help from a physiotherapist who is attached to your cancer team. Otherwise, a good experienced exercise professional may be able to help.

Help with exercise rehabilitation after cancer

Hopefully this section of the book has provided some ideas and guidance which will help to encourage physical activity in a realistic, enjoyable and fruitful way. The next challenge is knowing where and when to exercise to suit the individual lifestyles of the physically and culturally diverse population of cancer survivors. Some oncology units have a list of local facilities so it may be worth trying the local information room first. Our website cancernet.co.uk has tools (see exercise page) which allows users to search for local exercise recreational facilities based on their post code. It will provide locations and times of exercise groups, dance classes and community and private gyms. In some hospitals exercise rehabilitation classes have been initiated for the early stages after cancer therapies and again information should have been forthcoming from the local information centre. For those with physical disabilities it is appropriate to ask for a referral to a local physiotherapist or occupational therapist. Finally, the most exciting national scheme to help individuals exercise after cancer is and an expansion of the existing activity for life referral scheme:

The national exercise referral scheme

There are over 5500 community recreation centres in the UK so most people have one in their area. A scheme has already exist which enables doctors to refer people for exercise rehabilitation, supervised by appropriately qualified exercise professionals. Up until 2010 this included those with medical or physical conditions such as diabetes, obesity, bad backs and high blood pressure. In the autumn of 2010 we lobbied the government and submitted the standards to expand this scheme to include cancer rehabilitation. In addition, a course for exercise professionals has been established in order for existing exercise professionals to qualify as cancer rehabilitation trainers. This qualification, at the highest level of their training, provides them with the knowledge of how cancer and its treatments affect an individual's ability to exercise in order for them to design bespoke exercise schedules for their clients. Hopefully, as the scheme expands in 2011, all patients in the UK will be able to request their doctor to refer them to their local gym for a personal programme, usually 24 weeks, supervised by a qualified exercise professional.

Chapter Fourteen

Smoking and cancer
Evidence, harm, advice

Evidence: Smoking increases relapse risk

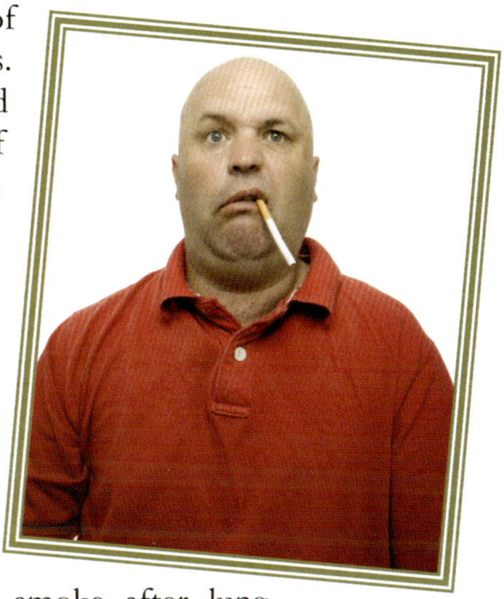

Smoking has been linked to the formation of more than 10 different types of cancers. Although the relationship between cancer and smoking is no longer in question, the effect of smoking during and after cancer therapies is less well known. As recently as March 2008 data from a publication in the European Journal of Cancer revealed an important oversight – that up to 30 percent of patients continued to smoke after their diagnosis. Data obtained from 25,000 patients with cancer have suggested that the cure rate at five years is at least 10 percent lower in smokers compared to non-smokers. This was even worse in female patients who continued to smoke after lung cancer. Likewise, patients with cancer of the head and neck area not only had a higher rate of their original cancer returning but the development of cancer elsewhere.

What makes smoking harmful?

Tobacco smoke contains over 4000 different chemicals, many of which are carcinogenic. The last chapters described the evidence for how these can reduce the chance of cure and increase side effects and complications of treatment. The four components of smoke which we know are particularly damaging are:

- **Carcinogens**
- **Nicotine**
- **Carbon monoxide**
- **Tar**

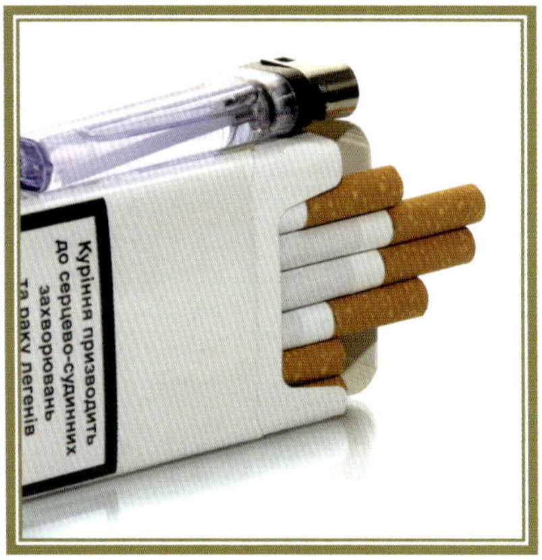

Carcinogens include benzene, pyridine, formaldehyde, ammonia, hydrogen cyanide, acetone and arsenic. These can directly damage the DNA of cells, causing the locked cancer genes to become active. They can also damage the immunity so that early cancers progress more rapidly. These chemicals have been shown to interact with the body's enzymes responsible for metabolising drugs used to treat cancer. For example, the biological agent erlotinib used for lung cancer is up to 25 percent less bio-available in smokers (This was proven to be caused specifically by an interaction with the enzyme called CYP1A). The chemicals in smoke have also been shown to interact with the bile production pathway in up to 40 percent of cases, which in turn can interfere with the excretion of a chemotherapy drug called irinotecan used for bowel cancer. This makes it difficult for the doctors to calculate which dose of chemotherapy to use in the treatment process, usually leading to under-dosing and therefore a worse outcome.

Nicotine is a powerful, fast acting and addictive drug. Most people who smoke are dependent on the nicotine in cigarettes. When a smoker inhales, nicotine is absorbed into their bloodstream and the effects are felt on their brain seven to eight seconds later. Nicotine also has many complex effects on the rest of the body. In small amounts nicotine stimulates nerve impulses in the central and the autonomic nervous system, but in large amounts nicotine inhibits these nerve impulses. The immediate effects of nicotine are:

- **Increased heart rate**
- **Constriction of the small blood vessels in the skin**
- **Increased blood pressure**
- **Increased metabolism**
- **Adverse effects on mood and behaviour**
- **Anxiety and tremor**

Carbon monoxide is a poisonous gas found in relatively high concentrations in cigarette smoke. It combines readily with haemoglobin, the oxygen-carrying substance in blood, to form carboxyhaemoglobin. In fact it combines more readily with haemoglobin than oxygen does, so up to 15 percent of a smoker's blood may be carrying carbon monoxide round the body instead of oxygen. Oxygen is essential for body tissues and cells to function efficiently. If the supply of oxygen is reduced for long periods, this can cause problems with growth, repair and absorption of essential nutrients. Carbon monoxide is therefore particularly harmful during pregnancy as it reduces the amount of oxygen carried to the uterus and foetus. Carbon monoxide can also affect the 'electrical' activity of the heart and, combined with other changes in the blood associated with smoking and diet, may encourage fatty deposits to form on the walls of the arteries. This process can eventually lead to the arteries becoming blocked, causing heart disease and other major circulatory problems.

Tar: When a smoker inhales, the cigarette smoke condenses and about 70 percent of the tar contained in the smoke is deposited in the lungs. Many of the substances in tar are already known to cause cancer (see below). Irritants in tar can also damage the lungs by causing narrowing of the bronchioles, coughing, an increase in bronchiole mucus, and damage to the small hairs (ciliostasis) that help protect the lungs from dirt and infection.

Passive smoking

Breathing the smoke from other people's cigarettes is called passive smoking. It consists of smoke from the burning end of the cigarette, called side stream smoke, and smoke inhaled and exhaled by the smoker. The US Environmental Protection Agency has declared passive smoking, or exposure to environmental tobacco smoke (ETS), to be a 'Class A Carcinogen, which means that it is capable of causing cancer in humans. Passive smoking may cause the following: irritation to the eyes, nose and throat in adults, babies and young children; increased acute respiratory illness in early childhood (including infections); headaches, dizziness and sickness; chronic cough, phlegm and wheeze; aggravation of asthma, and allergies; chronic middle ear lesions (glue ear); increased risk of coronary heart disease; reduced levels and capacity of lung functions; 10 percent to 30 percent increased risk of lung cancer for non-smokers, and increased prevalence of asthma, for those who are exposed to passive smoking over long periods.

Summary: risks of smoking:

- Premature ageing
- Skin wrinkles
- Coronary heart disease – smokers double their risk
- Heart disease particularly worse if overweight or high blood pressure
- An eight fold higher risk if associated with a high cholesterol or sedentary.
- Hardened arteries - strokes, peripheral vascular disease and gangrene,
- Damaged to major arteries causing aortic aneurysms.
- Increased anxiety and risk of depression.

- Cancer – lung, mouth, nose and throat, larynx, oesophagus,
- Cancer - pancreas, bladder, stomach, and kidney cancers.
- Lleukaemia, lymphoma
- Smoking 25 cigarettes a day means 25 times more likely to die from cancer.
- Chronic bronchitis, emphysema and other lung diseases
- Recurrent infections in the airways and general loss of efficiency in the lungs.
- Peptic (stomach) ulcers increase in incidence and the time they take to heal.
- Tobacco amblyopia (defective vision).
- Increased risk of osteoporosis – brittle bones that are liable to fracture.
- Infertility and earlier menopause.
- Increased risk of erectile dysfunction and vaginal dryness.
- In pregnancy, spontaneous abortion and low birth weight is more common.
- Blood clots – deep-vein thrombosis, pulmonary embolism, strokes.
- Macular degeneration and blindness.
- Dementia and memory loss.
- Psychological illness.

Advice and help to quit smoking

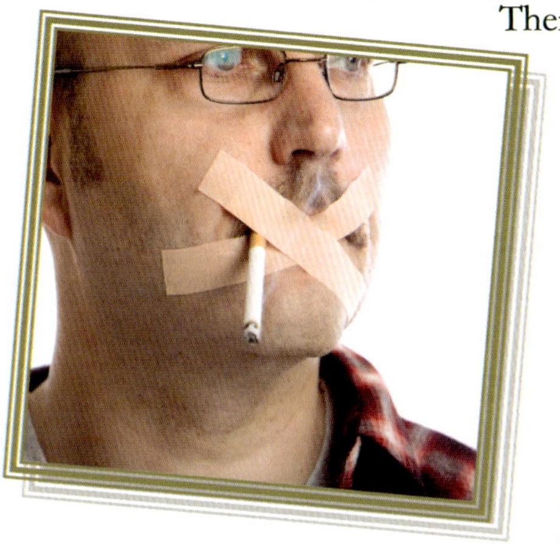

There is no quick and easy way to quit. Up to half of smokers continue to light up cigarettes after being diagnosed with cancer. You really have to want to stop smoking. Most smokers do want to stop, and it is the single most important thing a smoker can do to help reduce their risk of cancer, and live longer. At any one time, one in six smokers are trying to quit. Despite the strong addiction of cigarettes, more than 11 million people in Britain alone have become successful ex-smokers. Most of those who stop do so by themselves. Being determined is the vital ingredient. Deciding to quit and really wanting to succeed are important steps to becoming a non-smoker. It is helpful for smokers to have a plan to quit smoking. The following suggestions have helped some people to quit successfully.

Cutting down or stopping outright? Cutting down is less likely to work than simply stopping outright. Unfortunately, even if trying to cut down, the numbers tend to creep back up again. So, once the date has been chosen, it is better to stop outright.

Diet and physical activity. Both of these have an important effect on the body. Stopping smoking is a major change for the body to adapt to, and a healthy diet and regular physical activity at a suitable level of exertion is encouraged.

Reducing other peoples exposure. When smoking cigarettes other people around you are being exposed to its risk – this is called passive smoking. The US Environmental Protection Agency has declared passive smoking to be a 'Class A Carcinogen' which means that it is capable of causing cancer in humans. In addition, passive smoking may cause irritation to the eyes, nose and throat in adults, babies and young children; increased acute respiratory illness in early childhood; asthma, headaches, dizziness and sickness; chronic cough, phlegm and wheeze; aggravation of asthma and allergies; chronic middle ear lesions (glue ear); increased risk of coronary heart disease; reduced levels and capacity of lung function.

Extra help: For those who have tried to quit and have gone back to smoking again, there are other things that can help, including products to help you quit smoking; alternative therapies such as hypnotherapy or acupuncture; joining a 'stop smoking' support group.

Products to help you quit. There are many different smoking cessation aids on the market. It is important to check whether the product is safe and effective before spending time, energy and money on it. If in any doubt as to whether a product is safe to use, check with your doctor or pharmacist first. Some manufacturers claim very high success rates, promising between 80 percent and 90 percent effortless success. But there is no magic solution. To be certain that a product or method works, it has to be put through proper tests (clinical trials). If the product has an effect, it can then be compared with that achieved by another product. Not all the products available have been tested in this way. There are two main types of commercial aids available to help crack the smoking habit. Nicotine-containing replacement products and non-nicotine replacement products:

A smoking cessation aid cannot:

- Stop you smoking
- Make you WANT to stop
- Make it painless and easy

A smoking cessation aid can:

- Ease withdrawal
- Boost your confidence and morale
- Lessen the urge to smoke

Nicotine replacement products: These methods replace some of the addictive nicotine from smoke. Nicotine replacement therapy has been well researched and tests have shown that, if used correctly, it can double the chance of success. If you smoke your first cigarette within 30 minutes of waking, then it is particularly likely that you can benefit from nicotine replacement therapy. Nicotine replacement products are generally safer than smoking but if you have, or have had, a heart problem, check with your doctor or pharmacist beforehand. It is also important to use the product properly, so following the manufacturer's instructions is essential. In particular, you must stop smoking completely while taking nicotine replacement therapy. Nicotine replacement products may also affect the action of some drugs such as warfarin and beta-blockers. The forms of nicotine replacement commonly available include patches, gum, nasal sprays and inhalators. Your family doctor may be able to prescribe nicotine replacement products. Patches, gum and an inhalator are available from a pharmacist without a prescription. The patch gives a continual supply of nicotine at a low dose while wearing it – so patches cannot respond quickly to a craving or a stressful moment. The gum, nasal spray and inhalator deliver a higher dose quickly, which can respond to a craving with a 'quick fix', as with cigarettes. If you smoke mainly in response to cravings or stress the gum, nasal spray or inhaler might be particularly helpful if you miss the 'hand to mouth' action of smoking. Side effects of nicotine replacement products include nausea, headaches, dizziness and palpitations.

Non-nicotine replacement products: These are many and varied. They are easily available through mail order, newsagents, health shops or pharmacists. Often they do not require a license under the Medicines Act. Generally there is not enough firm evidence to say how effective they are. You need to be wary of claims of very high success rates. Non-nicotine replacement products include nicobrevin capsules, scented inhalers, dummy cigarettes, tobacco-flavoured chewing gum, herbal cigarettes and filters.

Complementary therapies: Although some therapies undoubtedly help many people, the results of research so far remains unproven. The two most popular forms of complementary therapies for stopping smoking are hypnotherapy and acupuncture. If you decide to try these therapies it is important to find a registered practitioner.

Support groups: Joining a 'stop smoking' support group can help you feel less alone in an attempt to quit. Being with other people who are also trying can provide mutual support, a sense of being understood and a sense of competition! They are usually run over a period of weeks, and take you through the different stages of giving up smoking. Specialist smoker's clinics can improve three-fold an individual's likelihood of stopping.

Summary – ten tips to quit smoking:

Make a date and stick to it: Commit yourself to a time and date. Most people who successfully quit smoking do so by stopping altogether, and not by gradually cutting down.

Keep busy: Keeping busy helps to take your mind off cigarettes. All ashtrays, lighters and unopened cigarette packets should be thrown away.

Drinking plenty of fluids: Keeping a glass of water or juice and sipping it steadily. Trying different flavours.

Get more active: Try walking or cycling instead of using the bus or car. Use the stairs instead of the lift. Physical activity helps relaxation and can boost morale.

Think positively: Withdrawal, irritability mood swings and poor concentration are common but keep reminding yourself they will disappear after a couple of weeks.

Change your routine: Try to avoid shopping in places where you have previously bought cigarettes. Avoid the pub garden or smoker's corner at work if there are lots of smokers around. Try doing something totally different. Surprise yourself!

No excuses: Don't use a crisis, or even good news, as an excuse for 'just one cigarette'. There is no such thing. The next will be craved and the next, and so on.

Treat yourself: This is important. Use the money that is saved to buy something special, big or small, that you couldn't usually afford.

Be careful of what to eat: Try not to snack on fatty foods. Instead try fruit, raw vegetables or sugar-free gum or sweets.

Take one day at a time: Each day without a cigarette is good news for your heart, your health, your family and your pocket.

PART 4

The symptoms of cancer and side effects of treatments

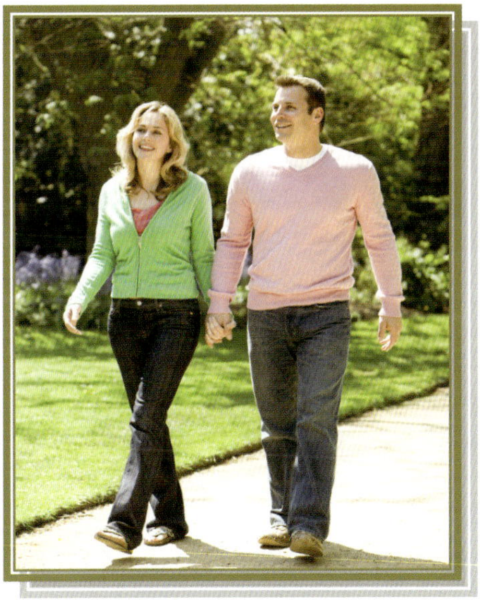

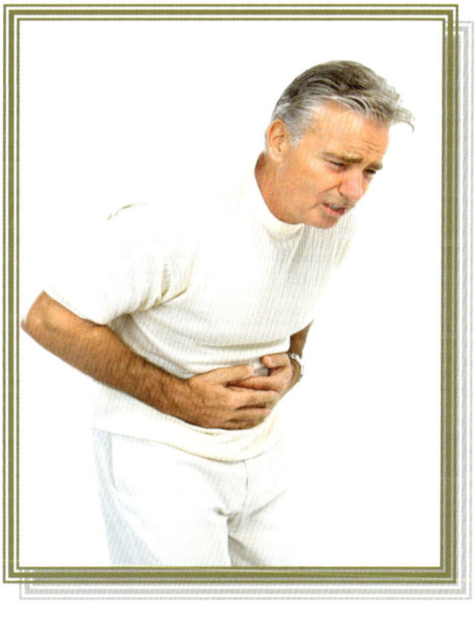

Advice and guidance for self help and empowerment

Background to this self help guidance

Changing your lifestyle after a distressing diagnosis such as cancer is not an easy task. There is enough to cope with between telling your family and employers, understanding the options, and remembering to be in the right place at the right time for treatments and investigations. No doubt there is a strong temptation to bury your head in the ground and put any thoughts of exercise and diet interventions in the back of your mind until treatments have finished. There is, however, strong evidence that straight-forward lifestyle strategies should be considered early as possible as they can reduce the chance of serious complications after surgery and during other active treatments such as chemotherapy, radiotherapy, hormones and herceptin. They can also improve the overall sense of well being create a sense of empowerment and control in this vulnerable time. Even though it is best to start early, lifestyle interventions can also help many months or years following the initial flurry of therapeutic activity, especially if ongoing anti-hormone therapies have been prescribed – so it is never too late to start. To make the advice clearer it has been simplified into the separate categories:-

Mind and body
- Fatigue and tiredness
- Mood, anxiety and depression
- Brain power and intellect
- Poor sleep pattern

Abdomen and digestion
- Exercise after abdominal surgery
- Poor appetite
- Sickness and vomiting
- Diarrhoea
- Constipation
- Bowel adhesions
- Rectal damage
- Indigestion and heartburn
- Pelvic floor exercises
- Incontinence

Chemotherapy and Radiotherapy
- Skin care and radiotherapy
- Skin care and chemotherapy
- Chapped lips and cold sores
- Sore mouth
- Blood clots (thrombosis)
- Nail damage
- Hair loss
- Hand foot syndrome

Other common concerns
- Breast tenderness
- Sexual function
- Joint pains and neck stiffness
- Hot flushes
- Bone density
- Secondary cancers

Chapter Fifteen

Mind and body
Background and advice

Fatigue and tiredness

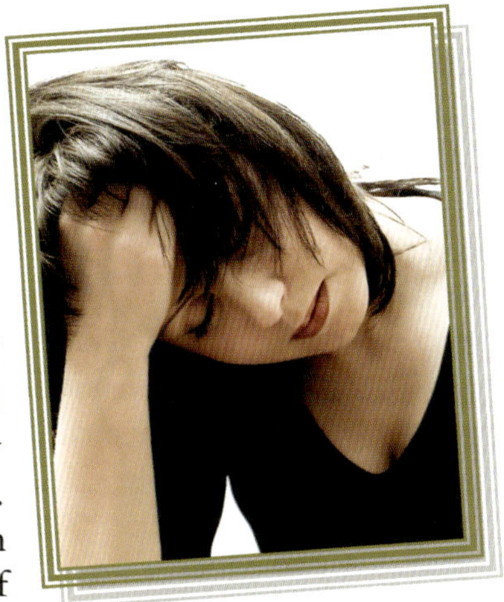

It is very likely that you have, or will have, experienced fatigue during your treatment, as studies have shown that the burden of fatigue has now overtaken nausea and pain as the most distressing symptom during chemotherapy. It has been described as tiredness, exhaustion, depression, feeling unwell, loss of motivation and limitation of mental state. Over 75 percent of patients complain of fatigue, and in up to a third of cases, this can be severe – considerably impacting on quality of life and ability to self-care. Fatigue can also have a negative impact on treatment by preventing the required dose of chemotherapy from being administered and it can also delay recovery for several months after treatments have finished. This post-treatments fatigue, as well as being distressing, can have a considerable impact on the ability to return to work or full time care of children, husbands, wives or other dependants.

Clinician awareness of the impact of fatigue is now improving, but not so long ago, in a survey of doctors from Philadelphia, only 20 percent felt their patients suffered fatigue, whereas in reality 70 percent of their patients said that it was the most significant side effect. Fatigue is common not just with chemotherapy, but with the other main cancer treatments such as radiotherapy, surgery, hormone therapy and the new biological therapies such as herceptin, erbitux, avastin, sutent and nexevar.

Medical interventions for these conditions may have a significant impact on well-being, so clinicians and patients should look out for these aggravating causes at each consultation and treat them appropriately. Anaemia, for example, responds to blood transfusion or injections of growth factors which stimulate the bone marrow to make more blood. A thyroid deficiency, more common after radiotherapy and prolonged chemotherapy regimens, can be easily corrected by thyroxine. Disturbed sleep may be helped with better pain control, or medication to avoid getting up to pass water in the night. In other situations, low dose steroids or stimulants can sometimes be given if fatigue is severe.

What can you do to help?

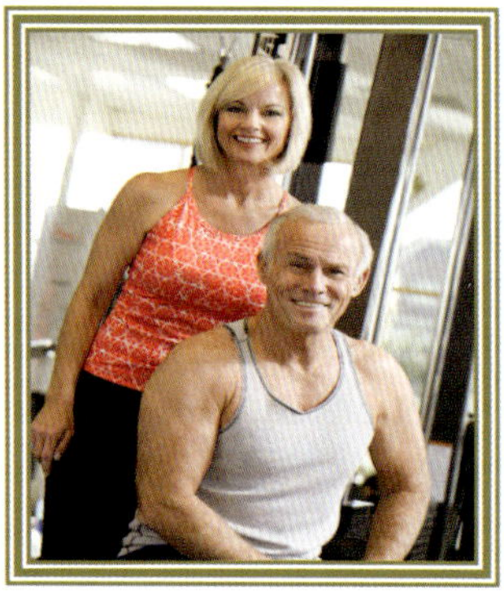

It is important to discuss fatigue with your doctor, as this is a genuine symptom which can seriously affect your quality of life. Try to get enough sleep at night or even consider a nap in the day. The sleep hygiene rules may help in this chapter. At other times try to embark on stimulating activities which can distract you from your fatigue, such as meeting friends or going for a walk in an interesting environment. Some people find going back to work is fulfilling and useful.

Exercise: There have been 48 published RCT's evaluating exercise interventions in patients with cancer-related fatigue. These include home based exercise programmes such as walking, jogging or cycling and supervised programmes such as aerobics, resistance exercises, stretching and a general "work out" in a gym or dance class. Studies have shown that the optimal level of exercise differs between individuals and the stages of their treatments:

A study involving patients with acute leukaemia receiving intense hospital based chemotherapy evaluated a three week supervised walking programme during chemotherapy. Participants walked five times a week for 12 minutes, in the hospital hallway. The supervised exercise programme was completed by 69 percent of the participants. No adverse events were reported and there was a moderate improvement in terms of fatigue.

A study from Michigan USA showed that women receiving radiotherapy who participated in jogging or brisk walking for 20-45 minutes 3-5 times a week had significantly greater haemoglobin levels (red blood cells) and experienced less fatigue. Another study in men with prostate cancer receiving radiotherapy showed a benefit from daily 15 minute aerobics exercise compared to sedentary controls.

The impact of exercise on the fatigue related to long term hormone therapies has been evaluated in men taking Zoladex (or equivalent) and in women taking tamoxifen, anastrozole (Arimidex) or the other hormone tablets. There was a reduction in fatigue, and performing aerobics exerciseses at home for 15-30 minutes per day, such as dancing, jogging or brisk walking, was more effective than weight lifting or resistance bands alone. Studies which involved a supervised exercise in a gym, dance or aerobics class had the best results with a combination of both aerobics and gentle resistance training being particularly effective. Five further studies evaluated the role of supervised exercise involving patients who were experiencing fatigue, which can last up to a year after chemotherapy. Aerobic exercises with stretching and resistance were supervised 2-3 times a week. Aerobic exercises were performed with an intensity of 40 percent - 80 percent heart rate max adjusted for age for 10-30 minutes. Exercise lasted at least 15-30 minutes per day. The programme was completed by 90 percent. The supervised exercise programme showed a significant reduction in CRF as well as improved muscle strength, sleeping patterns and quality of life in favour of the exercise groups.

Other lifestyle initiatives are summarised in the table below but regular light exercise is by far the most important self help strategy which you can carry out to reduce fatigue. It is also clear from the studies summarised here that a supervised exercise programme is better than doing it alone at home. If you are a member of a gym a suitably qualified exercise professional should be able to help you. Otherwise, you can ask your oncology team or GP whether a formal exercise rehabilitation programme exists in your area, either in the hospital or your local community gym as part of the national exercise referral scheme.

Summary – fatigue coping tactics:

- Acceptance – it's normal to get tried, so try not to get disheartened
- Eat a healthy balanced diet: fruit, berries, herbs, fibre and protein
- Eat slow energy releasing carbohydrates: pasta, bread, rice, quinoa, potatoes
- Avoid refined sugar in foods producing peaks and troughs in glucose levels
- Rest – allocate set times for rests, throughout the day between activities
- Aerobics exercise between 15-30 minutes per day, every day, if possible
- Try gentle resistance exercise (weights or exercise bands)
- Supervised exercise is ideal – ask for a national exercise referral
- Distraction tactics – maintain an interest and meet up with friends
- Stimulation tactics – listening to stimulating tapes or music
- Try to keep comfortable – avoid being too hot or cold
- Consider sleep hygiene rules – see sleep section
- Task avoidance – use energy saving aids: remote controls, lifts, etc.
- Task management – organise others to help with regular strenuous tasks

Mood, anxiety and depression

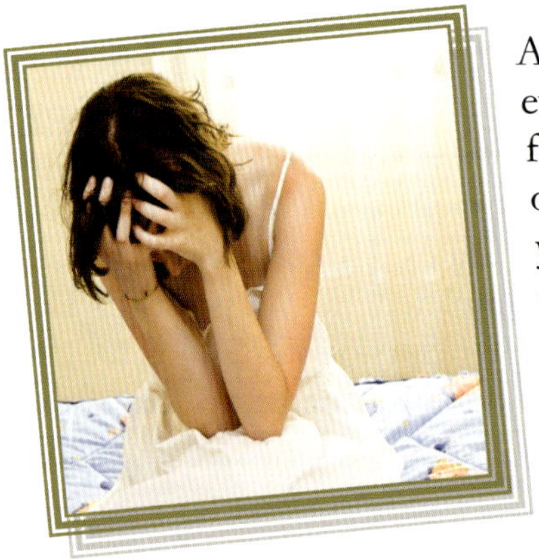

A diagnosis of cancer remains a devastating life event and the 'word' still strikes a deep sense of foreboding, even after the initial shock has worn off. It is very likely that there will be times during your treatment when you will feel 'low', anxious or depressed. A number of well conducted studies have shown that this occurs in over 40 percent of patients. What's more, these troublesome symptoms are frequently under-recognised and under-treated. Apart from being distressing enough on their own, of equal concern are studies which suggest that depressed patients have a reduced chance of cure compared to the psychologically healthy. A particularly risky period is shortly after the end of the initial course of intensive therapies, such as after the last cycle of adjuvant chemotherapy for breast or bowel cancer, where the sudden end to hospital support may make you feel at your most vulnerable.

What can you do to help?

If there is overt anxiety or depression, therapeutic intervention should be considered. Otherwise, consider asking your community doctor for a referral to a psychological counsellor, and help re-channel your negative energy or fear into positive enthusiasm for lifestyle and self-help strategies.

Exercise improves mood, a sense of well-being and studies have demonstrated reduced levels of depression and anxiety and an improved quality of life. For example, a review of the published literature printed in the Archives of Internal Medicine in February 2010 showed that regular exercise helped those who suffer from a chronic illness feel much less anxious. After analysing data from 40 studies on 3,000 participants who were previously sedentary but who were able to exercise in sessions of at least 30 minutes, researchers found that those who exercised had a 20 percent reduction in anxiety symptoms compared to those who did not exercise at all. Notably, exercise helped people no matter what kind of health problem they had including cancer, depression, heart disease, or fibromyalgia. Regular exercise sessions longer than 30 minutes were even better at providing relief from anxiety than sessions shorter than 30 minutes. So it looks like the more the better. The underlying reason for the benefit may lie in the release of positive brain chemicals (neurokins) that are similar to drugs, and which make people euphoric. Exercise is also generally fun, gets people out of the house – socialising and interacting with other people.

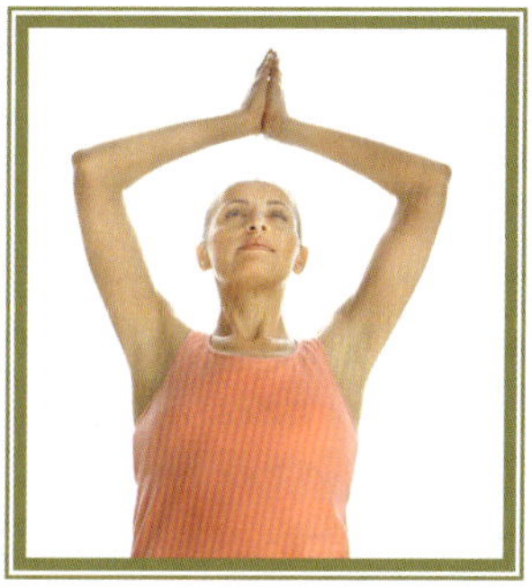

Relaxation techniques, especially those combined with exercise such as yoga or Pilates, are excellent remedies for anxiety and the muscle tension associated with it. Hands-on complementary therapies such as massage, reflexology and acupuncture have also shown improvement in anxiety in fairly robust analyses. Note that despite common folk lore, gentle massage is safe and there is absolutely no evidence that it "spreads cancer cells around the body".

Alcohol may initially make you relaxed, but like any drug there is an up and down effect. When the pleasant effect wears off, particularly if associated with a hangover, it can make you irritable, significantly lower your mood, or even make you depressed.

Some medications such as hormone therapies for breast and prostate cancer can also cause a reduction in your mood leading to depression. In this case, it is worth asking your doctor if there are any alternatives. Certainly our own research has shown that different brands of breast cancer drugs, even within the same category, can be tolerated differently from one person to another.

Smoking: Contrary to popular opinion amongst smokers, cigarettes greatly increase anxiety. It is a myth that smoking calms your nerves. This only appears to be the case because even a few minutes after smoking a cigarette, the body begins to 'withdraw', leading to tremors, sweating and anxiety which can only be relieved, momentarily, by another cigarette. This leads to an escalating spiral of increased cigarette dependence, followed by more anxiety and the only way to stop it is to give up. The same applies to other stimulatory drugs such as cannabis and most other illegal agents.

Summary – advice to improve anxiety and mood:

- Take regular light exercise
- Take part in regular social activities
- Maintain an interest or hobby
- Try to maintain good hygiene habits
- Consider investing in a psychological counsellor
- Avoid alcohol, coffee and strong tea
- Avoid cigarettes and other recreational drugs
- Review medications with your doctor

Brainpower and intellect

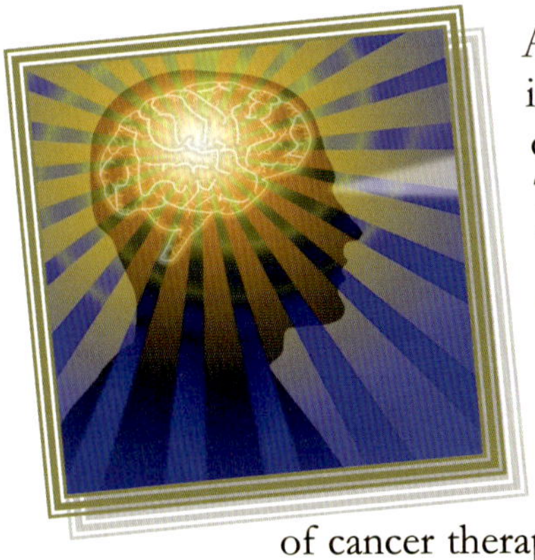

A number of studies have reported a reduction in intellectual ability or brainpower after surgery, chemotherapy or whilst taking hormone therapies. The official term for loss of brain power is 'cognitive impairment' and it can manifest itself as a loss of memory and the inability to concentrate. There are numerous underlying causes for this loss of brain power and patients often complain of being forgetful. In most cases this situation is temporary, returning to normal after completion of cancer therapies. For example a study published in the Journal of Clinical Oncology showed that after a year of taking tamoxifen women scored lower on tests of verbal memory functioning and other cognitive skills than before they started. They also showed that they generally scored better if taking another breast cancer drug, exemestane (Aromasin) rather than tamoxifen. Fatigue or drugs such as painkillers, sedatives or antidepressants, can also exacerbate the loss of brain power. One of the least stated but most important factors is the major disruption that cancer and its treatment has on your daily routine. It is very likely that you will not have the same intellectual stimulation previously received from the work place or social interaction with friends and colleagues. Fortunately, this lack of stimulation can be anticipated and can be corrected, although it may require a lot of hard work and intervention.

What can you do to help?

The golden rules apply to the mind as well as to the body – eat well, stop smoking and exercise. Exercise increases oxygen to the brain and also gets you out of the house, changes your environment and provides visual and intellectual stimulation. Alcohol is not a good idea. We are all aware of the muzzy headedness that occurs with even the mildest of hangovers.

The brain, like a muscle, gets stronger with use. Social interaction helps to stimulate the mind, especially when engaging in interesting conversation. Learning something new, or writing in a diary, will help you to think more creatively, help your memory and enhance your ability to make logical connections. Singing is a nice way to exercise your intellect, particularly those processes originating in the right side of your brain. I'm sure you have noticed that it's easier to rhyme when singing than when just speaking or writing. This is because the right side of the brain is better at pattern recognition, and also accounts for the phenomenon that stutterers can stop stuttering as soon as they start singing.

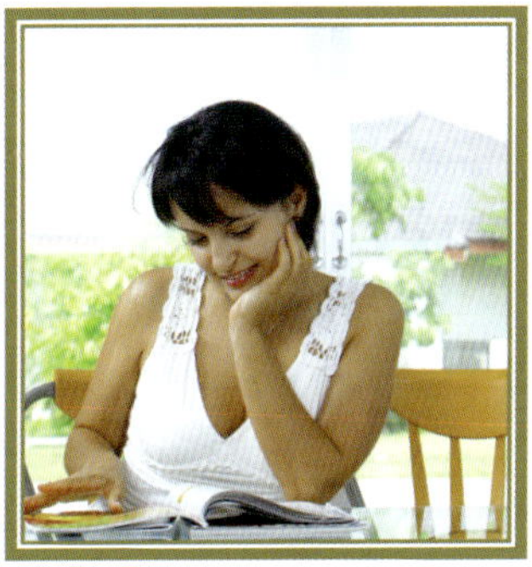

Various *brain exercise tools* are now available commercially – ranging from crosswords, Su Doku and riddle books to electronic brain-teaser gadgets. Brain training, however, doesn't have to stop if you don't have access to specific books or electronic gadgets. Imagination and day-dreaming exercises have been shown to improve brain power and can be performed anywhere. Imagine different rooms of the house and how they would look if decorated differently or, whilst looking out of the window, try to imagine how it would look during different seasons or when covered with snow. Ideally, try running slowly on a tread mill or in the local park and try to solve a mental problem – you will be exercising your mind and body at the same time.

Finally, you may be frustrated by a lack of concentration. However, this will improve with time, but in some cases recovery is hindered by anxiety or a pre-occupation with unconstructive thoughts. The relaxation tips highlighted in the anxiety section of this book may help, but otherwise try to dispel the negative thoughts which are sapping your ability to concentrate. When you are conscious of these thoughts they can often be resolved by discussing them with friends, relatives or your medical team. If not, meditation or psychological counselling may be useful.

Summary – advice to improve your brain power:

- Take regular exercise, stop smoking and reduce alcohol intake
- Eat a healthy, balanced diet with plenty of vitamins, antioxidants and fibre
- Take a fish oil regularly unless there is a contraindication
- Review your medication with your doctors – some may be sedating
- Use your brain – engage in conversation, socialise, visit friends and relatives
- Stimulate your brain – learn something new, read, listen to audio books.
- Exercise your brain – puzzles, singing, brain teasers, imagination techniques
- Use brain exercise gadgets – electronic challenges, chess
- Identify negative thoughts which may be sapping your concentration
- Try to establish a regular sleep pattern
- If you have memory loss and are on medication discuss with your doctor

Poor sleep pattern

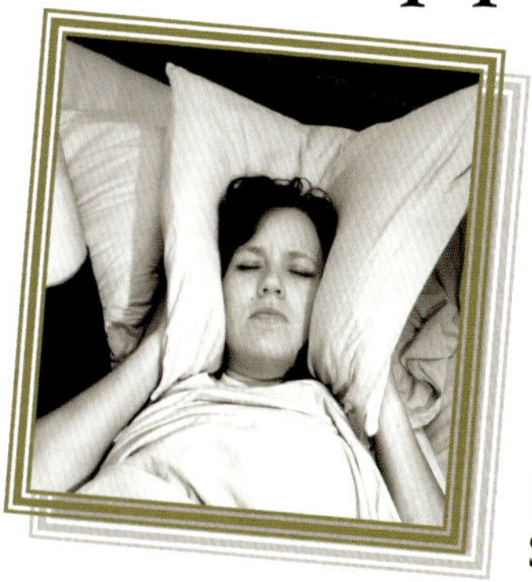

Everybody likes a good night's sleep, but after a diagnosis of cancer this is more of a dream than a reality. Several confounding factors conspire to keep you awake. It is normal to ponder over a diagnosis of cancer, and often this is at its worst in the early hours of the morning. A number of physical conditions can make night times uncomfortable; pain, indigestion, breathlessness, or having to pass water frequently. Steroids can keep you alert and agitated as can hormones for breast and prostate cancer which can also cause night sweats.

What can you do to help yourself?

It is helpful to try and accept that it is normal at an early stage to worry and have sleepless nights. This in turn means you are not worrying about the lack of sleep which will help break the self perpetuating cycle.

.

Summary – advice to help you sleep

- Establish a regular pattern of sleeping. Set a time to go to bed and get up
- Avoid temperature extremes and noise when in bed
- Ensure your bedroom is dark. Consider blackout curtains
- Avoid being uncomfortable or in pain. Consider taking painkillers
- Try not to watch TV or read exciting books in bed
- Exercise routinely, but try not to exercise within two hours of bedtime
- Reduce the intake of caffeine, alcohol and nicotine after mid afternoon
- Avoid drinking large amounts of liquids prior to bedtime
- Avoid food colourings and preservatives which can act as stimulants
- Avoid hunger or excessive eating prior to bedtime
- Sleep only as much as you need to feel rested and avoid taking daytime naps
- When taking steroid drugs, take them in the morning if possible
- Avoid sleeping tablets unless you are getting over a short-term issue
- If repeatedly awakened to pass water, discuss medication with your doctor
- Engage in a quiet, relaxing activity before bedtime
- If awake for 30 minutes, leave bed, perform a relaxing activity, then return
- If depressed, waking in a sad mood, discuss antidepressants with the doctor

Chapter Sixteen

Abdomen & digestion
Symptoms and advice

Exercises after abdominal surgery

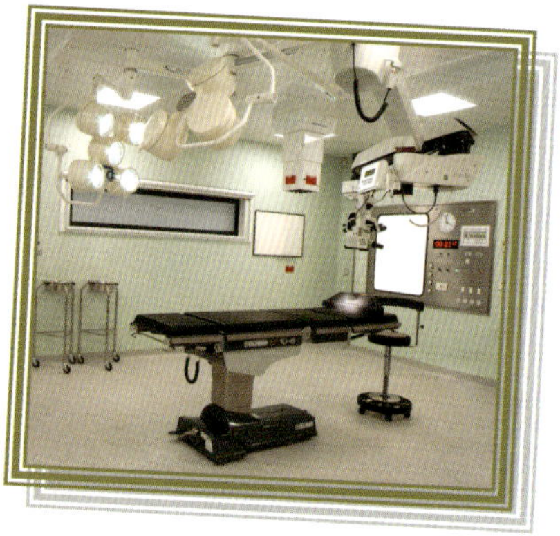

The surgeon will have had to cut through your stomach muscles and fibrous bands in the abdominal wall. This leads to an inherent weakness that not only creates a lax and less toned stomach, but increases the risk of hernia, either through the scar or elsewhere. Advice, including exercise, in the days and a week or two after the operation, is best sought from your surgical team and may change with local policies and techniques.

What can you do to help yourself?

After the acute period of recovery, abdominal exercises are helpful. The aim of exercise after abdominal surgery is to tone up the muscles and prevent a hernia. It would therefore be counter-productive to increase the pressure inside the abdomen during exercise, as this is would encourage herniation of tissues through the scar. The two most important rules when performing abdominal exercises are; '**do not strain**' and '**breathe correctly**'. These will be explained as we go along, but they essentially mean – no red faced squeezing and holding your breath!

Performing these exercises, in addition to getting generally fitter, will aid recovery, improve local symptoms and help prevent long term complications. Written information on these techniques is often provided by your surgical or oncology team and the specific advice provided here may differ a little from these but the fundamental principles should be the same. For optimal recovery it is important to perform these exercises regularly 2-3 times a day if possible for more than 5 minutes generally. If you miss a day try to make up for it the next day.

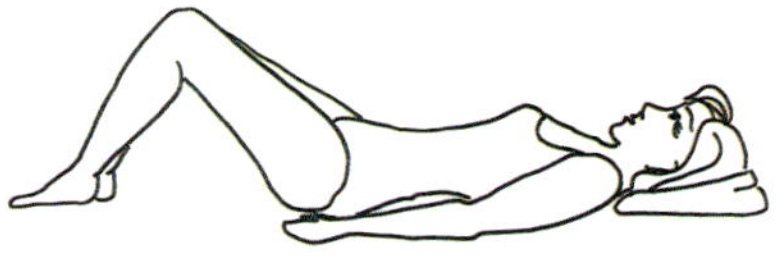

Pelvic tilting: Lying on your back, on a soft but level surface (exercise mat, towel or a carpet). Relax with the knees bent. Take a breath in and then push the lower back against the floor, tightening the stomach muscles at the same time. Each time the muscles are tightened, breathe out slowly for 5-10 seconds. Repeat 5-10 times. To help prevent backache, tighten your stomach muscles and pull them in, pressing your back down into the bed. Repeat 2 or 3 times a day.

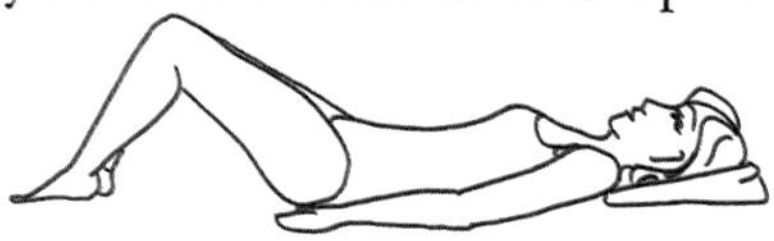

Knee Rolling: Hands by your sides – draw in your stomach muscles, and roll your knees over to one side. Slowly bring them up again, and roll them the other way.

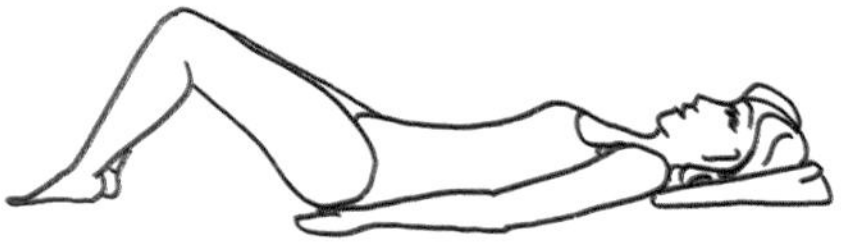

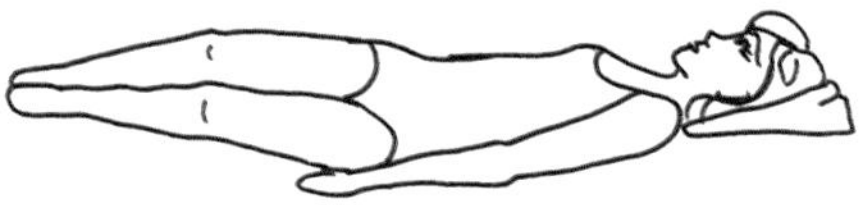

Bottom lift: Draw in stomach muscles. Lift your bottom up off the bed – lower slowly and relax

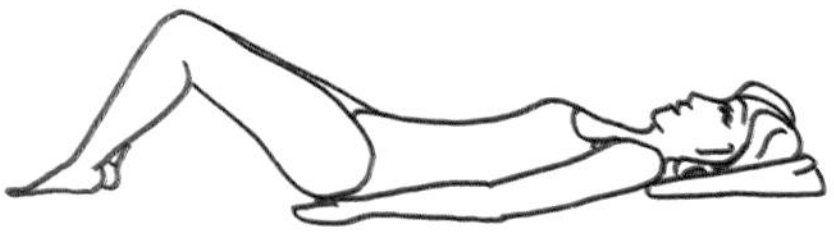

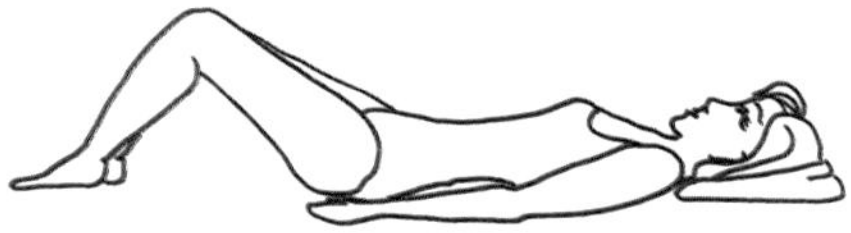

After 10-14 days, provided recovery is going well, try some gentle sit-ups. Lift your head and shoulders off the ground, hold for 2-3 seconds, and then repeat 10-20 times, three times per day. Keep your elbows back, with your hand behind your head, looking forward. Keep your lower back flat against the ground. It is most important to keep your mouth open, and breathe out slightly every time the head is lifted. This will prevent the pressure inside your abdomen increasing, whilst at the same time strengthening your abdominal muscles. Repeat the sit-ups with your legs twisted to the right, and then to the left.

Abdominal surgery may also affect the pelvic structures and the muscles which support the bladder and rectum. It would also be wise to start pelvic floor exercises regularly as soon as possible to prevent incontinence (see below for instructions).

Poor appetite

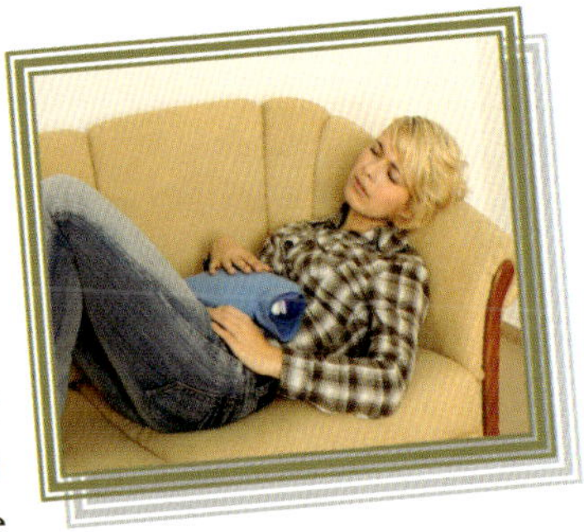

"Gone off your food?" or "Don't feel like eating?" a poor appetite is an annoying side effect, and can lead to weight loss and fatigue. There are several overlapping causes of a poor appetite; chemicals released from your disease itself; the function of your liver, brain or kidneys; compression on your gut or stomach; a salt imbalance such as high calcium; drugs such as pain killers. Chemotherapy and hormone therapies can cause a long term or transient loss of appetite. Your desire to eat may be impaired with recent surgery, mouth ulcers, depression and radiotherapy.

What can you do to help?

It is important to report a sustained poor appetite to your supervising medical team, so medication can be given. It is also worth seeing a trained dietician if a nutritional deficiency is suspected. Otherwise, if you are not eating as well as usual, the following tips may improve your appetite, and help you eat more of the foods that you need at this time. These foods may not be particularly healthy in the long term but this is not a priority at this time if a poor appetite is a prominent symptom. It is important, however, to revert back to a healthy diet once these short-term problems have subsided.

Summary – lifestyle advice for a poor appetite:

- Small and frequent meals and snacks every 2 hours are recommended
- Every mouthful helps, appetite comes and goes, so eat well in the good times
- You need not eat 'normal' foods at 'normal' times. Eat when you are hungry
- Try to relax and enjoy eating, eat slowly and chew your food well
- Try to rest before and after a meal
- A short walk before a meal may help increase your appetite
- If cooking is a chore, cold meals can be as nutritious as hot ones
- Experimenting with different foods, which you don't usually eat, adds variety
- Food and drinks should be as nourishing as possible
- A small glass of wine or beer may boost your appetite before a meal
- Friends & relatives may offer to help with cooking and shopping – Accept
- Short term use of convenience foods are a useful standby if chosen carefully
- Drinking with meals may make you feel full and spoil your appetite

Sickness and vomiting

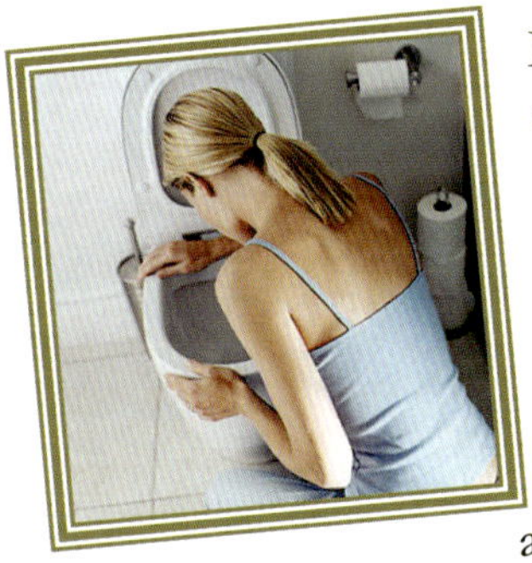

Loss of appetite is often the milder form or prelude to sickness and vomiting which, despite the great advances in anti-sickness medication, is still commonly experienced during a course of chemotherapy and to a lesser extent radiotherapy. Fortunately, only very rarely is this severe, but should be reported to your doctors nevertheless, as the underlying cause should be investigated. In addition to the factors affecting your appetite, investigations should look for salt and calcium disturbances, dehydration or, of more concern, liver, brain and gut metastasis.

What can you do to help?

Discuss nausea with your medical team; there are lots of effective treatments so your conventional medication could be changed to one which suits you. Otherwise the following advice may help.

Summary – lifestyle advice if feeling sick or nauseous:

- When feeling sick, it is not a good idea to 'insist' on eating
- It is important to keep fluid intake up to avoid dehydration.
- Clear, cold drinks may be better tolerated but avoid caffeine
- Sipping fizzy drinks such as soda water, ginger beer or lemonade may help
- Try sipping fluids slowly, using a straw – you'll get more down
- Solid food such as sorbet or jelly may be easier to manage
- Herbal, ginger or peppermint tea may soothe an upset stomach
- Food should be eaten slowly, followed by relaxation, but not lying flat
- Drinks should be taken 30 minutes after a meal, rather than with it
- Avoid a completely empty stomach – take regular small snacks
- A short walk in the fresh air before eating helps reduce nausea
- Tight-fitting clothes are not recommended
- Highly spiced, rich or fatty foods can make nausea worse
- Cold foods are better if the smell of cooking causes nausea
- If food smells upset you accept offers for others to cook
- Avoid the kitchen
- Eating slowly in a well-ventilated room is more relaxing

Diarrhoea

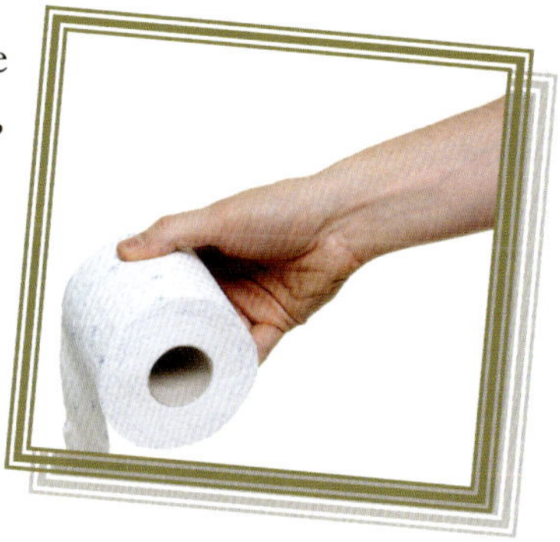

Radiotherapy to the abdomen and some chemotherapy agents cause diarrhoea, (capecitabine, florouracil, irinotecan). As well as the inconvenience of going to the bathroom, diarrhoea can have some more serious consequences. If left unchecked it can cause dehydration and damage the kidneys. If undergoing a course of chemotherapy, dehydration can concentrate the drugs in your blood stream, increasing the risk of a low blood count or infection.

What can you do to help?

The following tips may supplement the medication given to you by the hospital. Three separate trials have shown that probiotic (healthy) bacteria, found in some yoghurts and tablets, help reduce diarrhoea associated with radiotherapy, and a further trial showed improved bowel function during chemotherapy. Otherwise, it is important to avoid foods which aggravate diarrhoea in the short-term, but remember to resort back to a healthy diet once your diarrhoea has resolved:

Summary – dietary advice during episodes of diarrhoea:

- Eat small, frequent meals rather than binging on larger meals
- Drink plenty of caffeine-free fluids throughout the day
- Note which foods make you worse if you have diarrhoea, consider avoiding:
  - — Alcohol, strong tea, coffee, cola, fruit juice and malted drinks
  - — Spicy or highly seasoned foods e.g. chilli, curry and pickles
  - — Very 'fatty' foods e.g. fried foods
  - — Unripe fruit, pips, seeds, skins, nuts, raw vegetables and salads
  - — High fibre breakfast cereals and large amounts of dried fruit
  - — Very rich foods e.g. chocolate and cream, should be eaten in moderation
  - — Foods labelled as 'Low sugar' or 'diet' products are not advisable
- Foods to consider trying if you have diarrhoea:
  - — Sipping high energy drinks between meals
  - — Probiotic 'live' yoghurts or tablets
  - — Grilled, steamed, poached, boiled potatoes, white bread, pasta and rice

Constipation

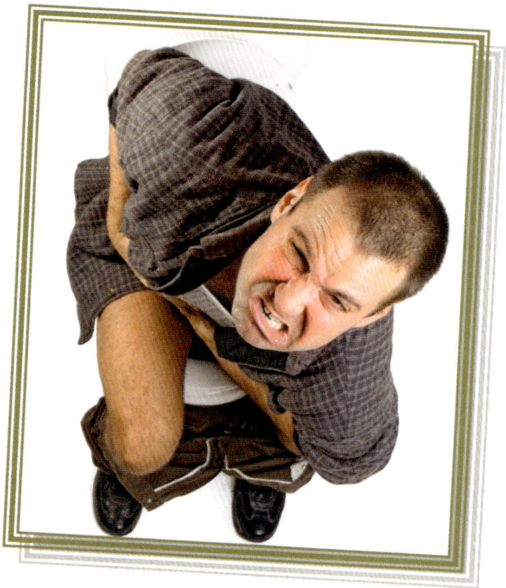

Constipation is a common complaint during and after cancer therapies. This is usually brought on by the general disruption of your daily routine and being less active. Anti-sickness medication such as ondansetron and granisetron can often cause temporary constipation but the biggest culprits are opiate pain-killers such as codeine, tramadol, and morphine. Other medication such as iron tablets can also disrupt the normal function of the bowel. Other non medicinal contributory factors include: not eating enough fibre; inactivity; bowel muscle weakness; recent abdominal surgery; haemorrhoids; or an anal fissure which can also make it painful to open your bowels.

We are all familiar with the common symptoms of constipation – discomfort, bloating and abdominal cramps – but a recent survey also reports how constipation can affect lifestyle in other ways:

- Fatigue, apprehension, irritability and being argumentative with a partner;
- Feeling less attractive, impacting on their social lives;
- Cancelling or leaving a social engagement early;
- Affecting sex lives either because they felt unattractive or are in pain;
- Reporting embarrassment due to the associated flatulence.

What can you do to help?

Despite the frequency of this complaint, it is often only addressed when it becomes a significant problem. Prevention is always better if possible. With some foresight constipation can be anticipated and appropriate action taken to avoid it. For example, if drugs such as fentynyl or other opiates have been prescribed, it is better to change your diet before the stools harden. Likewise, if a previous cycle of chemotherapy caused a period of constipation, consider a dietary change before the next cycle. Eating some ground linseeds, dried prunes or figs the night before, and the morning of chemotherapy, could help. Immediately after chemotherapy it is more difficult to modify diet as there is usually some impairment of appetite, but this way the fibre will already be in the system. Exercise and activity are very important. A brief walk or cycle ride around the park outside, in the evening after the chemotherapy, is also a good tactic. This may seem unusual, but will help keep your bowels moving and also help reduce nausea. At other times regular exercise, particularly jogging, walking, cycling and dancing all have a positive effect on the bowels.

Summary – measures that can be taken to avoid constipation:

- Eat plenty of fibre (bran, prunes, raisins, cereals, leafy vegetables)
- Eat a tablespoon of ground linseeds every day.
- Eat plenty of fruit and berries
- Drink plenty, but not excessive, quantities of water
- Have a regular routine in the morning – shortly after breakfast
- Try not to ignore the call to open your bowels. If you need to go – go!
- Take your time and try to stay until you have a good result.
- Exercise regularly – it reduces the time a motion takes to pass through
- Activity softens the stool and makes it easier to pass
- Avoid constipating medications if possible (codeine, opiates)
- Take a note of which activities constipate you
- Take a note of which foods work for you and keep in stock
- Prevention is better – anticipate constipation and change diet first
- If starting medications, increase fibre, or take a gentle laxative if necessary
- If necessary, use ointments or suppositories to relieve a painful anus

Bowel blockages – adhesions

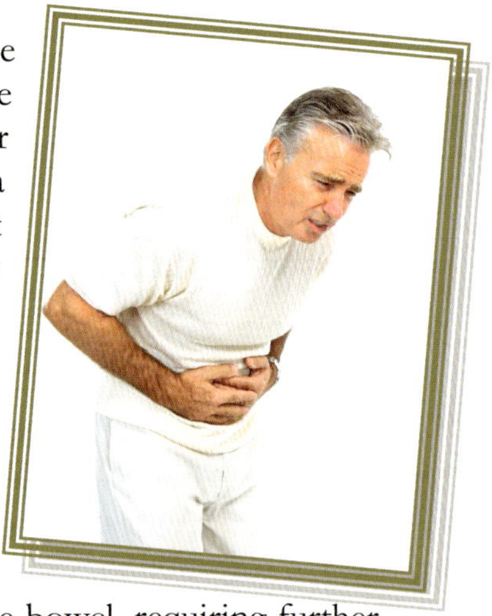

Surgery to the abdomen has a tendency to cause fibrous tissue to form between the loops of the bowel. Normally these loops slide smoothly over each other, expanding and contracting easily as a motion passes through them. Fortunately, in most cases, a small amount of fibrous tissue (or scarring) after abdominal surgery is not noticeable, but in some, it impairs the normal flexibility of the bowel, causing kinks and partial blockages. These physical barriers to the regular flow of a motion result in intermittent, colicky indigestion and bloating, leading to a general feeling of malaise and ill health. If severe these episodes can progress to partial obstruction of the bowel, requiring further surgery to remove the adhesions (fibrous bands). This of course, is a 'double-edge sword' because, although it relieves the immediate problem, it adds to the underlying cause of adhesions in the long term.

What can you do to help?

Physical activity and stopping smoking are the two most important activities. Smoking tends to thicken tissues, adding to the risk of adhesions. Exercise literally jigs your bowels around like worms in a bucket! Although this may cause some discomfort initially, it breaks down the adhesions between the loops of the bowel preventing further problems. As you can imagine, exercises that move the body around are particularly helpful – such as walking, running, dancing and cycling – but any activity that is performed regularly is helpful. Clearly, finding an activity that is convenient and enjoyable makes it more likely to be sustained.

Summary – prevent bowel adhesions:

- Exercise: walking, running, aerobics, dancing and cycling
- If you smoke, stop!
- Increase soluble fibre intake, keep the stool soft but not bulked (see fibre)
- Drink plenty of caffeine-free drinks
- Massage your tummy – or get someone else to do it
- If symptoms persist consult your doctor

Indigestion and heartburn

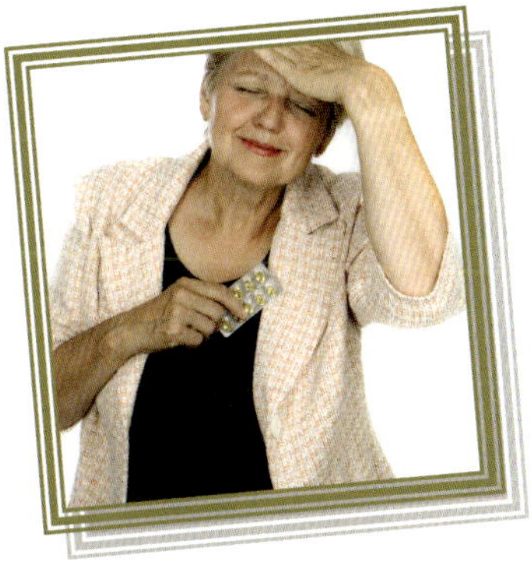

Indigestion and heartburn are common complaints often experienced during chemotherapy or after surgery. The cause of pain is usually gastric acid irritating the lining of the stomach or oesophagus. If there is too much acid, or if the sphincter doesn't work properly, it refluxes up into the oesophagus causing heartburn. It is aggravated by steroids and anti-inflammatory drugs.

What can be done to help?

You may be prescribed antacid medication and investigated with an endoscope to exclude an ulcer. Antacids can also be given temporarily to prevent damage whilst taking steroids. Indigestion and heartburn can also be helped by avoiding some foods, improving the way we eat and live.

Summary – diet and lifestyle advice if you have heartburn:

Foods to avoid:

- Very fatty foods should be avoided
- Too much coffee and alcohol should be avoided
- Sweet carbonated drinks (with and without caffeine) should also be avoided
- Fried food, or foods high in fat, only make matters worse
- Acidic foods such as citrus, onions and tomatoes may not help
- Peppermint and chocolate are usually sweet and can aggravate indigestion
- Try not to overeat and eat slowly

Other lifestyle changes:

- A journal could be kept of foods that trigger heartburn or indigestion
- Straining if constipated should be avoided
- Two or three hours should pass after eating before going to bed
- For reflux, raise the head of the bed - the chest is higher than your feet
- Wear looser-fitting clothing
- If overweight, some slimming would be a good idea
- At least two hours should pass after eating before exercising
- When exercising, breathe out slowly when tensing the stomach muscles

Pelvic floor exercises

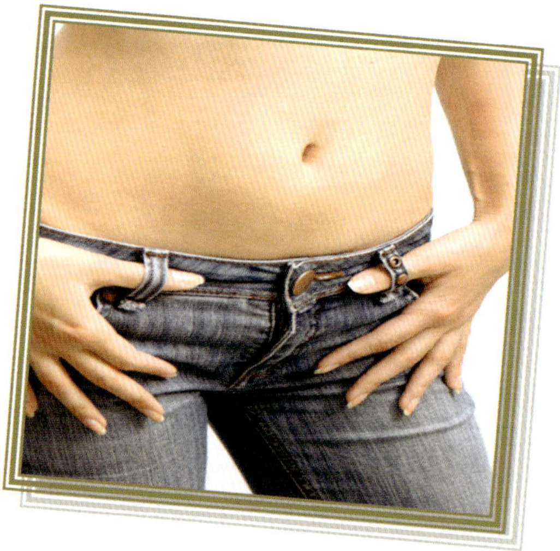

It's a good idea to include pelvic floor exercises as a routine part of your regular exercise program, especially because, as we get older, our pelvic muscles and ligaments generally become lax and weak. These exercises are particularly helpful if you are overweight, have had abdominal or pelvic surgery, or radiotherapy to the pelvis. Studies have shown that, if performed regularly, they can improve pelvic tone and muscle strength, which can benefit a number of urinary, sexual and bowel functions:

Stress incontinence refers to the complaint of urine leaking out when you cough, sneeze or laugh. This is more common in women, and it is particularly seen if the uterus is enlarged, or after a person has had pelvic surgery.

Urgency is the situation where there is a strong desire to pass urine immediately and you have very little notice before you lose control and become incontinent, i.e. there is an urgent need to find a toilet! Urgency can also apply to controlling a bowel motion. This can occur in men with prostate cancer after radiotherapy, which may have partially damaged the anal sphincter and at the same time irritated the lower rectal mucosa.

Sexual performance. Some advocate pelvic floor exercises to improve sexual performance – particularly in men – to control orgasm. In women, it is reported to increase sensitivity as it generally increases blood supply to the area if performed long enough.

Here's how to do it:

First of all find the pelvic floor muscles. Imagine trying to stop passing wind and urine at the same time. Tighten the muscles around the back and front passages, and lift them up. When doing this, you should be able to feel th pelvic floor muscles tightening. If you really concentrate it is possible to tighten and contract different parts of the pelvic floor group of muscles. Try the left side then the right side, then the front and back – this may seem hard at first by gets easier with practice.

It is very easy to use other muscles as well, so be sure to use only the right ones. Avoid the following:

- Do not pull in your stomach;
- Do not squeeze your legs together;
- Do not tighten your buttocks;
- Do not hold your breath.

Exercise 1 – The slow exercise. Tighten your pelvic floor and count to five, then relax. Repeat this at least ten times. Perform this exercise five times daily. When feeling confident with this regime, increase the tightening time for ten counts and include exercise 2 as well. Another way to do this is to tighten the PFM slightly, hold for 3 seconds, tighten further, hold for 3 seconds, really tighten (maximum force) for 3 seconds then relax and repeat

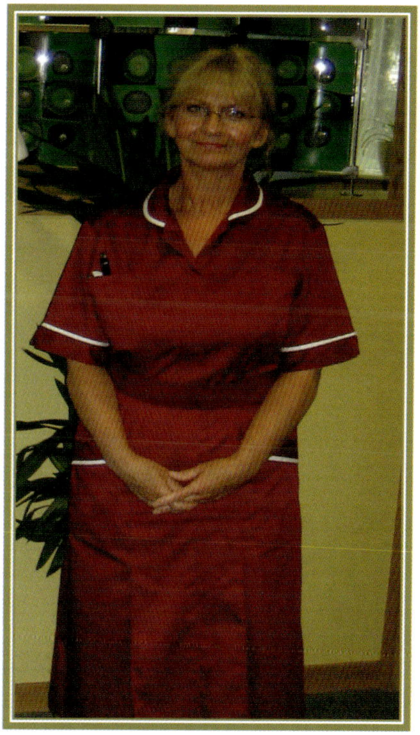

Exercise 2 – The quick exercise. This exercise works the muscles quickly to help them react to sudden stresses like coughing, laughing or exercise. Draw in your pelvic floor, and hold it for just one count before letting go. Repeat this up to ten times. Aim to perform this regime of exercises five times a day.

These exercises can be performed whenever you are feeling relaxed – either lying down, standing up, in the supermarket or in a bus queue. The level of exercise depends on your fitness level. A general rule is to attempt some form of exercise at least once or twice every day, for 5-10 minutes and to keep it going regularly. Some men and women have reported that it has helped them to meditate whilst performing the pelvic floor exercises so they can really concentrate on the correct muscles. Our nurses often demonstrate to patients that, if done correctly, there should be no visible signs that they are being performed.

As an extra form of discipline some men and women keep and exercise diary and tick off each day. It you miss a day, you can make up for it the following day so at the end of each week sufficient time has been spent on the pelvic floor muscles

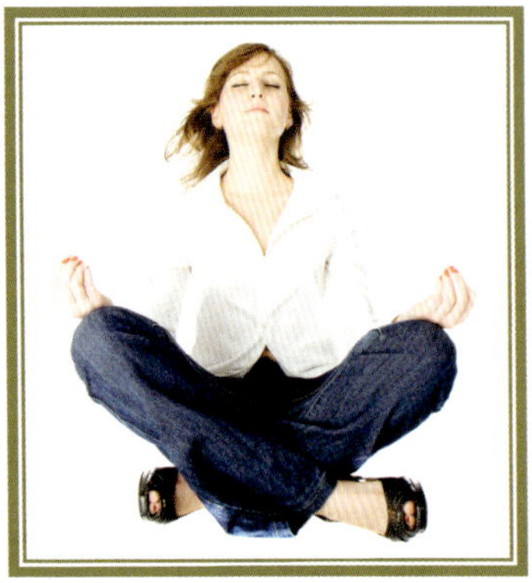

Finally, be aware that the benefits which were shown in the clinical studies only appeared after 5-6 weeks of daily pelvic floor exercises or sometimes longer and may take several months to peak. Most people give up after a week or so thinking they are not working, so it is important to keep going for at least 5-10 minutes a day every day and continue for at least 6 weeks – even if you are not initially seeing a benefit. Likewise, when a benefit does occur, don't stop; keep going as otherwise the benefits may be lost.

Chapter Seventeen

Chemotherapy Radiotherapy

Skin care during and after radiotherapy

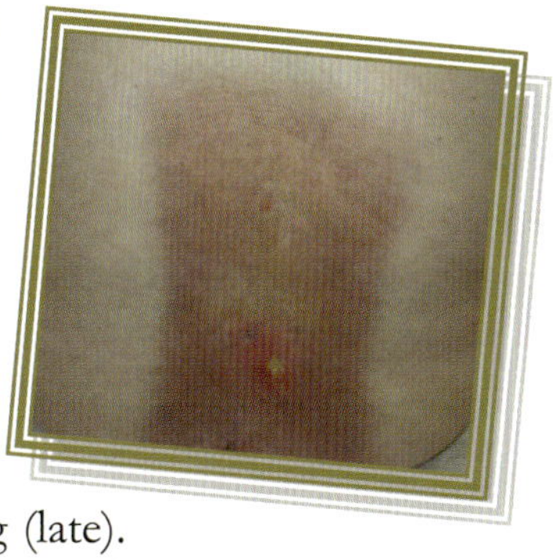

Radiotherapy can only affect your skin in the treated area. Most regimens have no obvious skin damage, as advances in techniques have significantly reduced the dose of the radiotherapy the skin receives. Those areas still most likely to be affected are the head and neck, and skin creases, such as under the breast, the groin and between the buttocks.

Radiotherapy side effects can occur during treatment (acute), or come later and can be life-long (late). Acute skin reactions may make your skin red, itchy and dry. If severe, however, the skin might break down and form superficial ulcers, known as moist desquamation. In this situation the skin can sometimes develop a secondary fungal or bacterial infection and treatment should be considered if the reaction is inappropriately severe or the redness spreads outside the actual treated area. In the vast majority of cases the skin heals completely and looks entirely normal, albeit with some reduced hair formation. In some cases long-term damage may occur and the skin could become thin, occasionally developing small, abnormal blood vessels (telangiectasia).The underlying tissues can thicken and be less supple. There is also an increased risk of skin cancer in the treated area, especially if you were to sunburn the skin within this area.

What can you do to help?

During radiotherapy, moisturising may improve the condition of your skin. It is particularly important not to rub or scratch the area even though you will be very tempted. If the itching becomes unbearable you should report this to your medical team who can prescribe a mild steroid ointment.

Smoking during radiotherapy will significantly increase the chance of an adverse skin reaction. If you cannot give up completely, at least don't smoke four hours before the radiotherapy and four hours after. This will avoid having a high concentration of the harmful smoke chemicals at the time of radiotherapy or when it is most active.

Moisturising the skin is important during radiotherapy. Many radiotherapy centres advocate aqueous cream or products similar to E45. These are non-perfumed and regarded as "simple". However they are petroleum based and therefore contain hydrocarbons. No trial has shown they are harmful but, on the other hand, no trial has shown they are helpful over nothing at all. There have been a number of trials comparing Aloe Vera creams with aqueous cream. Most showed there was no difference – one showed it was worse. As a consequence, Aloe Vera creams or gels are not recommended after radiotherapy despite their anti-inflammatory properties for other skin conditions. There has been one published randomised trial evaluating the benefits of calendula cream against a standard emulsifying cream commonly used in France called trolamine. Research found that 41 percent of patients using the calendula ointment suffered moderate-to-severe dermatitis, compared with 63 percent of those using the standard moisturising cream. Creams containing calendula are not generally supplied in UK oncology units but it may be worth buying your own supply.

If your skin worsens towards the end of the radiotherapy or even afterwards, particularly if there is cracking and oozing, your medical team can prescribe an anti-fungal cream. If there are signs of a bacterial infection, antibiotics can likewise be recommended. Sometimes the radiotherapy dose or technique can be modified. The skin care guidelines listed in the box below will help limit damage to the skin as the treatment progresses.

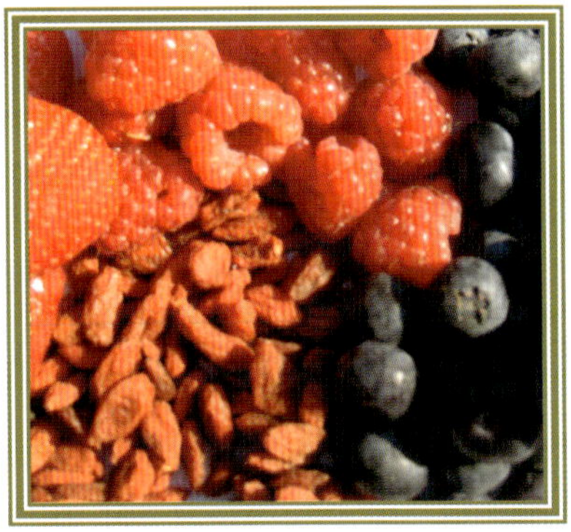

In the long-term certain lifestyle manoeuvres can improve the quality of your skin and underlying tissues, as well as reducing the risks of secondary skin cancers. A healthy diet of fruit and vegetables containing vitamins and antioxidants is important in order to protect your skin both from further damage and also the higher risk of skin cancer. Smoking, in particular, increases the thickness of skin (fibrosis) and contributes to on going pain and lymphoedema in the areas affected. Exercises generally improves well-being, which will show itself through your skin. It is important to perform the specific exercises relevant to the area of the body irradiated It is particularly crucial to look after your skin in the treated area by regularly stretching the tissues, which include the underlying muscles, tendons and joints.

Olive oil can offer protection, not just by adding it to your food, but by applying it directly onto your skin. This amazing oil, predominantly oleic acid (C18:1, n-9), has strong antioxidant and skin-protecting properties, including reducing sun damage, the risk of skin cancers, skin wrinkling and aging. For centuries, Greeks and Egyptians have used olive oil for skin redness. A good tip is to buy a high quality natural oil-based moisturising cream then add some extra virgin olive oil yourself, mix this into a paste and apply to the skin and massage for 5-10 minutes before a shower or bath, which will then wash off the excess oil leaving the skin soft and smooth.

Summary – advice to help the skin during radiotherapy:

During radiotherapy:

- Gently wash in warm water with a mild, non-perfumed soap
- Do not use a washcloth, bath oil or bubble bath
- Rinse thoroughly, then air dry or dab with a soft, clean towel
- Wear loose fitting clothing, preferably made with a natural fibre e.g. cotton
- Clothes should not rub, chafe or cause friction in the treated area
- Use a mild detergent to wash clothing
- Avoid friction, including rubbing, scratching or massage in the treated area
- Avoid the use of adhesive tape (e.g. Elastoplast) in the treated area
- Avoid extremes of heat in the area: ice packs, hot water bottle hairdryers
- Only use recommended skin creams (aqueous cream or E45)
- Avoid using aftershave, perfume, deodorant and make up in the area
- Avoid swimming in a chlorinated pool during radiotherapy treatment
- Swimming in the sea is fine but avoid clothes rubbing
- Eat a healthy diet
- Do not smoke or at least avoid 4 hours before or after

To reduce the risk of long term damage after radiotherapy:

- Stop smoking – bad during radiotherapy and for late thickening
- Eat a healthy balanced diet, avoiding excessive alcohol.
- Exercise regularly & regularly stretch the tissues in the treated area
- Avoid sun burn in the treated area
- Massage olive oil based creams into the treated area before a shower

Skin care during and after chemotherapy

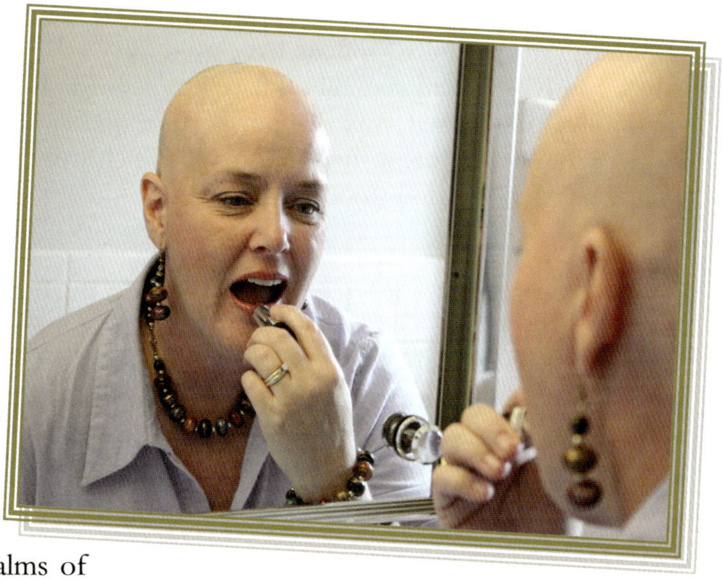

Chemotherapy can affect the skin in several ways and with varying degrees of severity. At the very least it can make skin dry and blotchy. Not uncommonly red rashes may also appear. Some chemotherapy and biological agents (e.g. capecitabine, caelyx, sunitinib and sorafeneib), can particularly affect the palms of your hands or the soles of the feet (see 'Palmer-Planter Syndrome' below). Some chemo-therapy agents affect the nails (see nail changes below), whilst others affect the lips (see sore lips below). Your doctor may give additional medication for these conditions or reduce the dose for a while, to allow your skin to recover. Other drugs, such as erbitux (cituximab) for bowel cancer, can cause acne. In this situation topical anti-acne creams or antibiotic tablets may be prescribed. Most chemotherapy drugs will also make your skin more sensitive to the sun during their administration, but some drugs such as bleomycin, capecitabine and fluorouracil can increase the risks for several months afterwards.

What can you do to help?

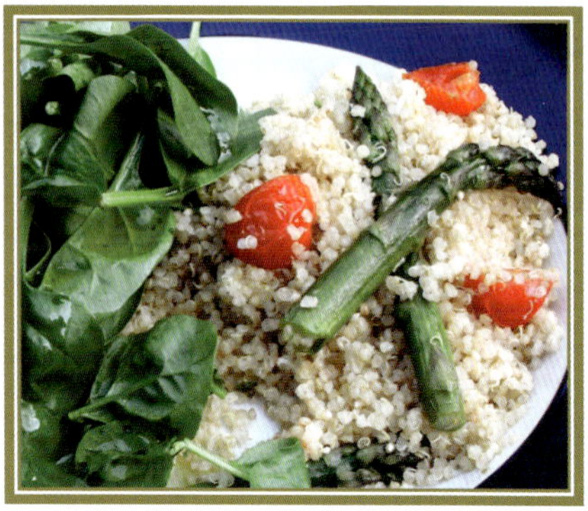

For a more general lack of lustre, dryness or blotchiness the basic four principles apply; stop smoking, eat well, exercise and oil the skin. As a rule, people who are healthy tend to look healthy. Smoking, for example, reduces oxygen to the skin and increases ageing (thinning, reduced flexibility and age spots). The amount of haemoglobin carrying carbon monoxide instead of oxygen is increased, and this produces a grey/brown pallor particularly on your face and around your eyes. There has to be a degree of common sense when it comes to sunlight. Light sun exposure is encouraged as it increases vitamin D levels, helps bone health and may also have a direct anti-tumour effect.

Summary – skin care advice during chemotherapy:

- If you smoke – stop. It is the worst thing you can do for your skin
- Avoid excess alcohol, especially hangovers, as this can dry the skin
- Take extra care in the sun – many chemotherapy agents photosensitise skin
- Eat a well balanced healthy diet with plenty of oily fish and antioxidants
- Gently wash in warm water with a mild, non-perfumed soap
- Avoid harsh "drying" shower gels and detergents
- Do not use a coarse washcloth, bath oil or bubble bath
- Rinse thoroughly, then dab with a soft, clean towel
- Wear loose-fitting clothing, preferably made with a natural fibre e.g. cotton
- Clothes should not rub or cause friction
- Use a mild detergent to wash clothes that will be next to your skin
- Exercise and stretch regularly
- Swimming in chlorinated pools can dry the skin rinse off properly
- Swimming in the sea is good but avoid rubbing
- After swimming shower and apply oils
- Use chemical free natural oils (e.g. nature-medical natural oils)*
- If healthy oils are not available use extra virgin olive oil before a shower
- Oiling the skin will be soften and moisten but stop if they cause irritation
- Massage your skin gently when applying oil
- Massage is safe - despite the myths

* see www.keep-healthy.com for details of natural and essential oil based skin creams

Chapped lips and cold sores

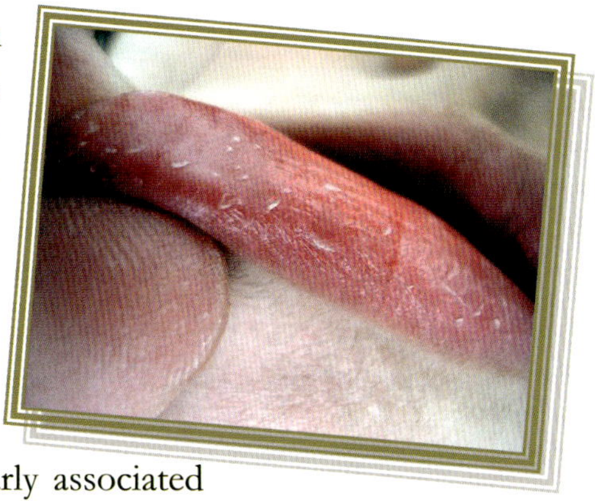

Chapped lips refer to a common condition in which the lips become dry, cracked and sore. If marked, this can lead to bleeding and secondary infection. Lip soreness during chemotherapy is an understated symptom as it is common and can cause considerable distress and an unfavourable appearance to the sufferer. It can also cause or aggravate sore lips including overexposure to the sun or cold wind, dehydration, particularly associated with alcohol intake, and drugs which cause oral dryness including codeine, morphine-like pain killers, anti cholinergics, steroids and aromatase inhibitors. Some people can also irritate their lips by habitually licking them or applying heavily perfumed lips creams.

Despite being so common, sore lips are generally regarded by medical teams as a trivial condition and are rarely mentioned in patient information materials. Likewise, within oncology units, there is very little advice on how to prevent or alleviate soreness. We conducted a study to find out more about how much sore lips affected 100 individuals during chemotherapy. The incidence of soreness more than doubled among patients during chemotherapy. Sixty-six percent self-medicated with lip salves and there was a strong perception from patients that non-petroleum based lip creams were better than petrol based creams. Although the number of people having cold sores did not increase, those who did get them said the episode was worse than normal. There appeared to be an association between sore lips and cold sores as 82 percent of the patients who were prone to cold sores also had regular episodes of chapped lips as opposed to 22 percent who did not have a history of cold sores. This association does suggest that preventing the chapped lips may also prevent cold sore episodes among vulnerable individuals. Other strategies to prevent an acute episode have so far been unsuccessful but topical or systemic anti-viral agents such as acyclovir, or valacyclovir, have been shown to shorten the length of the attack if used early in an episode.

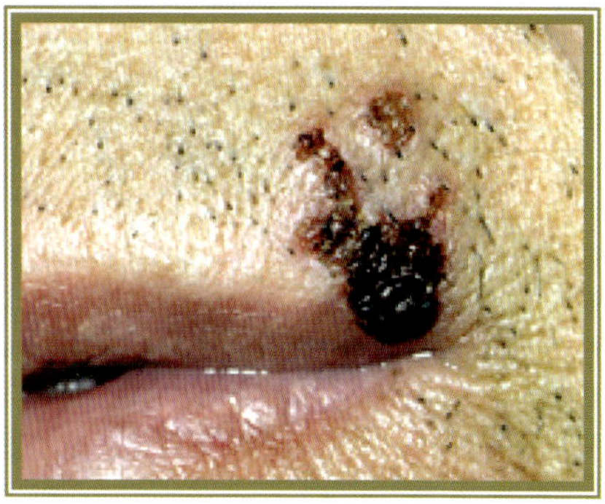

So why does the prevalence of chapped lips increase after the start of chemotherapy? There may be many causes, ranging from dehydration to the dry air in hospitals, but the most likely reason is that chemotherapy damages the rapidly dividing basal cells in the deep layers of skin (vermillion boarder) of the lips. This means that the skin on the lips does not grow fast enough to replace the skin which is shed or rubbed off through everyday activities such as eating, speaking and breathing. The lips become thin and more vulnerable. On top of this, between chemotherapy cycles the skin-producing cells recover but can then go into overdrive, producing too many skin cells, which pile up and thus cause scaling and cracking leading to secondary infection.

What can you do to help?

Understanding that lips can get sore and chapped during chemotherapy is important so basic preventative precautions, listed below, can be made. These precautions should start from the beginning of chemotherapy to prevent soreness happening in the first place. It is always more difficult to treat chapped lips once they have started. There is an association between dental treatment and an exacerbation of cold sores so it may be worth applying topical anti-virals after a visit to the dentist if you have a history of cold sores.

Summary – advice to help avoid chapped lips and cold sores:

- Avoid dehydration – drink regularly and often (unsweetened drinks)
- Avoid licking and rubbing the lips
- Avoid wind and excessive cold
- Avoid excessive sunlight
- Apply a sun block when outside
- Particularly use blocks when walking, cycling, skiing or on summer holiday
- During chemotherapy use a natural oil based lip salve daily*
- If you have a history of chapped lips or cold sores apply more often
- If you are prone to cold sores ask for an oral and topical antiviral
- Apply topical antiviral and start tablets as soon as the tell-tails signs appear
- Natural oils based salves appear better than petroleum based salves
- Avoid salves containing colours, perfumes, hydrocarbons or preservatives

* see www.keep-healthy.com for details of natural and essential oil based salves

Blood clots – Thromboembolism

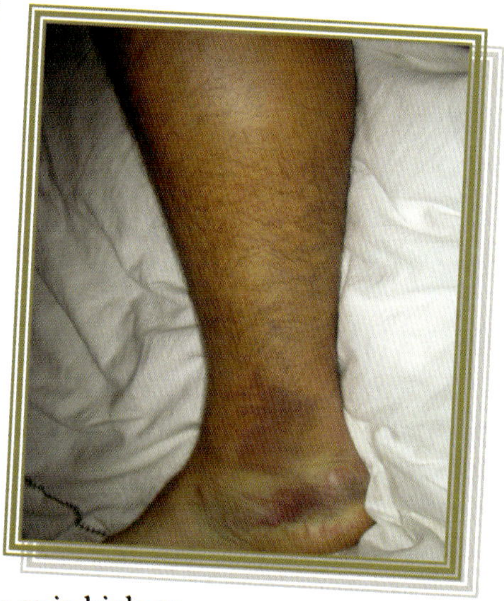

After cancer there is an increased risk of blood clotting in your deep veins (thrombosis), especially if you have recently had a recent operation or disease involving the lower abdomen or pelvis. The risk is also greater if you don't exercise, are overweight, smoke, have a previous history of thrombosis, have varicose veins, are receiving chemotherapy or have had long periods of immobility. Everybody talks about plane journeys but one memorable patient developed one after being stuck on a motorway in a traffic jam for just a couple of hours. Individuals are also more likely to form clots if their platelet count is high or they have a hereditary abnormality of the blood. Blood can clot in the deep or superficial veins. Signs to look out for include:

Superficial vein damage and thrombosis: You may experience a darkening of the veins in your hands and arms after chemotherapy. This is normal. The veins usually don't hurt and the dark colour should fade once your course of treatment has been completed. Of more concern is that during your chemotherapy course, some veins start to feel hard and 'cord-like'. This is caused by blood clotting in the superficial veins of the hands or arms. This can be associated with painful inflammation and may prevent the oncology nurse from finding a good vein for your next chemotherapy session. This thrombosis may take several months or, rarely years, to resolve. Fortunately, although uncomfortable, this sort of thrombosis is localised and does not result in clots embolising to the lung or elsewhere.

Deep vein thrombosis (DVT): The most common veins affected are those in the back of the legs causing a DVT. Thrombosis can occur in a number of deeper veins; these include the axillary vein following insertion of a central line, the Inferior Vena Cava associated with kidney cancer or even within the head causing a stroke. In the leg, the DVT tends to cause swelling, redness and discomfort. The danger with DVT is that a clot could break off and travel through the venous system to the lungs where it gets trapped (pulmonary embolus), which can cause considerable damage or even be fatal.

What can be done to help?

Medical strategies such as warfarin and low molecular weight heparin are important. If the risk of thrombosis is high, ask the doctor to consider an injection of heparin before travelling. Although the evidence is not particularly good, unless you have a history of aspirin allergy or stomach ulcers take 75mg of aspirin before you make a long car, coach or plane journey. In terms of lifestyle, stopping smoking and exercising are the two most important factors to reduce the risk of thrombosis. Other factors can also reduce the risk of this potentially life-threatening complication:

Summary – advice to prevent blood clots:

- Previous history of clots – discuss preventative medicine with your doctor
- Walking; this pumps the legs – try to walk briskly for >20 minutes every day
- Other exercise – all activity reduces the risk; consider cycling or aerobics.
- Compression stockings are recommended when travelling
- Whilst in a car keep the legs moving and avoid being cramped
- Whilst travelling, if possible, take regular breaks to walk and stretch
- In airports walk around for as long as possible before boarding the plane.
- Prolonged periods of immobility should be avoided,
- Avoid confined spaces for long periods of time
- Smoking – stop immediately. It is dangerous to smoke if you have cancer

For the arms (superficial thrombosis):

- Exercise arms – it is important to get blood pumping through your veins
- Exercise hands – a specific hand grip device or use a tennis ball or sponge
- Oil and moisturize – rub pure olive oil into your arm gently, every day
- Gently massage your skin and veins at the same time as applying the oil

Hand foot (palmar-plantar) syndrome

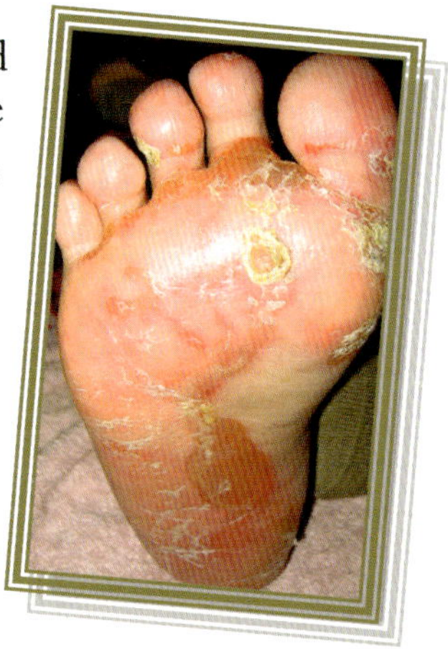

This strange side effect of chemotherapy is characterised as reddening of the palms of the hands and soles of the feet. Although the mechanism is not completely known, one theory this that the small blood vessels of the extremities are damaged, which then causes the chemotherapy to leak into the tissues. It can range from mild cracking of the skin around the tips of the fingers to swelling, deep cracks in the skin with secondary infection and loss of the nails. On the feet, as there is more friction from walking, so the skin tends to slough off creating raw painful blisters.

The most common causative chemotherapy drug is capecitabine (Xeloda) but it can occur with fluorouracil, particularly if it is infused. It is common with caelyx and is now emerging as a problem with some of the biological agents for renal cancer. If the condition is marked the oncologist will reduce the dose of the responsible agent, usually with no loss of effectiveness; otherwise keep the hands and feet clean and moisturised with a good quality natural oil based cream.

Summary – advice to treat hand-foot syndrome:

- Keep clean by gently washing in warm water and non-perfumed soaps
- Do not use a washcloth, bath oil or bubble bath and avoid soaking
- Rinse thoroughly, then air dry or dab with a soft, clean towel
- Avoid strong chemicals e.g. when washing clothes or dishes
- For the rest of the body wear loose fitting and soft natural fibre clothing
- Clothes should not rub, chafe or cause friction in any areas
- Avoid friction, including rubbing, scratching or massage in the treated area
- Avoid the use of adhesive tape in the treated area
- Avoid extremes of heat; ice packs, hot water bottle or hairdryers
- Avoid swimming in a chlorinated pool – the sea is fine
- Stop smoking and eat a healthy balanced diet, avoiding excessive alcohol
- Exercise and regularly stretch the tissues in the treated area
- Avoid sun on the hands and feet.
- Moisturise with a natural oil based cream daily from the start of the chemo

* see www.keep-healthy.com for details of natural & essential oil based creams

Nail damage and chemotherapy

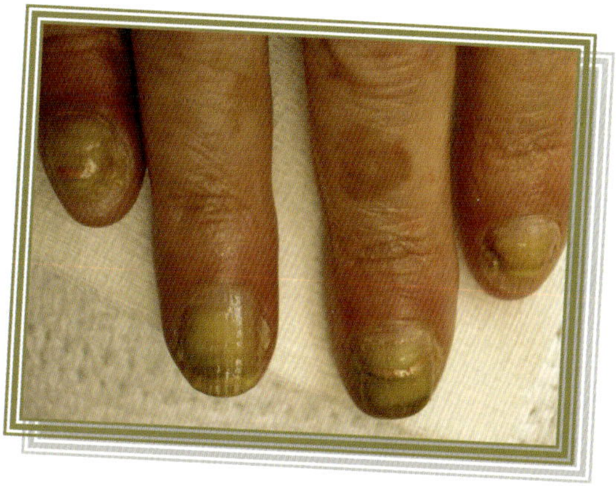

It is common for the quality of nails to be affected by chemotherapy. In most cases a pale ridge appears across the nail each time a cycle is given. As the course proceeds, several ridges appear at regular intervals, like the rings of a tree, corresponding to each intravenous cycle, as you can see towards the cuticle of the nails in the adjacent picture. These are called Beau's lines which are not uncomfortable and can be easily covered by nail varnish.

Unfortunately the damage does not stop there, especially with chemotherapy drugs called taxanes (paclitaxel and docetaxel). The nails of up to 44 percent of those patients receiving them become severely damaged. It begins with discolouration, brittleness and splitting but later in the chemotherapy course the nails lift off the nail bed, which can be very painful. Secondary infection usually sets in at this stage, so the surrounding and underlying skin becomes red, inflamed and seeps pus. Nasty and distressing!

If the nails get this bad, all you can do is soak regularly in salt water, keep them as clean as possible and wait for the nails to fall off. It is much better to limit damage to the nails in the first place. It is known that cold treatment of the scalp can reduce hair loss by reducing the blood flow during the chemotherapy administration where blood levels are at their highest. It is not particularly widely known that the same technique can be used on the nails. A study from France used cooled gloves during taxane chemotherapy and reported a significant reduction in nail damage. Unfortunately, these are not widely available in the UK or elsewhere in Europe. However, in true "Heath Robinson" style we have published a case report of a simple self-made cooling system:

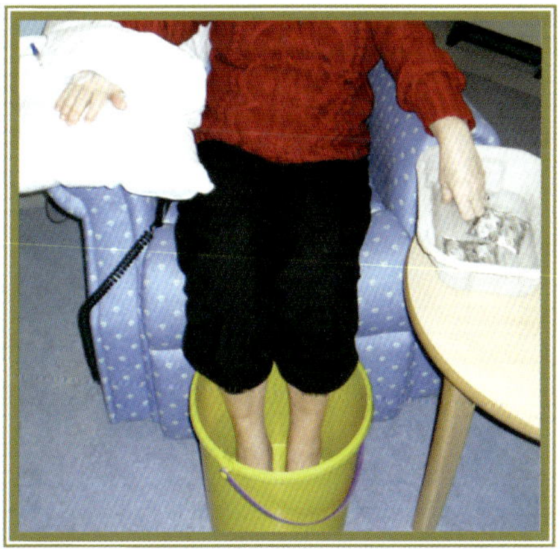

Mrs S is a 64 years old lady with breast cancer undergoing docetaxel administration as part of her chemotherapy treatment. We set up two buckets of cold water, one for her right hand and the other for both feet which were immersed immediately prior to the start of her infusion, during her 90 minutes infusion and then for 30 minutes afterward, for each of her four cycles. The water was kept cold by the addition of frozen gel packs, which were replaced when necessary, in order to keep the fingers comfortably cool while being careful not to over-cool the hand. Mrs S complained of marked discomfort in the right finger nail but not the left hand or her feet following cycle two and for six weeks after her fourth cycle. Furthermore, she developed separation of the nails in her right finger nails but not the nails of the left hand. A photo was taken 4 weeks after the end of the fourth cycle of docetaxel administration which clearly showed damage in the right hand but not the left.

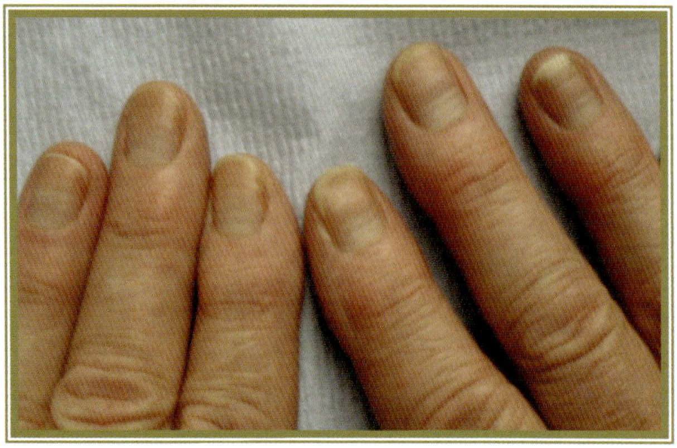

If it is not too late for you, it may be worth asking the chemotherapy nurse to set up a similar "bucket system" although within a busy crowded oncology suite this may not always be feasible.

Summary – tips for nail damage during chemotherapy:

- Keep nails clean and cut short
- Avoid trauma so protect them when washing dishes or gardening
- Avoid excessive cold – wear gloves in the winter
- For women, wear nail vanish as this can help reduce chemotherapy damage
- For men a clear varnish may help
- Moisturise the nails beds with a natural oil based creams*
- Stop smoking and eat a healthy diet
- During the chemotherapy infusion, cool the nail beds
- Ask the chemotherapy nurses for pots of iced water or bring your own

* www.keep-healthy.com for details of natural & essential oil based nail creams

The mouth and cancer treatments

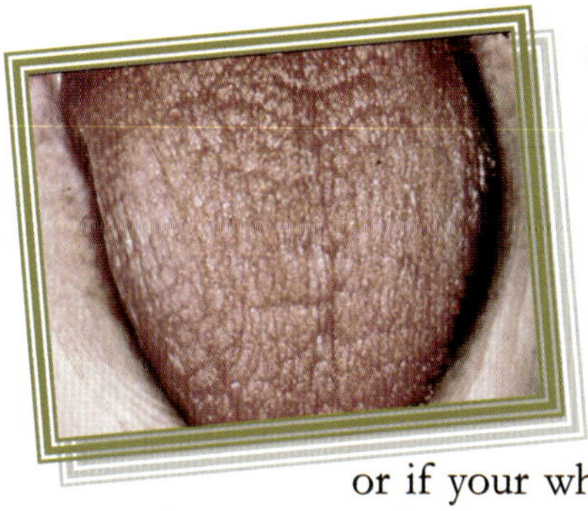

Chemotherapy and radiotherapy can affect the rapidly dividing normal cells of the lining of the mouth. The most common and understated result is an alteration in taste. As well as disconcerting, this symptom can contribute to a poor appetite and weight loss. In more severe cases inflammation and ulceration (mucositis) can cause pain and discomfort. In this instance, or if your white cell count is low after treatment, you will be susceptible to oral infections such as thrush (candida). Oral mucositis can often be painful, and this in turn can make it difficult to eat and drink. Radiotherapy in or around the area of your mouth, particularly involving the major salivary glands, can make it dry and sore, which may be permanent.

What can be done to help?

See a dentist before treatment starts. Inform your medical team if you develop a sore mouth, particularly if you have red areas, blisters, white spots, coated tongue or bleeding. They will often prescribe an anti-fungal lozenge or tablet. If severe they may also reduce your chemotherapy dose at the next cycle.

Summary – advice for mouth care:

- Clean teeth thoroughly but gently after each meal and before going to bed
- If the gums are delicate use a soft toothbrush (baby/infant)
- Suck ice/ice-lollies immediately prior to and during chemotherapy
- Mouthwash with salt water after meals (5 mls salt: 500 mls tepid water)
- Swill around the mouth for two to three minutes but do not swallow
- Strong antibacterial mouthwashes can damage the lining of your mouth
- Some mouthwashes can also stain the teeth (read the label)
- If mouth is dry, try sucking soft sugar-free sweets (too many cause diarrhoea)
- Be careful of boiled sweets as they can cut your mouth leading to ulcers
- Spicy foods are not harmful but can be uncomfortable
- Use plenty of fluids, e.g. gravy, yoghurt, sauces, to keep foods moist
- See a dietician if your appetite is impaired, consider a protein supplement
- Use a straw for drinking if the mouth is sore
- Avoid tobacco and alcohol

Hair loss

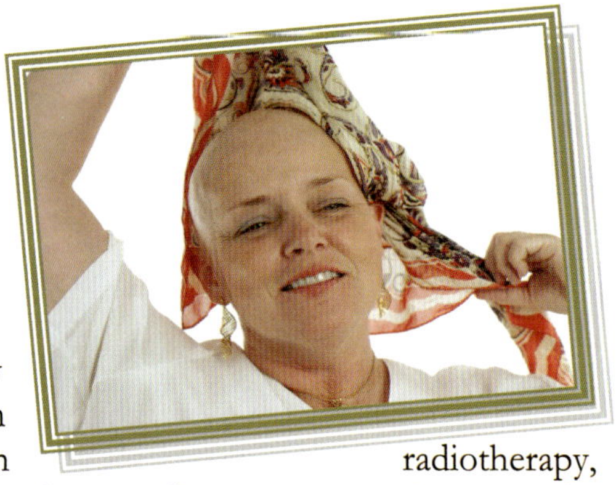

Chemotherapy often causes hair loss, otherwise known as alopecia. This is because the cells in hair follicles grow fast and chemotherapy damages fast growing cells. Hair loss with chemotherapy is not permanent, and it will grow back once your treatment has ended, although it may be slightly different from before treatment started in terms of colour and texture. With radiotherapy, hair loss occurs in the treated area only, and it may be permanent. For example, women having their armpit irradiated never have to shave there again. Not all chemotherapy agents cause hair loss, some just cause thinning, while others cause dramatic hair loss, including body hair and eyebrows. Furthermore, different people have different tolerances to the drugs. Occasionally, some people lose their hair when it is not expected, and sometimes no hair loss occurs when it is expected. The table below will give you an idea of whether hair loss will occur. The cold cap system works best for the middle group:

Usually causing hair loss	Sometimes hair loss	Usually no hair loss
Adriamycin	Amsacrine	Methotrexate
Etoposide	Cytarabine	Carmustine(BCNU)
Irinotecan (Campto)	Bleomycin	Mitroxantrone
Cyclophosphamide	Busulphan	Mitomycin C
Epirubicin	5 Fluorouracil	Carboplatin & Cisplatin
Docetaxel, (Taxotere)	Melphalan	Capecitabine
Paclitaxel, (Taxol)	Vincristine	Procarbazine
Ifosphamide	Vinblastine	6-Mercaptopurine
Vindesine	Lomustine(CCNU)	Sreptozotocin
Vinorelbine	Thiotepa	Fludarabine
Topotecan	Gemcitabine	Raltitrexate (Tomudex)

Hair loss can start at any time, from the first few days after chemotherapy, to within a few weeks. It usually begins growing back within a few weeks of the last cycle of chemotherapy but can surprise many people when it starts growing back before that. Don't be concerned – this does not mean the chemotherapy is not working. At first the re-growth is quite fluffy, fine and usually more curly, but as the months go by it resorts back to its former glory. Many say it is more grey but that is actually because it is no longer dyed.

What can you do to help?

Most oncology centres can partially prevent hair loss by cooling your scalp during administration of chemotherapy. The availability and types of cold cap vary between hospitals. The cap is put on before chemotherapy and is kept on for up to 1-2 hours after chemotherapy. This will extend the time spent in the oncology department. Not everyone can tolerate wearing the cold cap. Not wearing it has no effect on the outcome of treatment. In some situations (e.g. leukaemia) doctors may advise against using a cold cap. There are a wide variety of wigs and head scarves available from most oncology centres. Wigs can be made from either synthetic or human hair, or a combination of both. Wigs made from human hair often require a specialist shampoo and set, whereas synthetic ones can be shampooed at home and, when dry, fall naturally into place. They are also cheaper than human hair wigs.

Summary – advice for coping with hair loss:

- Before undergoing treatment your hair can be cut into a shorter style
- Thinning hair causes an itchy scalp – try cool showers, gently moisturising
- Avoid harsh chemicals and shampoos - they increase dryness & itchiness
- A perm should be avoided for at least six months after treatment
- Avoid irritating and scratching your scalp. If it is tender, use a soft hairbrush
- Cotton is a good alternative to nylon pillowcases which may irritate
- Hairdryers and rollers can further damage brittle hair.
- Avoid sleeping with rollers
- If underarm hair has been lost, avoid deodorants – try unscented talcum
- If some long stringy hairs remain on your scalp, cutting them off looks better
- As your hair starts growing, clip it short so it grows back the same length

Wearing a wig:

- A well fitted wig should stay in place by itself. If not, consider replacing it
- If a little loose, a hypo-allergenic double-sided tape is available
- If the lining irritates your scalp, wear a thin cotton skullcap underneath
- Your wig may need to be adjusted, as more hair is lost

Chapter Eighteen

After breast surgery
Side effects & advice

After breast surgery

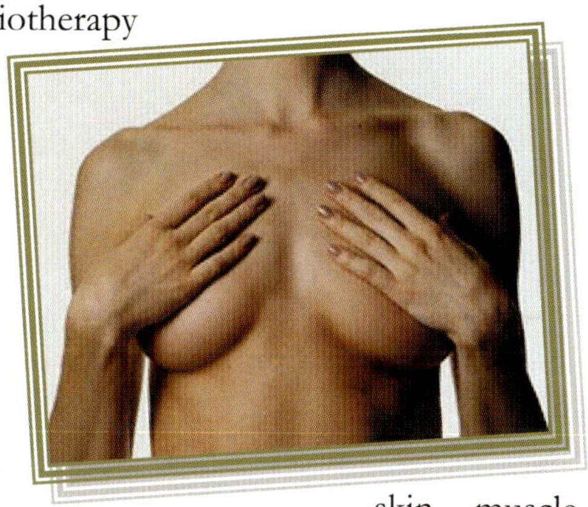

Advancements in breast surgical and radiotherapy techniques have substantially lowered the complication rate. Most cases in the UK involve a procedure called senetil node biopsy, which has lessened the number of cases requiring more extensive surgery to the armpit. This has reduced the number of women suffering from lymphoedema following breast and armpit surgery. It is still very important to practice a few simple exercises regularly, to reduce the risk of shoulder stiffness, skin, muscle and underlying tissue thickness (fibrosis), particularly if radiotherapy has also been given. Exercises should start as soon as feasible after surgery to alleviate post-operative pain and promote a good recovery. At this early stage, however, exercise advice is best sought from the individual surgical team, and it may alter according to local healthcare policies and techniques. The following may then be helpful:

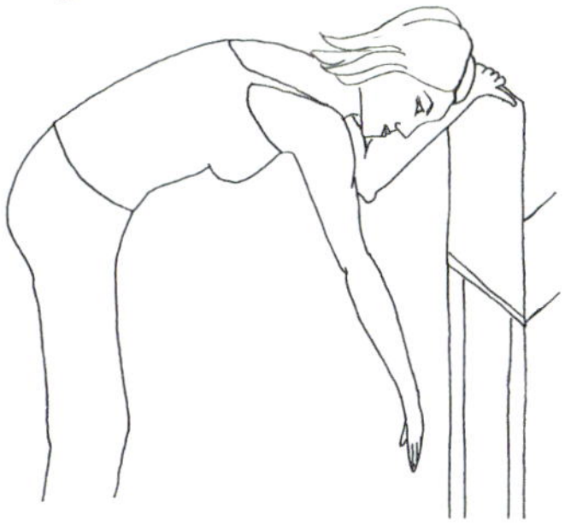

The monkey swing: Stand squarely and bend forward at the waist leaning on a chair/table. Circle entire arm clockwise, then anti-clockwise. Swing forwards and then backwards. Swing arm sideways, away from the body, and back again – particularly good in the early weeks after surgery.

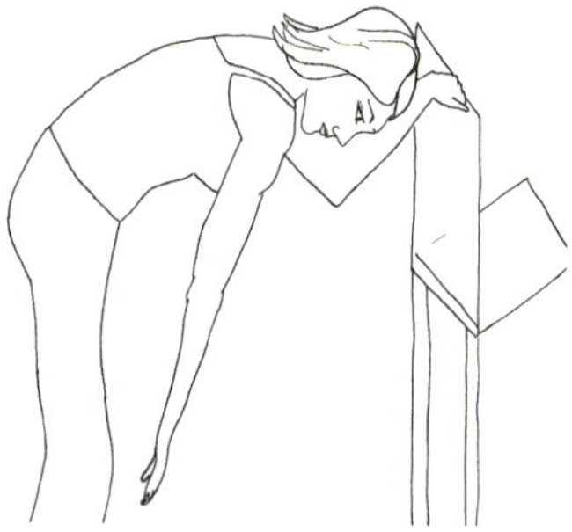

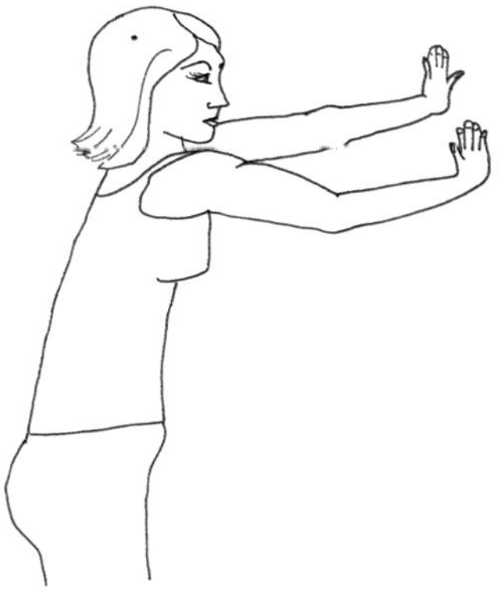

Walk the wall: Stand straight facing a wall. Stretch upright as far as comfortable.
Place your hands on a wall, ensuring a comfortable stance. Walk your hands up then down the wall. Repeat ten times.

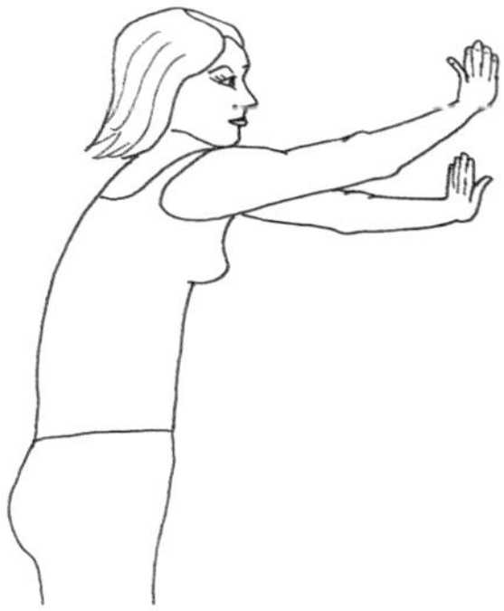

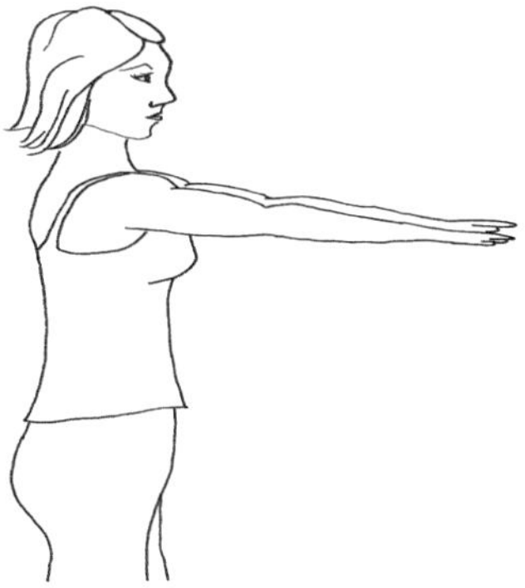

The fan: Put your hands out horizontally in front of your body. Take them up above your head as far as possible. Drop them down to the waist.

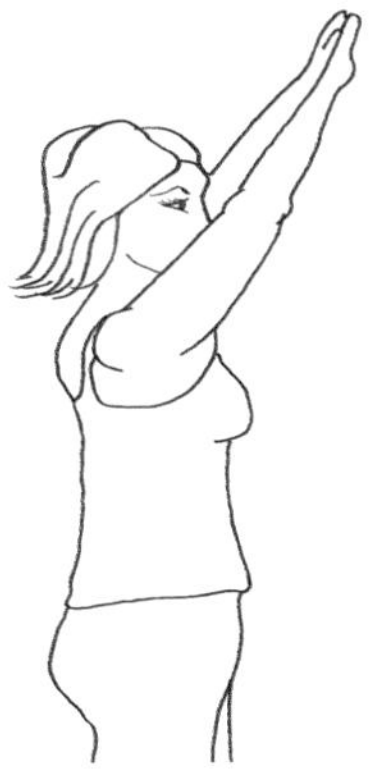

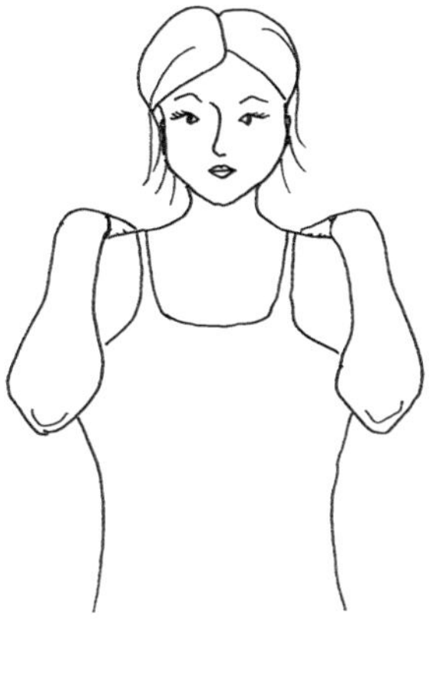

The praying mantis: Place your hands on your shoulders (or at the level of your shoulders). Move the elbows forwards and upwards, then down and inwards. Repeat each movement ten times.

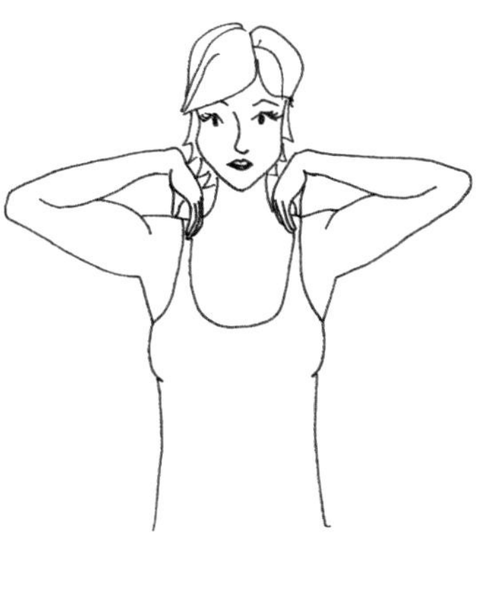

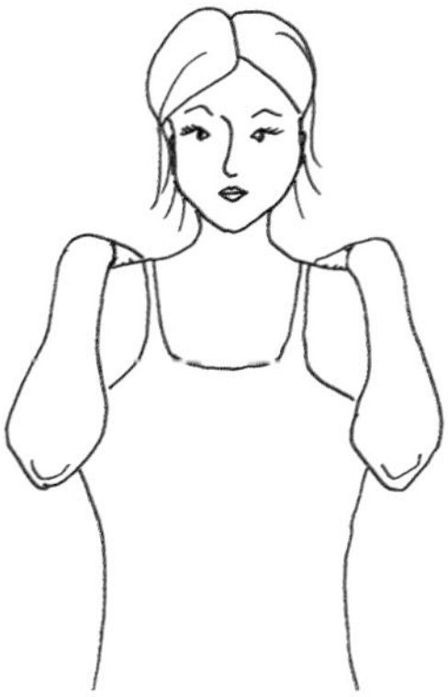

Small bird: Place your hands on your shoulders. Move your elbows sideways and upwards, then back down. This should look like a small bird flapping its wings slowly. Repeat ten times

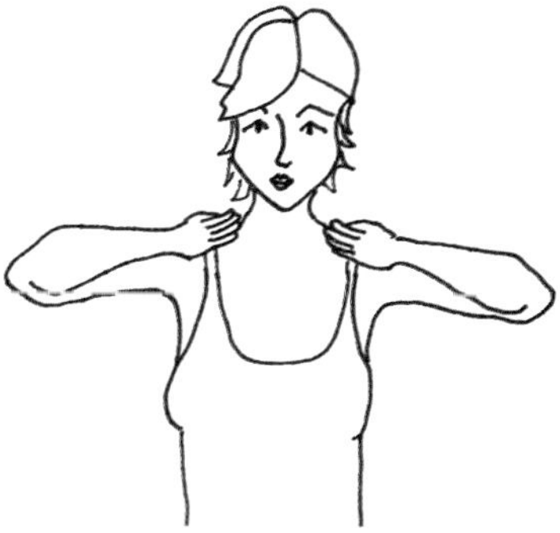

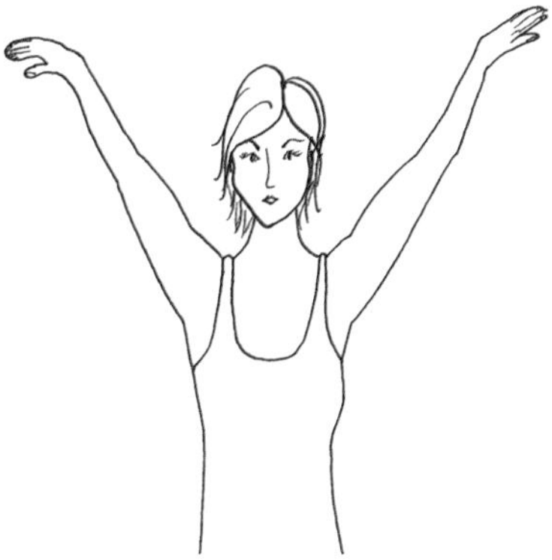

Big bird: Place arms by the side of your body, standing upright. Raise and lower your straight arms as high as possible. This should look like a big bird flapping its wings slowly. Repeat ten times.

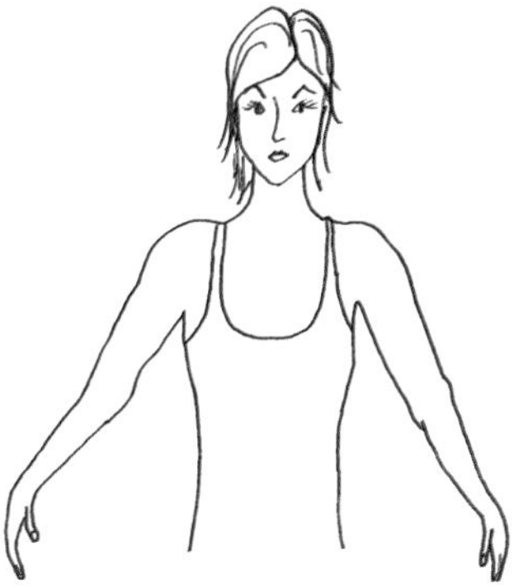

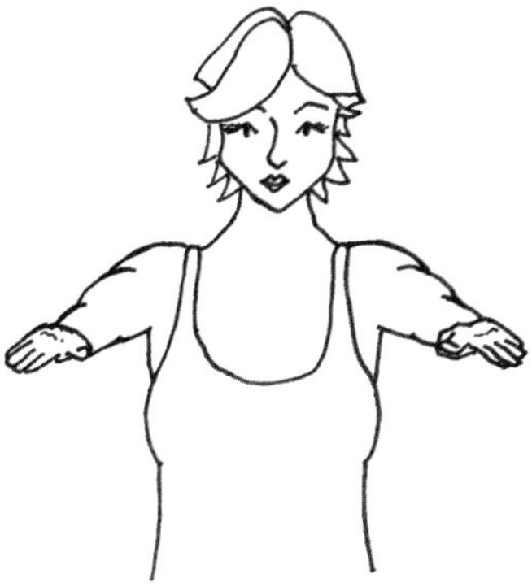

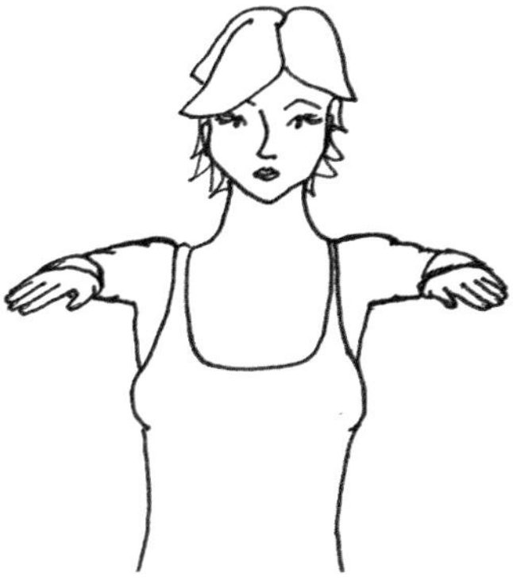

Show me the money (front): Raise the arms straight out to the front of your body, from the shoulders. Rotate the palms of your hands to face upwards then downwards. This should look like asking for money to be put in the hand. Repeat ten times.

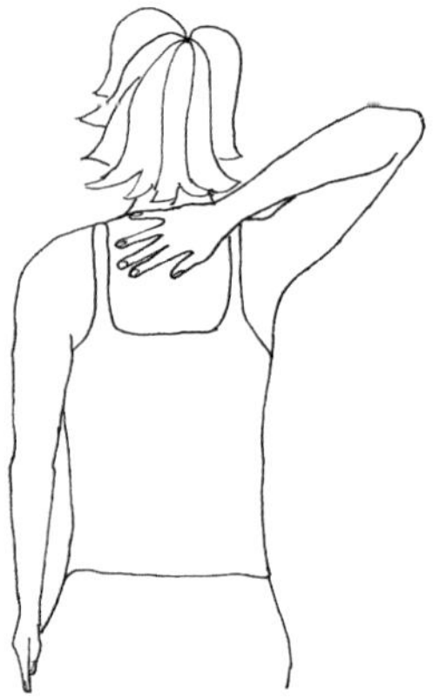

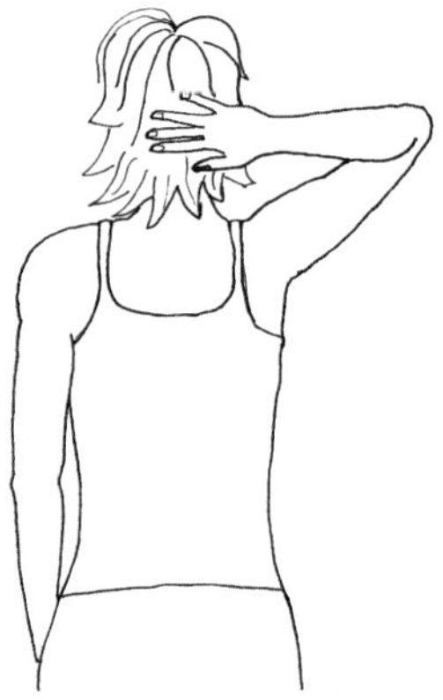

Finger walking (neck): Stand straight, with your head slightly bent forward. Take each hand to the back of your neck alternately. Walk fingers down your spine as far as comfortable. Walk them back up to your head. Repeat ten times.

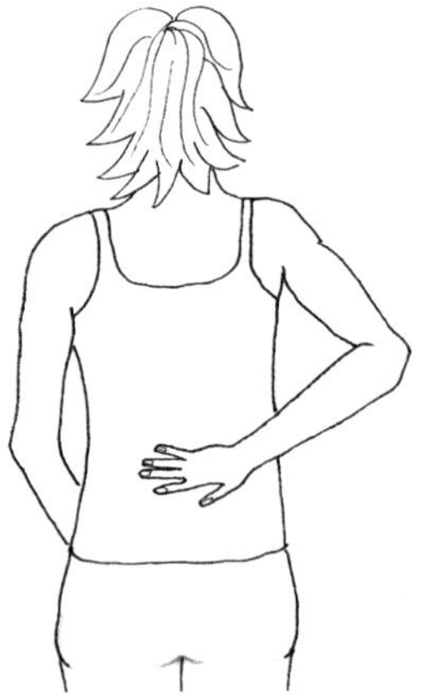

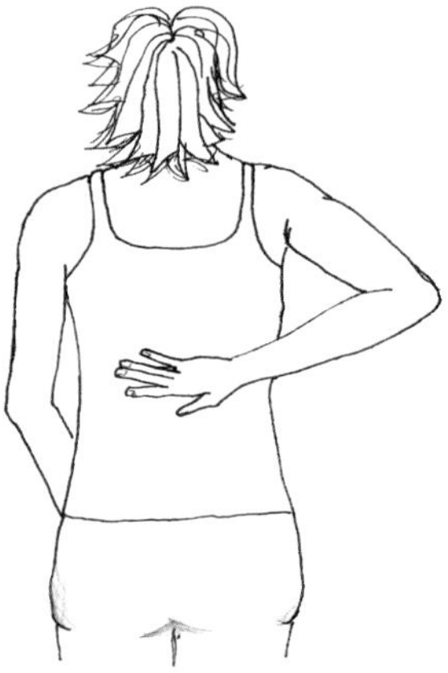

Finger walking (back): Now do the same thing to the lower back. Lower your hands to the base of the spine. Walk your fingers up the spine, to bra level. Walk them back down. Repeat ten times.

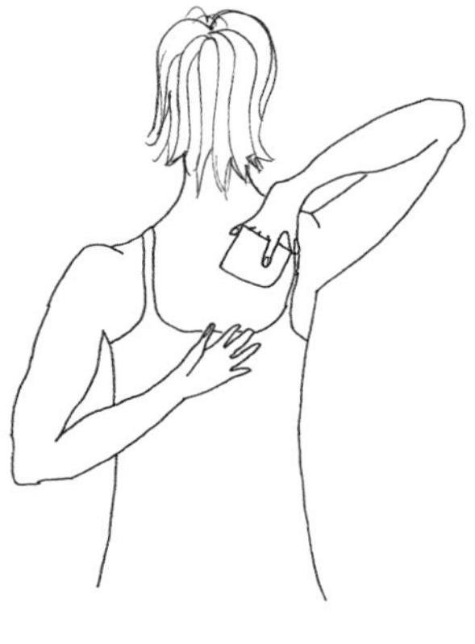

The hand over: Put your right hand behind your back. Pass a small, light object across your back, over your left shoulder to the other hand. Repeat and swap hands. The ability to do this may depend on your previous flexibility.

In addition to these exercises and stretches, which concentrate on the chest and shoulder, it is worth considering the neck exercises described in the joint pains section below. Furthermore, now is the time to start generally exercising the whole body in order to help recovery from the surgery, reduce the risks of blood clots, improve overall well-being and reduce the risk of cancer returning.

Breast tenderness

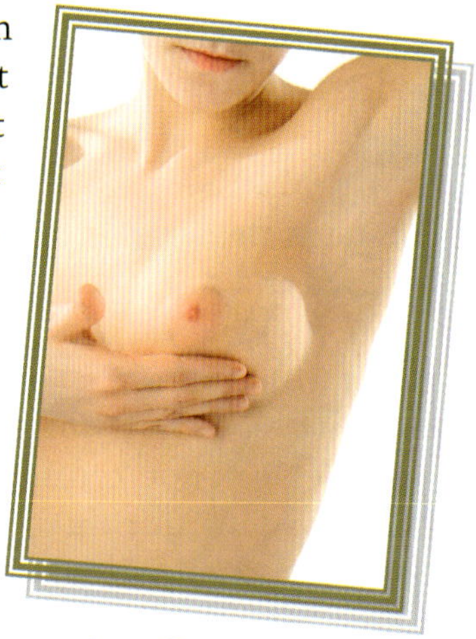

Women who have been treated for breast cancer often have the added indignity of experiencing breast tenderness or pain. There are a number of different underlying causes, producing a variety of different types of pain. The tumour itself, along with surgery, would have disrupted the normal architecture of the breast, disturbing the flow of fluid around it. Not only will this cause a throbbing, aching discomfort in itself, but it also makes the breast heavier and hotter, straining the underlying muscles. Surgery also cuts the minor nerves in the breast and under the arm, often causing numbness. When these attempt to repair themselves, the numbness usually gives way to a burning, over-sensitive pain (hyperaesthesia), which can last for several years. As well as all this, the disrupted nerves, not infrequently, send sharp, lightening, jabbing pains into the breast. These neuralgic pains may only last a few seconds, but they are enough to make your toes curl! If these neuralgic pains get severe, medication can be prescribed

During radiotherapy your skin can also become red and itchy and, in the long-term, it can contribute to the underlying thickening and fibrosis of the tissues. Some of these pains can still be cyclical, exacerbated at different times of the month as your hormone levels go up and down even if the periods have finished.

What can you do to help?

It is important to gently break up scar (fibrous) tissues, which have accumulated in the breast tissue itself or the surrounding skin, muscles, joints and nerves. Stretching particularly helps to improve the mobility and compliance between the breast tissue and the skin, and the underlying muscle and ribs. At first moving your arm or upper chest is often associated with an aggravation of the pain, because the tissues do not glide smoothly across each other. Sometimes even a tearing sensation is felt. Regular exercise and stretching, however, is the best way to break down these scar tissues, particularly those that affect your shoulder and armpit. Following the specific exercise instructions in the breast section as much as possible will help tremendously – but they have to be continued as often as possible for the rest of your life, even when the tenderness appears to have resolved. Dietary healthy oil supplements such as evening primrose and cod liver have been said to help, and some clinicians prescribe these for their patients, but similar oils can be found in oily fish, avocado and nuts. It has long been acknowledged that ginger is a natural anti-inflammatory and, if you like the taste, it may be worth adding more of this to your cooking. It almost goes without saying, but smoking significantly increased the fibrosis and thickening of underlying tissues, particularly the breast glands.

Massaging the skin gently on the breast and surrounding tissues is helpful. Although this should be avoided during radiotherapy, where the skin may be a little red and sore, there is no evidence at all that massage is harmful or should be avoided after a diagnosis of cancer. Use a natural oil, such as extra virgin olive oil, rather than commercial oils containing perfumes and additives. Apply the oil with the fingers gently, trying to roll the skin over the ribs – you should be as firm as possible but not causing any pain or bruising, as this would be counter-productive. At first there will not be any noticeable improvement, but with daily persistence the pain and mobility will improve. As an added bonus, let your partner have a go, which leads us onto the topic of sexual function.

Summary – tips to help breast tenderness:

- Regularly perform local breast exercises
- Regularly perform shoulder and neck exercises
- Consider physiotherapy if self measures fail
- Consider medication for neuralgic (shooting) pains
- Improve your fitness, but wear a good fitting bra when exercising
- Gently massage your breast with olive or another natural oil,
- Gently massage the skin around your breast and armpit
- If you smoke stop as this increases thickening in the breast
- Consider a diet rich in healthy oils e.g. cod liver and evening primrose
- Ginger is a natural anti-inflammatory agent – increase your dietary intake

Lymphoedema

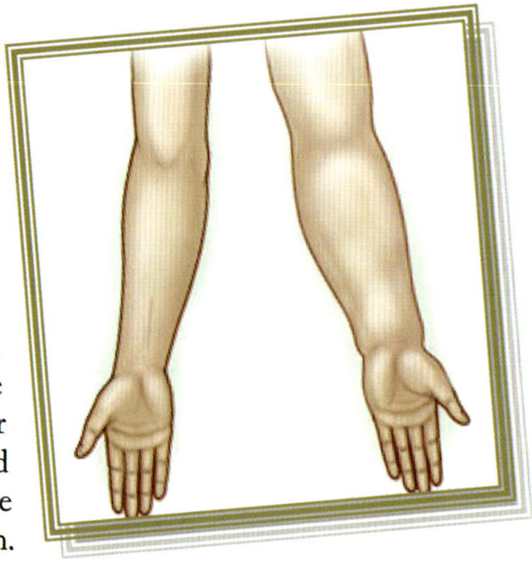

To understand how lymphoedema occurs, it is helpful to know a bit about the lymphatic system. Your body's tissues are bathed in lymph, a colourless, watery fluid. It contains lymphocytes, a type of white blood cell, which help your body to fight infection and other diseases such as cancer. The lymph travels along tiny channels called lymph vessels or lymphatics which, like blood vessels, join together to form larger channels. Eventually the lymph is filtered through a number of lymph nodes before draining into the into the bloodstream. The job of the lymphatic system and the nodes is to collect and filter out unhealthy matter such as bacteria, other micro-organisms and cancer cells. These are carried in the lymph through the nodes, where the lymphocytes will try to attack and break them down before they are carried away by the bloodstream and filtered out along with other body waste. If lymph nodes trap an infection or cancer, they will usually swell. With infection the swollen nodes are usually hot, painful and tender to touch. With cancer, however, the nodes are often painless and do not cause any discomfort when touched. Painless swollen nodes should be viewed with suspicion.

The presence of cancer in the lymph nodes of the armpit is the most important prognostic factor in breast cancer, and thus the removal and evaluation of these lymph nodes are integral components of breast cancer management. However, removal of the lymph nodes can result in a number of side-effects, including lymphoedema. The more lymph nodes that are removed, the higher the risk of developing the condition. Fortunately, the risk of lymphoedema is significantly less with the development of better surgical techniques such as sentenil node biopsy.

Lymphoedema usually manifests as a swelling to the affected arm, but can also occur in the hand, trunk and breast. It can develop immediately or many years after treatment. Whenever it develops, lymphoedema is a chronic, debilitating condition that can cause severe physical and psychological morbidity as well as a reduction in quality of life. If you have lymphoedema you should be referred to a specialist unit for evaluation and therapy, which will include the fitting of compression garments and sleeves. Massage is an important part of the treatment of lymphoedema but it is essential to use the correct technique. Deep, firm massage, for example, is harmful as it stimulates blood flow and increases the amount of fluid produced. The aim of massage is to stimulate or move the excess fluid away from the swollen area so that it can drain away normally. This type of massage is called manual lymphatic drainage (MLD) and because it is a specialised form of massage it should be given by a trained therapist who should be trained in one of the Vodder, Foldi, Leduc or Casley-Smith methods.

What can you also do to help?

A review of the evidence has shown that various self help strategies can help prevent and treat lymphoedema. The main interventions include: protecting the arm, weight reduction, aerobic exercise, weight lifting, stretching and massage.

Protect the arm: Breaks in the skin can allow bacteria to enter your tissues causing infection which can be more severe and cause lymphoedema to start or deteriorate if already present. Reduce your risk of scratches and cuts by being aware of this extra risk. For example, if you are washing dishes with a pan scourer, gardening or playing with the cat, always wear gloves. If you shave your armpits, use and electric razor as there is less chance of nicking or cutting your skin. If you need to have an injection, or have a blood sample taken, ask to have the needle inserted in your other arm.

Weight reduction: A study from Royal Marsden Hospital compared women with early lymphoedema who had weight loss counselling against a group who continued their normal diet. After the 24-week period of dietary intervention there were notable differences in the mean body weight, BMI, skin fold thickness, and percentage body fat between the control group and both the weight-reduction and low-fat groups. There was a significant reduction in excess arm volume in women who had lost weight. Several other studies have also been published which show that maintaining a healthy weight and avoiding obesity is one way to help avoid and treat lymphoedema.

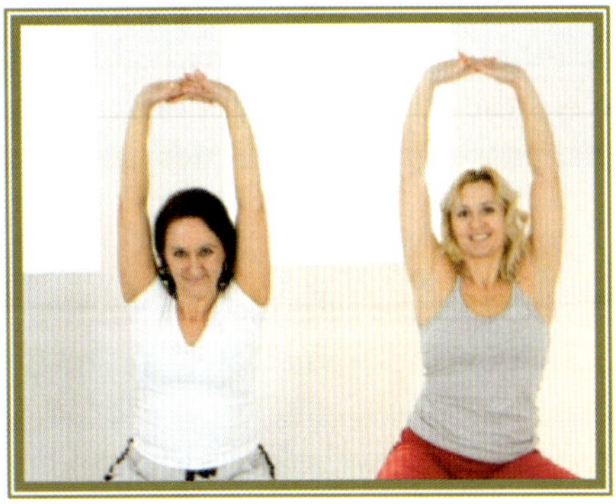

Stretching: A study published in 2006 compared a group of women who had no intervention with a group who were taught stretching exercises to increase range of motion. Stretching did not make the lymphoedema worse and the range of movement and comfort improved.

Aerobic Exercise: A study in 2000 found that two hours of steady exercise increased lymph clearance rate five-fold in the first 15-minutes, while the rest of the time it was increased 2–3 fold. This was supported by a further study in 2005, which demonstrated increased lymphatic clearance in the hands of healthy women who performed arm crank ergonometry for five-minutes each day. Studies of vigorous aerobic exercise such as running, group fitness and dance have all been shown to be safe and effective.

Exercise combined with compression garments: Two studies in 2004 examined the outcomes of anaerobic and resistance exercises while wearing a compression garment. Both studies demonstrated a reduction in arm volume of and no harmful effects were reported.

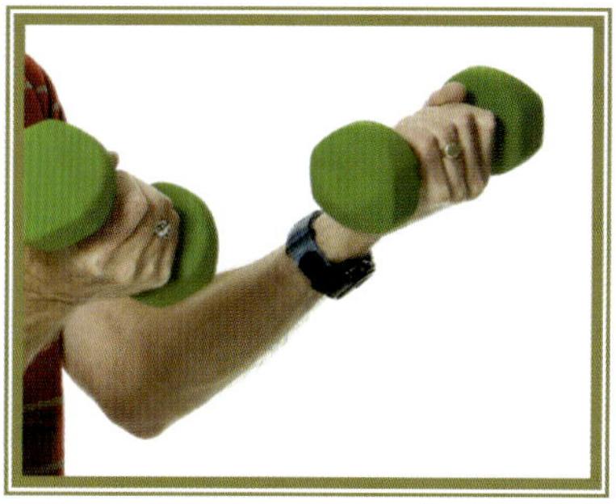

Weight lifting: A review of the published evidence in 2008 concerning the safety of weight lifting among ladies with lymphoedema concluded that a wide variety of strenuous exercise can be undertaken by those at risk of developing lymphoedema and those who already have the condition without adverse effects. The latest and most convincing evidence for the benefits of weight lifting were published in 2009 in the prestigious New England Journal of Medicine. One hundred and forty one women with breast cancer were randomised to a supervised weight lifting programme of control. They all had received an axillary node clearance and had completed adjuvant chemotherapy or radiotherapy. Both groups received standard lymphoedema advice. The intervention group received twice weekly supervised exercise sessions for six months. Weight lifting started with a warm up and warm down which included particular stretching exercises. The initial weight and escalation was determined at each session by a certified exercise professional. At six months there was a significant difference in the number of lymphoedema flares which required acute intervention (either infection or sudden deterioration in upper limb circumference).

A combination of aerobic and weight lifting exercises are ideal but there are many other exercises that may help you, depending on your fitness and preferences. What is right for you depends on your agility and general condition. Ideally, seek help from a qualified person before starting an exercise programme.

Massage: In addition to massage by a lymphoedema specialist, self massage can helpful and convenient. The skin should be moved by gentle, circular movements of your fingers (if the skin becomes reddened the movement is too hard). Use

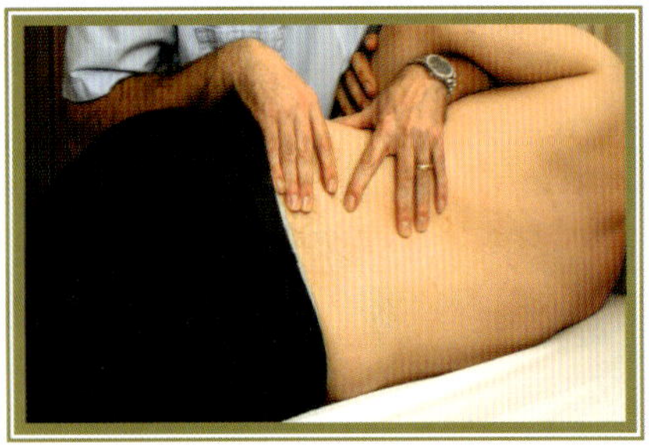

your fingers in a relaxed scooping movement pushing gently towards the head or the direction of the unaffected side. Start on the non-swollen tissue as close as possible to the swollen area, often in the armpit, then move down the limb. Move the skin across and then release the pressure to allow the skin to come back. Repeat this technique with a slow and gentle rhythm. Start the massage at position one and repeat five times. Remember to be careful with rings or sharp nails as these could damage the skin.

Hand-held massagers can also be particularly useful for people who have restricted movements of their hands, perhaps due to arthritis. They are not as effective as using your hands, because it is not easy to achieve such a light touch. They are available at most large chemist's shops. There are some basic rules to follow. Aim to use it for at least 15 minutes a day; don't use harsh oils or creams; don't use the heat setting; use a gentle circular movement covering the areas of the body described for self massage; avoid abnormal or broken skin.

Summary – tips to prevent and improve lymphoedema:

- Reduce your risk of scratches and cuts that could cause infection
- If you are washing dishes with a pan scourer, always wear rubber gloves
- Be careful with pets and gardening
- If you shave your armpits, use an electric razor to avoid nicking your skin
- If you need to have an injection, or blood sample avoid the at risk arm.
- Ensure you are referred to a specialist lymphoedema expert
- Loose weight if over weight
- Stop smoking if you smoke
- Don't take diuretics (water tables) for this purpose as they do not help
- Take regular aerobic exercise
- Regularly and gently stretch the shoulder, elbow and wrist of the limb
- Increase your overall exercise levels
- Embark on a regular supervised weight-training programme

Chapter Nineteen

Other common concerns
Advice and guidance

Sexual function

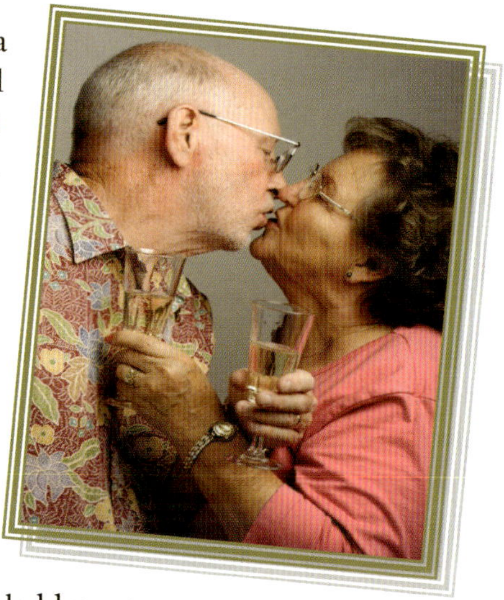

Cancer and its treatments can often have a profound effect on libido and sexual function. In males this also usually means erectile dysfunction, and in women vaginal dryness or soreness. In both sexes the desire for sex can be impaired, even if the *machinery* still works. Both partners therefore can miss out on the physical, psychological and bonding benefits of a sexual relationship. This can put a strain on even the most loving of partnerships.

The are several physical causes including trauma to the pelvic region or spinal cord, or surgery on the prostate, bladder or rectum, which can damage veins and nerves needed for sexual function. To a lesser extent radiotherapy can have an adverse affect on the nerves to the penis, and can certainly cause vaginal dryness. Drugs given for prostate cancer can reduce male hormone levels, the most common culprit being LHRH modulators (e.g. zoladex), but other drugs for depression and high blood pressure can also compromise sexual function. Erectile dysfunction (ED) has also been reported after taking drugs to improve the waterworks (e.g. tamsulosin). In women, drugs such as tamoxifen can cause vaginal discharge, and aromatase inhibitors (arimidex, aromasin and femara) can cause dryness.

Psychological well-being is very important for a healthy sex life. Depression, lack of self-esteem, low mood, guilt and anxiety all contribute to loss of libido and erectile dysfunction (ED). If a man experiences loss of erection, he may worry that it will happen again. This can produce anxiety associated with performance, and may lead to chronic problems during sexual intercourse. This is called performance related anxiety and is perfectly treatable.

What can you do to help?

If you have received radiotherapy to the pelvis, or you are taking dugs which cause dryness, consider regular vaginal dilators with plenty of lubricants or, if possible, have sexual intercourse regularly. In men, medication such as the PDE5 inhibtors viagra and cialis can, help not only physically, but also aid anxiety associated ED. If a man has the reassurance that he can get an erection with medication, just the thought of having them available is often enough. They work particularly well if "there is some life in the old boy". Partial erections or erections which are not sustained are usually restored to normal after these tablets but if there has been *no flicker of life* they are often unsuccessful. In this case some surgeons recommend taking them every day (whether you are having sex or not) for a month, as this seems to help in the longer term. It is worth asking for a referral to a specialist urologist or nurse who may be able to offer a number of other interventions ranging from penile pumps to intra-penile injections. For women, lubricants and pessaries are certainly helpful. It may not always be advisable to take oestrogenic pessaries if you have had breast cancer (discuss this with your doctor).

The penis is very sensitive to changes in oxygen and blood supply. In fact, ED is often the first sign of hardened arteries, and can precede angina by two years unless intervention has taken place. Lifestyle interventions should aim to improve the blood supply to your pelvis and include the usual culprits: stop smoking, as this also aggravates vaginal dryness and hot flushes, exercise, lose weight and eat a balanced diet. Pelvic floor exercises are useful as these directly stimulate the muscles around your penis or vagina. If performed correctly these can be a great help. The problem is that most people give them up after a few days or are very sporadic. They need to be performed correctly (see previous chapter), for at least 10 minutes a day indefinitely. Even then an improvement only usually starts appearing after six to eight weeks – it is important to keep going.

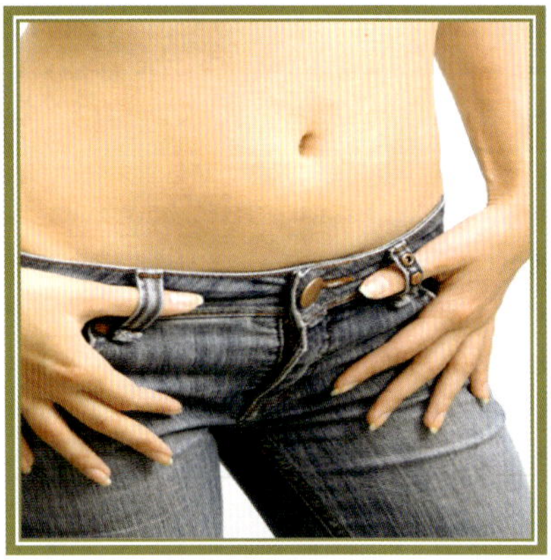

There may be some indirect truth in the aphrodisiac properties of oysters, which contain zinc and selenium, important for a number of the enzymatic functions, including those in the fertility pathways. Some people get the selenium and essential minerals checked so they can adjust their diet accordingly.

Xenoestrogens are contaminants that have oestrogenic properties which affect sex hormone activity. They are found in pesticides, herbicides, polychlorinated biphenyls (PCB's) and food containers. There is no direct evidence that they interfer with sexual function but there is a potential mechanism of harm if taken in excess. You may wish to consider organic foods. Also excessive alcohol intake and recovering from hangovers can compromise erectile function and reduce libido. Psychological factors in impotence are often secondary to physical causes, and they magnify their significance. The advice generally given to improve psychological well-being, described previously, certainly applies to sexual function.

Summary – advice to help preserve sexual function:

- Discuss medications with your doctor (including blood pressure tablets)
- For men consider extra medications, such Viagra, Cialis etc
- For men, if ED continues, ask to be referred to a specialist urologist
- In women simple lubrication may help
- If this does not work get referred to a specialist gynaecologist
- Look after your general health;
- Stop smoking,
- Eat well,
- Lose weight
- Exercise regularly
- Perform pelvic floor exercises correctly
- Perform pelvic floor exercises regularly and indefinitely
- Avoid excessive environmental and dietary xenoestrogens
- Avoid excessive alcohol or other recreational drugs
- Reduce general anxiety – see the 'anxiety' section
- Women discuss medications such as aromatase inhibitors
- Consider seeing a sexuality counsellor

Incontinence and urgency

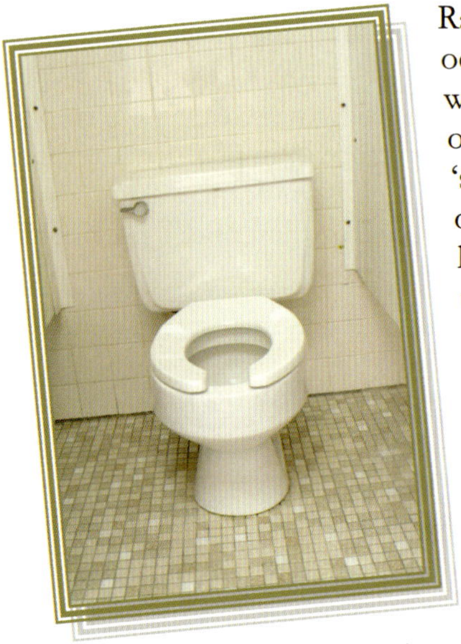

Radiotherapy or surgery to the pelvis can occasionally impair your ability to hold your water. Of course this can also happen as you get older anyway. It can be broadly divided into 'stress incontinence' referring to the complaint of urine leaking out when coughing, sneezing or laughing, and 'urgency incontinence' where there is a strong desire to pass urine immediately and you have very little notice before you lose control and become incontinent, i.e. there is an urgent need to find a toilet. This symptom is more common in women, and it is particularly seen if the uterus is enlarged, prolapsed, after pelvic surgery, or if you are overweight. It can happen in men with prostate or bladder cancer, particularly following surgery such as prostatectomy or even TURP (transurethral resection of the prostate). It can also occur after pelvic radiotherapy.

Urgency incontinence can also apply to faeces from the back passage, especially if high-dose radiotherapy has been given to the lower rectum or there has been surgery to the anus. Occasionally, the rectum can prolapse out of the anus, usually following years of constipation and straining to open your bowels. Fortunately, whatever the cause, this is very rare.

What can you do to help?

If there is a sudden onset of incontinence, particularly if associated with a burning pain (cystitis), a temperature or passing water frequently, this could indicate an infection. In this case a sample of the urine should be tested and the appropriate antibiotics taken for treatment. For men with prostate problems, tablets can be given, such as alpha blockers. These relax the muscles at the entrance to the bladder allowing the bladder to empty correctly. Sometimes, especially after a period of catheterisation, the bladder control has to be re-learnt. In this case your specialist urology team would perform a flow test and usually an ultrasound of the bladder after you have passed water. A trained specialist nurse can then issue specific advice depending on your individual deficit. In addition to these measures, a number of lifestyle factors can improve the ability to hold your water.

If you are overweight, try to slim down. Constipation can aggravate incontinence. Piles, rectal damage and a full pelvis can reduce the capacity of the bladder. Too much tea and coffee, especially in cold weather can cause urgency and sometimes incontinence.

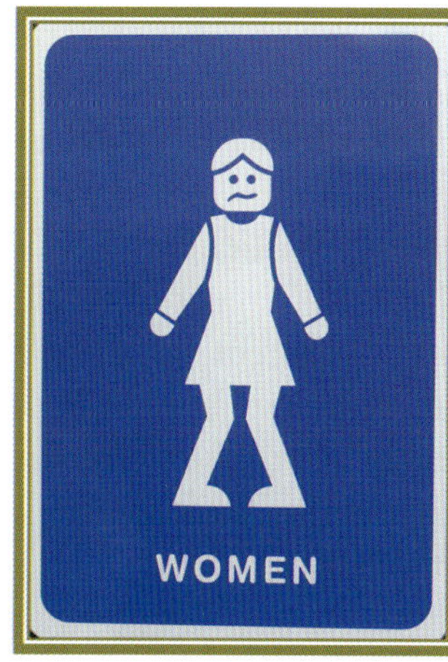

Exercise in general has been shown to help, not only by making you lose weight, but also by toning the abdominal and pelvic muscles. It is important to remember, however, that when exercising the abdominal muscles, you should breathe out slowly when tensing, for example, during a 'sit up'. This avoids increasing the pressure inside your abdomen (intra-abdominal pressure), which can aggravate incontinence by putting pressure on the pelvic muscles. The most important and relevant exercises to improve incontinence are those which strengthen the pelvic floor – pelvic floor exercises. These exercises can also improve muscle tone around the anus, helping piles, bowel urgency or rectal prolapse. Pelvic floor exercises also improve sexual performance. The level and intensity of pelvic floor exercises depends on the general fitness and abilities of the individual. A general rule is to attempt some form of exercise at least once or twice every day, and to keep it going regularly. Benefits usually only appear within two to three weeks, and may take several months to peak. The previous chapter explains how to perform the quick and slow versions of pelvic floor exercises correctly.

Summary – advice to help incontinence:

- Test urine and treat urinary infection if present
- At the end of urinating try to ensure the bladder is empty
- Avoid stimulants which aggravate urgency – strong tea, coffee and alcohol
- Slim down especially if overweight
- Exercise generally to increase muscle tone
- Perform regular pelvic floor exercises every day – keep them going
- Avoid holding your breath when tensing the abdominal muscles when lifting
- Avoid straining when opening the bowels
- Avoid constipation
- Seek medical attention if these fail

Joint pains

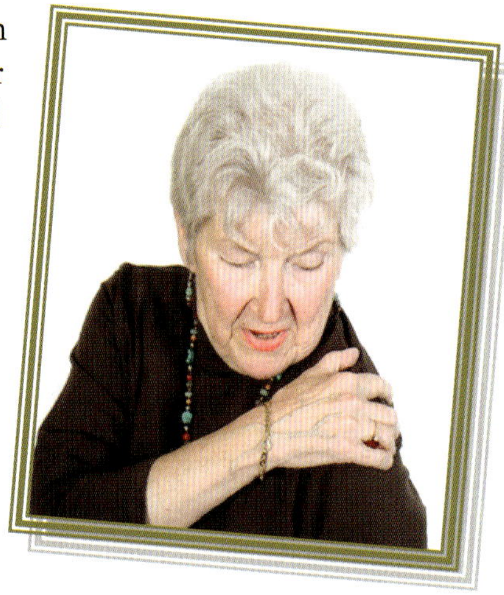

There is a risk that you could develop aches in your joints during or following cancer therapies. Fortunately these are mostly mild and usually wear off within a few weeks. This can be a problem with some chemotherapy agents, particularly those called taxanes. About 12 percent of women taking tamoxifen and 35 percent on aromatase inhibitor drugs are troubled by joint pains and this can persist for the entire duration of this medication and sometimes for months afterwards.

What can you do to help?

Excluding specific medical conditions, arthralgia (joint discomfort) is often associated with changes in our general sense of wellbeing. We are all familiar with aching joints when we get a cold or flu. Likewise, ingested toxins are thought to get caught in the micro-vessels of our joints. These toxins not only cause direct irritation themselves, but can also trigger an immune attack from the body, which causes collateral damage to delicate joint tissues. For these reasons a diet low in man-made chemicals is certainly well worth a try. This includes carefully washing fruit and vegetables, or considering organic foods to avoid pesticides and processed food, or excluding commercially packaged snacks, fizzy and sugary drinks or sweets in the diet to reduce your intake of preservative, colourings and flavourings. Cod liver oil and glucosamine supplements have been shown to help some people and the evidence for these has been reviewed in the specific supplement section. Regular fresh ginger can act as a natural anti-inflammatory agent.

Losing weight will help prevent further wear and tear, particularly on the large weight-bearing joints such as your hips, knees and back. Bad posture in particular leads to neck, lower back and shoulder pains. You may be more prone to postural problems after chemotherapy, not helped by its associated fatigue and weight gain. Most of us do not even know we are slouching until someone points it out, or we see a video or photograph of ourselves. Simply being aware of a deterioration of your posture is a good start, as most of us know what to do – walk tall, chin in, shoulders back and stomach in. It may be worth undergoing a short course of osteopathy to get things started.

Exercise may seem incongruous if joint pains have already set in, but especially when combined with stretching, it is a fantastic way to help immediate pain and prevent further progression. Imagine the hinges of an old door – if it is only opened and closed half way each time, only half the hinge will stay smooth; the other half will rust over, creek and strain if an attempt is made to open the door fully. Stretching may be a little more difficult at the beginning, because even if you stretched before treatment, there may be a degree of re-training required. It is well worth putting aside ten minutes every day for stretching in a fairly regimented programme, either alone or in a group, which ensures all your joints are stretched. Start from the neck down, extending and flexing your joints into the fullest range possible without causing pain. Move down your body, via the shoulders, back, hips, knees, hands and feet, to develop a system that works amazingly well.

If time and local facilities allow, major benefits can be achieved by attending a yoga or Pilates class. Pilates and yoga are not just for flexible young females; they benefit everyone at any age even if you cannot even touch your toes. You don't have to be a contortionist to participate, as a good class should cater for all levels. Instructors are usually highly qualified and really understand the exercises which strengthen the core muscles to enable you to improve your posture. Pilates and yoga stretch the joints, tendons, ligaments and muscles around them, which, although sometimes uncomfortable at the time, will improve the health of the joints, increase flexibility and reduce long term swelling and pain. The first step is to find a convenient class close to you. Next is to discuss with the instructor your level of fitness so you can join the relevant class. The third, and most difficult, is to attend regularly! Although classes are cheaper, if you are self-conscious, lack time or cannot find a suitable local class, a personal trainer should provide motivation, exercise and stretching guidance all in one.

Neck and shoulder exercises

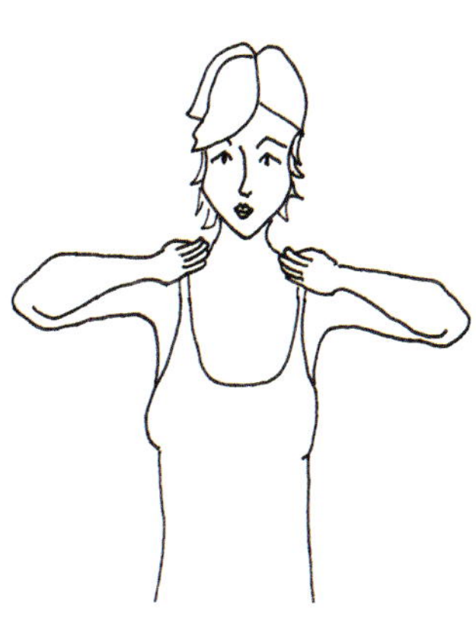

Neck stiffness is fairly common following cancer therapies, for a variety of reasons. Steroids may have impaired core strength and posture, chemotherapy and some hormonal therapies can generally cause joint discomfort, particularly with aromatase inhibitors. During radiotherapy, patients have to hold their neck straight during treatments which can cause some stiffness. Finally, as we all get older, our neck becomes very prone to stiffness and pain. The neck being a complex series of joints, which if weakened or inflamed can cause muscle spasm, pains down the arms and discomfort radiating up the back of the head – a not infrequent cause of headaches.

Exercise 1. (see pictures below). Stand straight and as upright as possible, stretching your arms towards the ceiling, as high as possible. Hold for 3-4 seconds, then bring your arms to the horizontal position, and push your elbows back. At the same time keep your chin towards your chest – this should arch the upper thoracic spine and straighten your neck. Repeat three times.

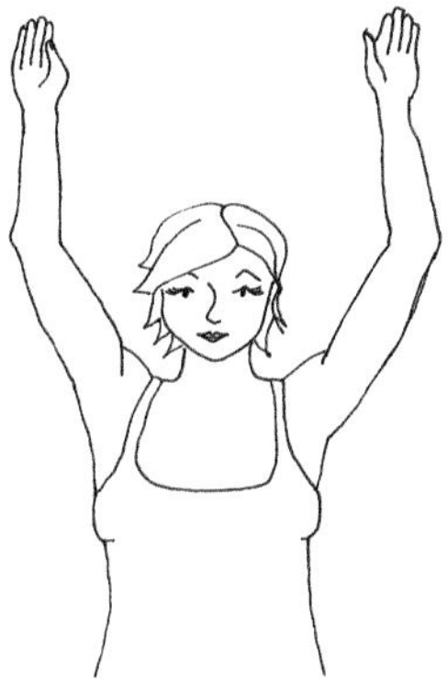

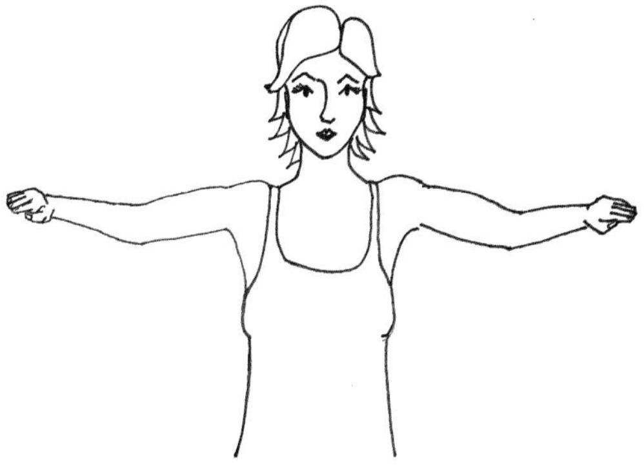

Exercise 2. Facing straight ahead, look up as high as possible. Hold for three to four seconds, and then look down as low as possible (hold for three to four seconds). Repeat three times.

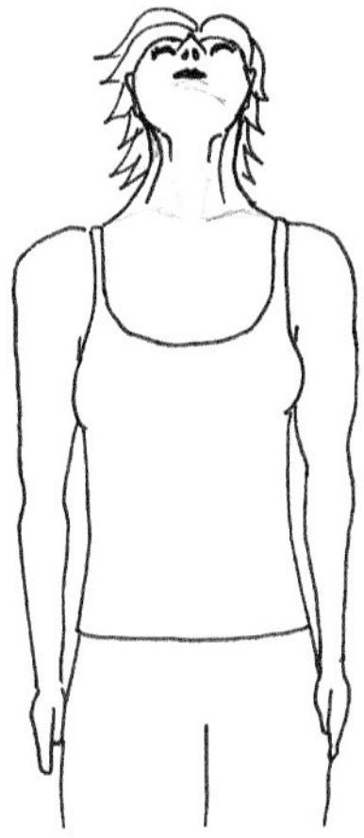

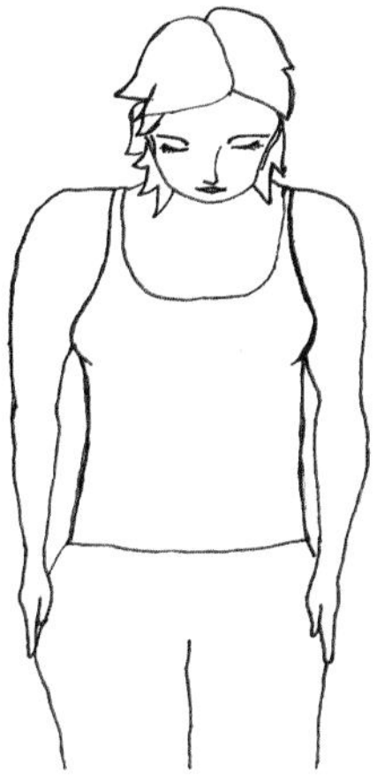

Exercise 3. Facing straight ahead, turn your head to the right as far as possible (hold for three to four seconds), and then move your head slowly up and down for ten nods. Then turn your head to the left, and repeat three times:

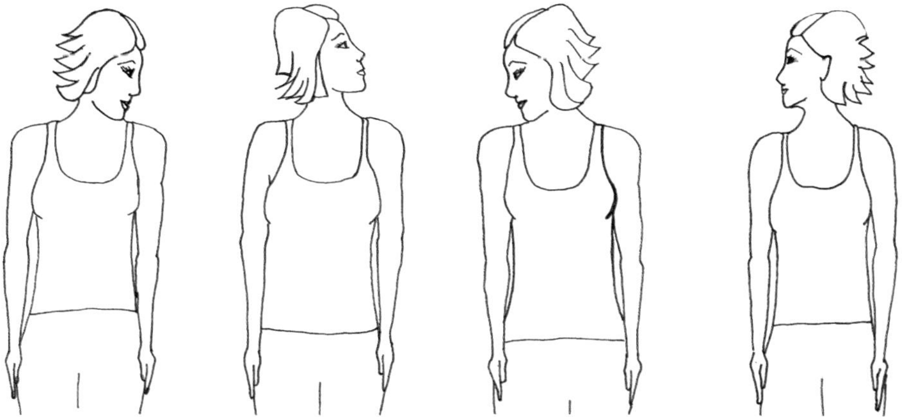

Exercise 4. Facing straight ahead, tilt your head to the right, as if trying to put your ear on your shoulder. Hold for three to four seconds, and then repeat on the left. Repeat on both sides three times.

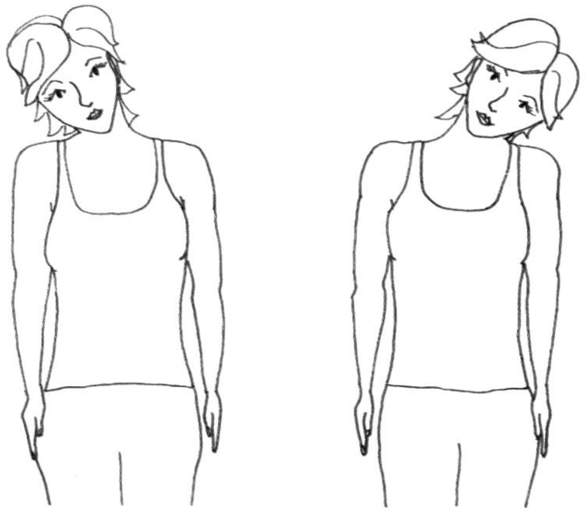

These neck stretches can be combined with the breast exercises above, or other good shoulder exercises, such as shrugging. To do this, sit or stand squarely. Bring your shoulders up towards your ear. Relax and repeat. Sink your shoulders downwards. Relax and repeat. Ease shoulders forwards. Relax and repeat. Pull shoulders back. Relax and repeat each movement five-ten times.

As with any exercises and stretches, it is very important to get into a routine and perform them every day – even if only for 10 minutes. It is also a good idea to perform neck exercises in front of the mirror, in order to achieve the optimal posture.

Summary – advice to help joint pains:

- Eat healthily, with plenty of vegetables and fish, and not too much meat
- Keep a diary of what foods can make your joints worse
- Reduce calories if you are overweight
- Use fresh ginger as much as possible
- Consider supplementation with cod liver or other healthy oils
- Avoid food additives, pesticides and particularly sulphites
- Avoid excess alcohol
- Avoid smoking
- Exercise and stretch your joints everyday
- Improve your posture and consider joining yoga or Pilates classes
- Review medications with your doctor

Hot flushes

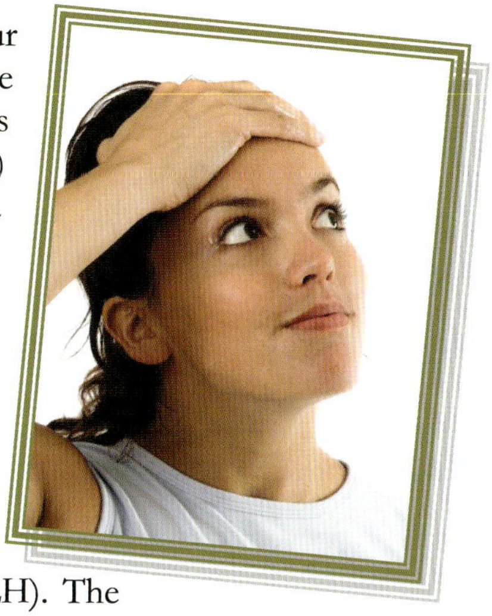

A troublesome consequence of reducing our natural levels of oestrogen and testosterone (the sex hormones), is an imbalance in the body's cooling system, causing hot flushes (flashes) and night sweats. These are described as a sudden and unpleasant sensation of burning heat spreading across the face, neck and chest. They normally start at the time of the menopause in women. In this situation the oestrogen levels fall dramatically and hormones from the pituitary gland in the head rise (this is what is tested when a blood test is taken to confirm a woman is post-menopausal i.e. low oestrogen, high FSH & LH). The severity of hot flushes can range from a mild intolerance to a change in temperature to prolific sweating throughout the day and night, causing fainting and exhaustion.

In pre-menopausal women and men, hormone levels can be impaired after cancer treatments earlier than expected naturally. The main causes of damage to the ovaries or testes are surgery, chemotherapy, radiotherapy, and hormone therapy (e.g. granisetron or zoladex). In post-menopausal women, aromatase inhibitors lower oestrogen even further. In both groups, tamoxifen commonly causes hot flushes via its ability to bind to the oestrogen receptors. Some other drugs, such as the bone hardening drugs (bisphosphonates) can cause or aggravate hot flushes by a completely independent mechanism.

What can you do to help?

In the first instance, it is useful to keep a diary of your hot flushes, in order to prepare for or, better still, avoid the common trigger factors. If lifestyle changes fail, it is worth discussing with your doctor a trial of different versions of the initially prescribed hormone drugs, or the addition of other drugs such as progesterone, clonidine or antidepressants (venlaflexine).

Acupuncture may be worth considering, as a recent study suggests that it is at least as effective as antidepressants. Yoga and relaxation classes have had limited success. Studies have also shown that women who have diets high in phyto-oestrogens generally have fewer hot flushes or other menopausal symptoms. Other studies show that eating phyto-oestrogens regularly for several weeks reduced blood oestrogen levels, despite the higher intake of the plant oestrogen. On the other hand, a well conducted scientific trial examining the effects of phytoestrogen supplements in breast cancer patients with hot flushes, showed no benefit. Of more concern is the fact that many oncologists around the world are not comfortable with recommending phytoestrogen supplements, or indeed herbal remedies such as ginseng, black cohosh, dong quai, lavender, fennel, false unicorn root, wild yam or sage (a natural anhidrotic which reduces sweating), as in theory they could stimulate residual cancer cells. There is no evidence for this in humans but some animal studies have shown that phytoestrogen supplements can stimulate the lining of the uterus. There are numerous ongoing studies to help decide whether phytoestrogens can be used to help hot flushes or whether prolonged use could be harmful but, in the meantime, it is probably best to avoid supplements in tablet form and stick to whole, healthy foods instead.

Summary – advice to help for hot flushes:

Clothes and environment

- Wear cotton clothing rather than polyester or other man-made fibres
- Wear layers of clothes that can be taken off or put on quickly
- Use layers of bedclothes (natural fabrics) that can be removed as required
- An electric fan placed on a desk or table helps to lower skin temperature
- Adopt sleep hygiene tactics, if you are not sleeping because of the flushes
- Avoid warm or stuffy rooms as they can make flushes worse
- Take plenty of cool baths, showers and saunas (cooling down afterwards)
- Use sprays or wipes to help lower skin temperature

Diet and liquids

- Avoid spicy foods, especially at night, if you find that they cause hot flushes
- Avoid large meals and excess sugar
- Hot drinks can trigger a flush. Open a window and loosen some clothes
- If you are overweight, it is more difficult to regulate your body temperature
- Alcohol and caffeine in coffee or strong tea can trigger a flush
- If sweating a lot, drink plenty of healthy fluids e.g. water and fresh fruit juice
- Evening primrose oil, Vitamin E and B6 supplements may help

Exercise and complementary therapies

- Regular exercise significantly helps to reduce the severity of hot flushes
- Stress: relaxation techniques, massage, reflexology and aromatherapy are safe
- Acceptance – hot flushes are normal, most people don't even notice them
- Acupuncture has been shown to help but needs to be done regularly

Bone health (Bone density, Osteoporosis)

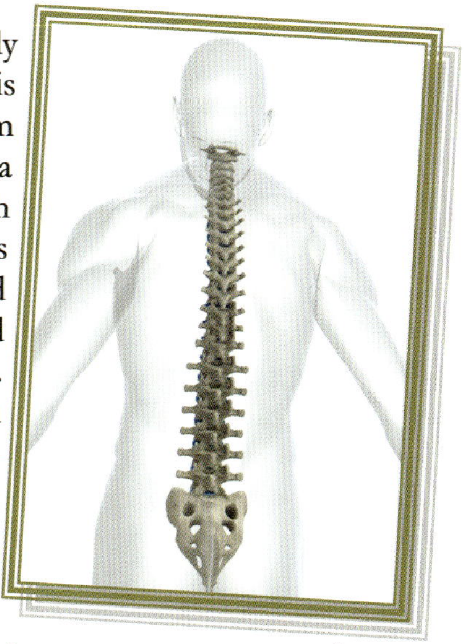

The health of your bones may be adversely affected after a number of cancer therapies. This may range from a mild reduction in calcium density, measured on a bone density scan, to a moderate reduction called osteopenia, through to a significant bone mineralisation loss with its associated risks of collapsed vertebrae and fractures. This latter condition is called osteoporosis and requires immediate treatment. The most significant risk to bone health is in women who have been made prematurely post-menopausal either by surgery (removing the ovaries – oophorectomy), radiotherapy to the ovaries, hormones or chemotherapy. Certain drugs also increase the risk of bone loss. The most notable are the aromatase inhibitor group given to post-menopausal women with breast cancer (arimidex, letrozole and exemestane). Likewise, prolonged use of zoladex in men with prostate cancer significantly increases the risk of bone loss.

In many instances, the risk of bone loss is so significant that it is advisable to have bone density scans (dexa scans – dual energy X-ray absorpiometry) at regular intervals after cancer therapies. These usually provide scores of bone mineralisation in the hips and spine although some scanners measure the wrist and bones in the feet. This is called the T-score and can be adjusted to that expected for your age at the time of the scan. Other medical conditions which are associated with osteopenia include thyroid disorders, prolonged intake of warfarin, phenytoin and corticosteroids. Lifestyle factors which increase the risk of osteoporosis include a low calcium intake, low protein diet, lack of physical activity, smoking, excessive alcohol intake and being too thin.

This section reviews the evidence that lifestyle factors may influence the prevention, development, progression or severity of impairments of bone mineral density among cancer survivors. It categorised self-help lifestyle strategies into exercise including: home-based aerobics; walking and resistance programmes; diet, including plant proteins, soya product and fibres; other lifestyle factors, including avoiding excessive alcohol intake and smoking.

What can you do to help?

Bone is not a solid lump of calcium, but a dynamic organ constantly remoulding itself. This explains why bone is strongly influenced by environmental and lifestyle factors, and of these exercise is the most prominent. Put a man in space, for example, and within six weeks he has osteopenia, due to a lack of weight-bearing stimulus to the bone. In a less dramatic but similar way, a sudden change to a sedentary lifestyle will result in bone thinning.

Exercise: Fortunately, weight-bearing and resistance exercise will do the opposite. It sends signals to the cells in the bone to lay down more calcium and harden them. This has been demonstrated in several well conducted trials. For example, the impact of aerobics and resistance training on bone mineral density (BMD) was tested in a randomised controlled trial (RCT) involving 66 women with breast cancer. Women randomised to the home-based aerobic exercise intervention were instructed to choose an aerobic activity they enjoyed (e.g. walking, jogging) and exercise for 15-30 minutes four days per week for the duration of the study, at a such a symptom-limited, moderate intensity that they were breathing hard but able to talk.. Resistance exercise subjects were instructed to exercise at home four days per week using resistance bands and tubing. The average decline in BMD was significantly less in the aerobic exercise group (0.7 percent), adequate in the resistance exercise group (4 percent) but in those who didn't exercise there was a 6.5 percent reduction. Pre-menopausal women had even greater benefit. Another study in 2009 evaluated the efficacy of a strength and weight training programme in 223 post-menopausal women who had completed breast cancer treatment (except tamoxifen and aromatase inhibitors) at least six months earlier. These women, randomised to exercise or not, also took vitamin D and a bone hardening drug called risedronate. Participants who were 50 percent or greater adherent to exercises were significantly less likely than participants on medications alone to lose BMD at the total hip and femoral neck.

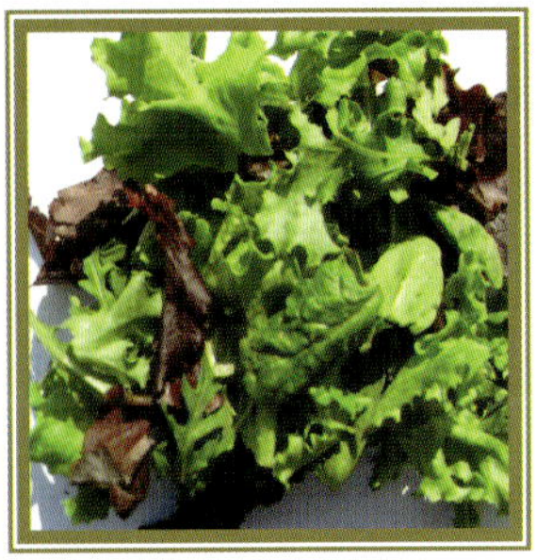

Diet, plant proteins and fibres: In 2005 a Dutch scientist performed a sub-analysis of the European Prospective Investigation into Cancer and Nutrition (EPIC) Potsdam study which included 8,178 females and examined the association between protein intake, dietary calcium and bone structure. He and his research team found that high consumption of animal protein was unfavourable, whereas higher vegetable protein was beneficial to bone health. These results support the hypothesis that high calcium intakes, combined with adequate protein intake based on a high ratio of vegetable to animal protein, may be protective against osteoporosis. Indeed, evidence has demonstrated the relationship between lower incidence of osteoporosis in Asian women and vegetarian populations due to a diet rich in vegetables and fruit. Furthermore, a large-scale dietary modification intervention of 4883 post-menopausal women showed that an increased consumption of plant proteins and fibres from fruits, vegetables and grains reduced the risk of multiple falls and had slightly better hip BMD.

Two other scientists further highlighted the benefits of plant proteins and fibres on bone health in two reviews where a positive link between a high consumption of fruit and vegetables and bone health has been demonstrated. In the first report it was found that fruit and vegetables had beneficial effects on bone mass and bone metabolism in men and women across the age ranges, whilst in the second review it was concluded that although the impact of a vegetarian diet on bone health is much more complex than merely being related to diet, vegetarians do tend to have 'normal' bone mass.

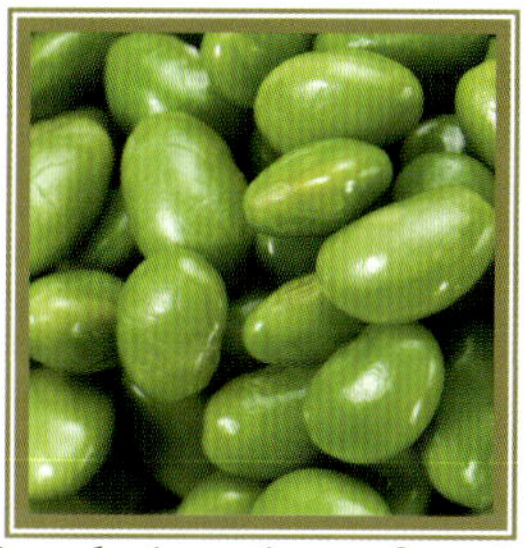

Soya products In 2008 a randomised, double-blind, controlled trial was published which evaluated the action of the soya derivative genistein aglycone and its effects on bone health amongst 389 women with breast and endometrial cancer. Bone mineral density increases were greater with genistein for both femoral neck and lumbar spine, compared to placebo. There were no differences in discomfort or adverse events between groups, the conclusion being that after 3 years of treatment, genistein exhibited a promising safety profile with positive effects on bone formation in this cohort of osteopenic, post-menopausal women.

Alcohol: Greater bone density was found in men consuming seven or more alcoholic beverages weekly than in non-drinkers, highlighting the potential benefits of low to moderate alcohol consumption. On the other hand, men with high alcohol intake had a worse BMD.

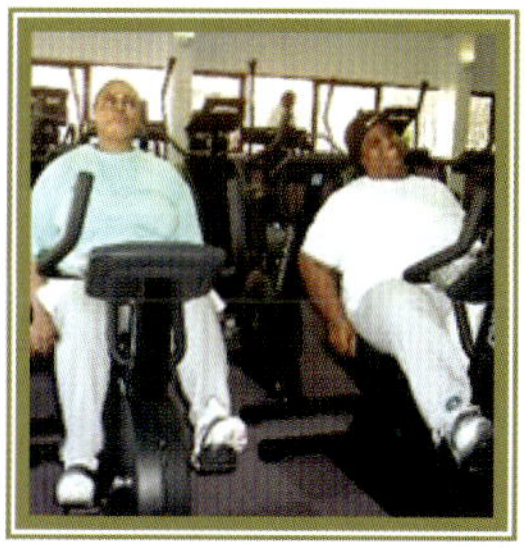

Body weight: In 2007 in a US study, involving men with prostate cancer, osteopenia or osteoporosis was detected in two thirds of the men. A positive association between body mass index (weight) and bone density of the hip was observed, suggesting that a higher BMI is protective of bone density loss in men with prostate cancer and that weight loss could increase risk of osteoporosis. The same authors, in another study, also reported that among breast cancer survivors, smoking and being underweight (BMI less than 19) were associated with lower BMD.

Calcium, vitamin D and sunlight supplement use, in one study, was associated with greater bone density measurements. Dietary calcium is not found just in dairy products such as milk, yoghurt and cheese, but also in a wide range of less fatty foods such as sardines, broccoli, almonds and salmon. Vitamin D serves several important functions in relation to calcium metabolism and is vital for the development of healthy bones. It helps to increase calcium absorption from the gastrointestinal system and the kidneys, and assists with the deposition of calcium into the bone. The body's main source of vitamin D arises from its manufacture in the skin upon exposure to sunlight. Research has found that people from some cultural groups are deficient in vitamin D due to more time being spent indoors. Only 10-15 minutes of exposure to outdoor sun is necessary to start the production of vitamin D. Dietary sources of vitamin D are limited, but sources often arise from foods fortified (boosted) with vitamin D such as milk, soy products and cereals. It is also found naturally in liver, fish (tuna, salmon, sardines, herring and mackerel) and egg yolk.

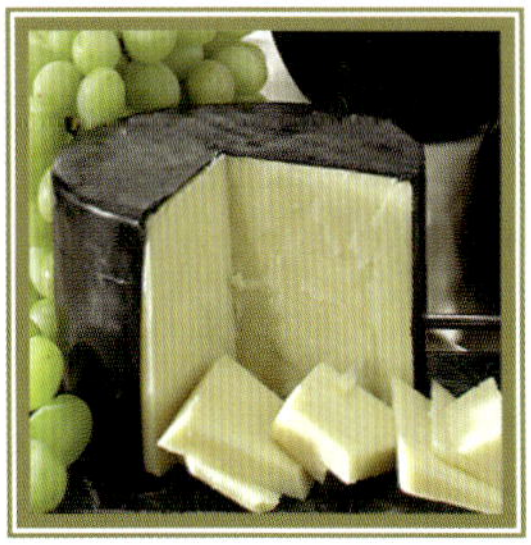

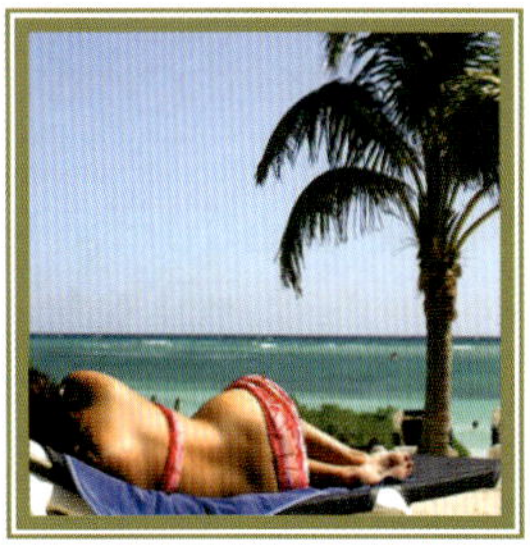

Summary – advice to protect bone density:

- Perform regular aerobic and resistance exercise in formal programmes
- Incorporate more physical exercise within the activities of daily living
- Stop smoking, and avoid excess alcohol or daily intake
- Increasing your exposure to low intensity sunlight
- Eat foods containing calcium and vitamin D
- Eat adequate but not too much animal protein in your diet
- Increase plant based proteins in your diet such as pulses and grains
- Increase Soya based foods diet; soya (beans, miso, tempeh, soy milk, tofu)
- Eat a diet rich in vegetables, fruits and salads
- Avoid being too underweight (BMI < 19)
- Avoid sugary carbonated drinks, and too much caffeine
- Have regular dexa scans
- If your T-score is low take a calcium & vitamin D supplement
- If your T-score is very low - take a bone hardening drug (bisphosphonate)
- Review your medication from your doctor

Secondary cancers

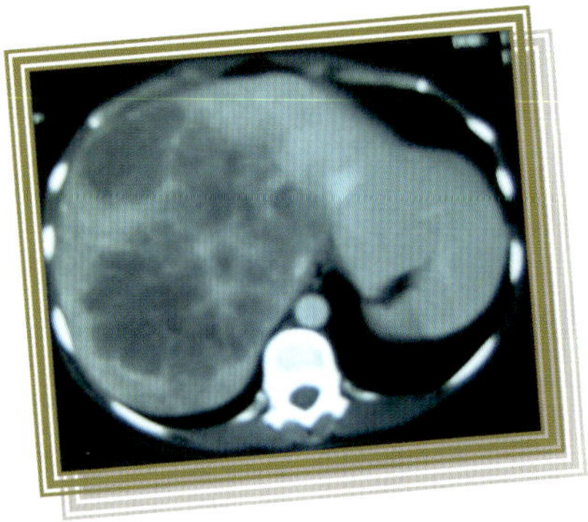

It is an unfortunate reality that radiotherapy and chemotherapy themselves can increase the risk of a new cancer, sometimes years after your initial treatment. This risk may have been discussed with you as part of the decision making and consent process. Fortunately, the risks are very low, for example, following breast, prostate, bladder, lung and rectal cancers, but women who received radiotherapy to their chest area before 25 years of age have almost twice the risk of breast cancer later in life. Likewise, young men with testicular cancer who had received radiotherapy to their abdomen have an increased risk of bowel cancer.

The chance of this happening is also likely to depend on other environmental factors. Workers who have been exposed to asbestos, for example, have four times the normal risk of developing cancer of the lining of the lung (mesothelioma). Those who have also smoked have a 10 times increased risk. This synergistic affect has also been identified in survivors of the Nagasaki and Hiroshima nuclear bombs, who were exposed to significant, but initially non-fatal, radiation outside the blast zones. Two groups were identified, and their lifestyles studied and followed for several years. The group that had a healthy lifestyle had an incidence of cancer similar to the general population. The group with an unhealthy lifestyle had more than 20 times increased incidence of cancer. A logical interpretation of the evidence from these two studies is that you can increase or reduce your genetic or acquired risk of second cancers by the way you live.

What can you do to reduce your risks?

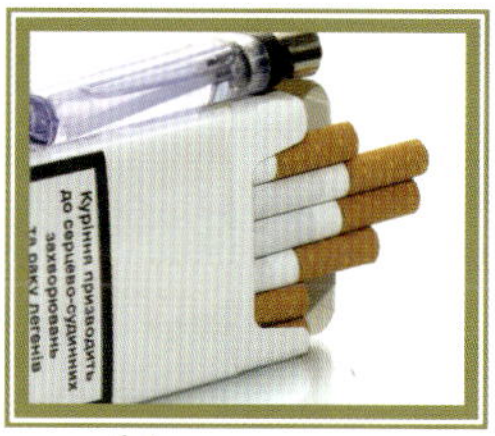

Firstly, reduce your exposure to other factors which further cause genetic damage, such as smoking, excessive sun exposure, and environmental and dietary cancer-inducing chemicals. Secondly, increase activities which have been shown to stabilise or help repair a genetic defect. Olive oil, for example, is reported to help repair DNA damage. An experiment in mice highlighted the major benefits of olive oil on skin: two groups of nude mice (without fur) were kept in a comfortable environment and exposed to ultraviolet light during the day. One group had olive oil massaged into their skin every evening. At six months the olive oil group had dramatically fewer skin cancers and fairly normal skin for the age of the mouse, compared with the others which were covered in skin cancers, dry, thin, aged and cracked skin – just like humans who over-expose themselves. Further tests demonstrated that the oil had repaired the DNA damage caused by the sun, before it had time to do any harm. For humans, as the risks of skin cancers are higher after cancer treatments, it makes sense to treat your skin with more care.

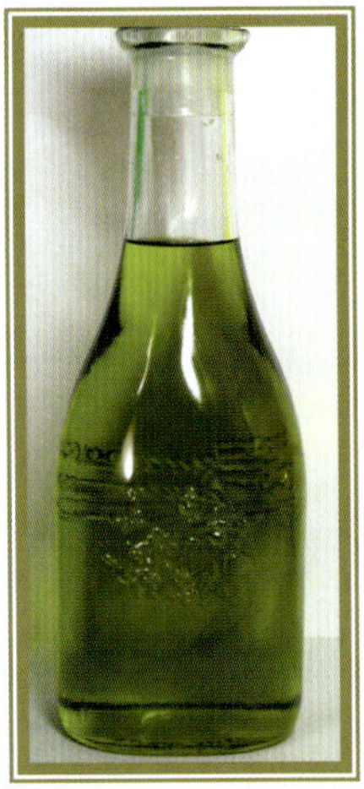

As well as healthy dietary measures, a good tip is to massage olive oil over sun-exposed or previously irradiated skin for five minutes before taking a shower, especially if you have been in the sun. This will also improve the general condition of your skin. The Roman gladiators had a great idea: they used to go into their steam baths and smother themselves with olive oil, then scrape it off into pots to be sold to admiring housewives. Most good gyms have a steam room, although it is probably not a good idea to massage oil into your skin in the room itself. Instead, consider making a habit of taking some oil into the shower after exercising, and applying it before going to the steam room, to avoid people slipping on the floor after you.

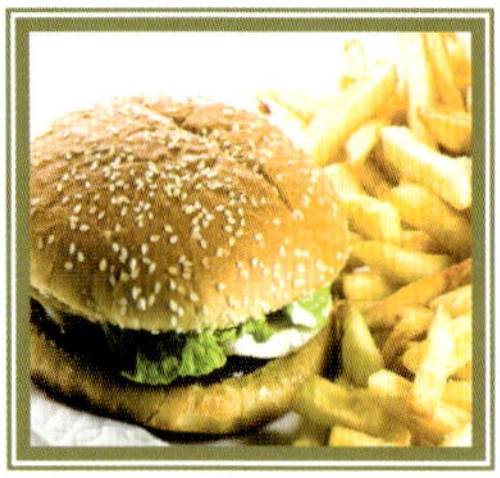

Summary – reduce the risk of treatment-related second cancers:

- Stop smoking – if you do
- Reduce exposure to harmful chemicals in the diet or environment
- Avoid excessive sun exposure and sun burning
- Avoid excessive alcohol
- Increase your levels of exercise (ideally greater than 2.5hrs)
- Eat more antioxidants, healthy oils, fibre, essential vitamins and minerals
- Consider nutritional testing to optimise levels of essential micronutrients
- Eat healthy fats and avoid unhealthy ones
- Sun bathe sensibly
- Attend for screening – e.g. breast mammograms and cervical smears
- After bowel cancer have regular colonoscopies
- Use olive oil on your skin before showering, sauna or steam bath

Chapter Twenty

Complementary therapies
Advice and guidance

Despite the lack of evidence from well conducted studies there is still a strong desire for supportive and complementary medicine from patients. This may reflect the emotional distress and side effects which have not been relieved by conventional medicine, or simply a desire from patients to be more holistic and be involved in their own management, decisions and destiny. The whole subject of complementary medicine is a vast, historic subject and to give it full credit is certainly outside the scope of this book.

Massage

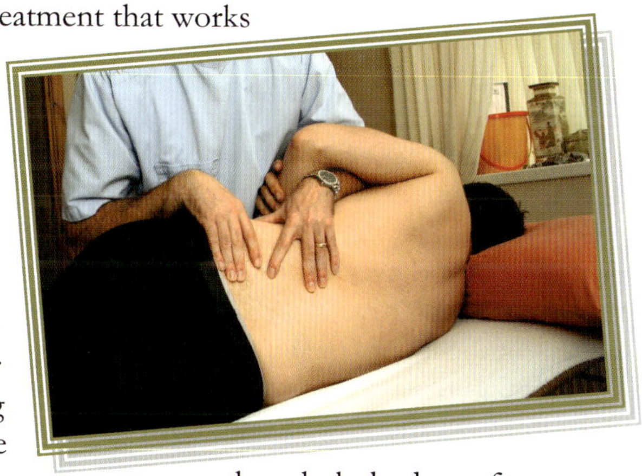

Massage therapy is a system of treatment that works by stroking, kneading, tapping or pressing the soft tissues of the body to relax it physically and mentally. Massage therapy involves the manipulation of the soft tissues and may concentrate on muscles or on acupuncture points. It can vary from simply holding someone or light touching and stroking through to deep, intensive kneading and probing. It may cover the whole body or focus on a particular area. It can be used with or without oils and lotions.

There are many differing types of massage but the most common are;

- Swedish massage – most common of all types of all-over body massage.
- Deep tissue massage – used for long standing, deep muscular problems.
- Sports massage – used before or after sport or to help heal sports injuries.
- Neuromuscular massage – helps balance the nervous system and muscles.

Massage has been used for thousands of years to promote healing and well-being. Along with its relaxing and soothing properties, there is reasonably good evidence that it helps:

- Reduce stress and anxiety.
- Provide a human touch.
- Elevate mood and reduce depression.
- Alleviate muscular pain.

All these benefits mean that many people with cancer may well find massage a help in coping with their condition. It does not suit everyone but could be a safe, positive addition to conventional treatments, although there is no evidence that it actually helps in curing or controlling cancer in any way.

Is massage safe?

There is an ill informed urban myth that massage has safety issues in people who have had cancer. This stems from an idea that massage might increase the spread of cancer cells around the body. There is no evidence at all for this. On the contrary, people who have had radiotherapy or surgical procedures such as mastectomy greatly benefit from massage combined with stretching and exercise as this helps break down fibrous bands and adhesions which cause restriction of movement and pain. Furthermore, gentle massage for lymphoedema of the limbs can often relieve the discomfort and reduce the amount of fluid in the limb. Lymphoedema massage, known as manual lymphatic drainage, MLD, is best performed by an experienced professional.

Side effects and precautions?

Most people don't have any side effects from having a massage. You may feel a bit light headed, tired or thirsty afterwards. Your massage therapist may offer you a glass of water when your treatment has finished. You should not be hurried into getting up and leaving until you feel comfortable. Massage therapists say you should drink plenty of water after your treatment to get rid of toxins released from the body tissues during massage. If you have just received radiotherapy and the skin is still red, avoid rubbing this area, which includes massage. Also avoid massage to any part of the body where the skin is broken, bleeding or bruised.

Tips on finding a good masseur

It is very important that you have your treatment with a qualified therapist. Some cancer centres and hospitals in the UK now offer patients different types of massage therapy and you should ask if this option exists at the hospital where you are having treatment. If the massage is not available they may have information on voluntary organisations that offer complementary therapies, free of charge or at reduced cost. If none of the above is available, information on private therapists may be obtained from the unit, but it is most important that you use only qualified therapists.

Currently there is no single professional organisation that regulates the massage profession in the UK. Therapists can join several associations but there is no law to say they have to. Nor do they have to finish any specific training, but most reputable masseurs will belong to one of the recognised organisations.

It is better that the person who massages you is properly trained and qualified. The best way to find a reliable therapist is to:

- contact one of the professional organisations and ask for a list of therapists or masseurs in your area.
- ask the therapist how many years of training they have undertaken
- How long they have been practicing
- Have they treated cancer patients before
- Ask if they have indemnity insurance

Homeopathy

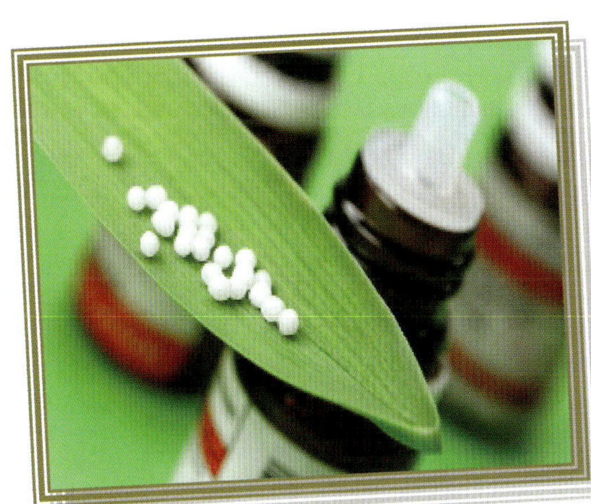

Homeopathic remedies are water (and sometimes alcohol) based solutions containing small amounts of certain naturally occurring plants, minerals, animal products, or chemicals. The term "homeopathy" comes from the Greek words "homoios" (similar) and "pathos" (suffering).

Some practitioners claim homeopathy can help cancer patients by reducing pain, improving vitality and well-being, stopping the spread of cancer, and strengthening the immune system. Some claim it can relieve certain side effects of radiation, chemotherapy and hormone therapy, such as infections, nausea, vomiting, mouth sores, hot flushes, hair loss, depression, and fatigue.

What is the evidence?

Two laboratory experiments published in 2006 found that homeopathic solutions had no effect on breast or prostate cancer cells growing in laboratory cultures. In a recent overview of all available clinical homeopathic trials conducted at the Royal Homeopathic Hospital in London a number had reported psychological improvement including increased hope and optimism. No study showed an actual direct anti-tumour effect. One study, involving extract of calendula, showed it reduced skin reaction during and after radiotherapy.

What does the treatment involve?

On your first visit the homeopath will ask you general questions regarding your health, medical history, lifestyle and diet. They might ask you about your moods, emotions and sleeping patterns. All the gathered information about you will help them to decide on the appropriate remedy for you. Homeopathic remedies come in the form of tablets, granules, powder or liquid and can be taken by mouth or as creams or drops. Your therapist will explain you how to take your remedies and when to come back for the check up. If you decide to use homeopathic treatment, *it is important to let your specialist doctor know about your intention to do so.* And your homeopath must be aware of your cancer ongoing cancer treatments.

Side effects and risks

Homeopathic remedies are generally safe. The main criticism of homeopathy is that a few misguided individuals rely on this type of treatment alone, and avoid or delay undergoing conventional medical care, which may have serious health consequences. Another potential adverse effect is the price. It is a good idea to ask how much a homeopathy consultation will cost before you book it and to get some idea of how much the remedies are or whether the price is included in the consultation charge. You can get free treatment in one of the UK NHS homeopathic hospitals, but you will have to pay for the remedies.

Finding a practitioner

To get more information about how to find a reliable qualified therapist contact one of the following organisations who can supply you with a list of registered professionals and hospitals that practice homeopathy. They can give you advice on how and where to get homeopathy treatment both privately and on the NHS:

- The British Homeopathic Association
- The Council of Organisations Registering Homeopaths

You will need a referral from your local doctor to get the treatment in one of the UK NHS Hospitals which include:

- Bristol Homeopathic Hospital, Cotham Hill, Cotham, Bristol.
- Glasgow Homeopathic Hospital, Great Western Road, Glasgow.
- Liverpool Homeopathic Hospital, Park Avenue, Liverpool.
- Royal London Homeopathic Hospital, Great Ormond St, London.
- Tunbridge Wells Homeopathic Hospital, Church Road, Tunbridge Wells.

Reflexology

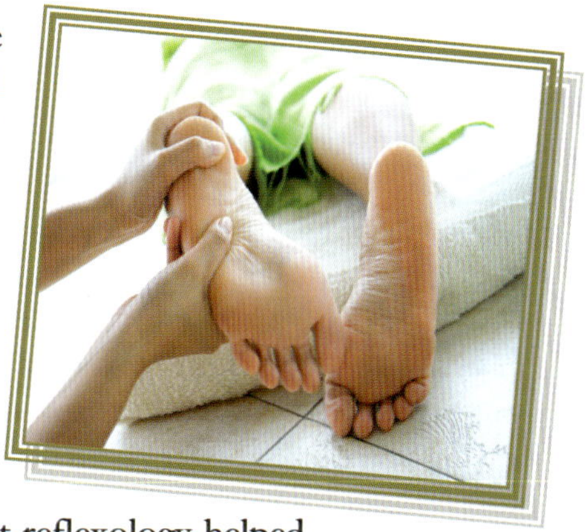

Reflexology originates in traditional Chinese medicine and consists of identifying and treating energy imbalances in the body through massage of reflexology points in specific areas of the feet or hands. The alternative theory is that reflexology enhances a relaxation response which has been shown to improve quality of life, reduce muscular tension and enhance mood.

A small randomised trial showed that reflexology helped reduce anxiety before and during chemotherapy. Other studies have demonstrated a benefit for premenstrual syndrome including irritability and anxiety. The largest and best conducted trial of reflexology was published in the European Journal of Cancer in 2010 and was co-ordinated from Hull University and involved 183 women with breast cancer. Post surgery they were randomised to six weeks of weekly reflexology, or head massage or routine self care. The results showed a significant benefit from both reflexology and head massage in terms of quality of life as well as feeling relaxed and in a good mood. The reflexology appeared to benefit all groups of patients including those receiving radiotherapy, chemotherapy, hormones and herceptin.

Reflexology is not routinely available in oncology units, although some have volunteers from time to time. Perhaps with this benefit demonstrated in well conducted trials health care providers need to consider it as an integral part of the management of breast cancer. In the meantime, there are numerous private reflexology practitioners available throughout the UK but it would be wise to ensure they are suitably qualified and experienced.

Herbal therapies

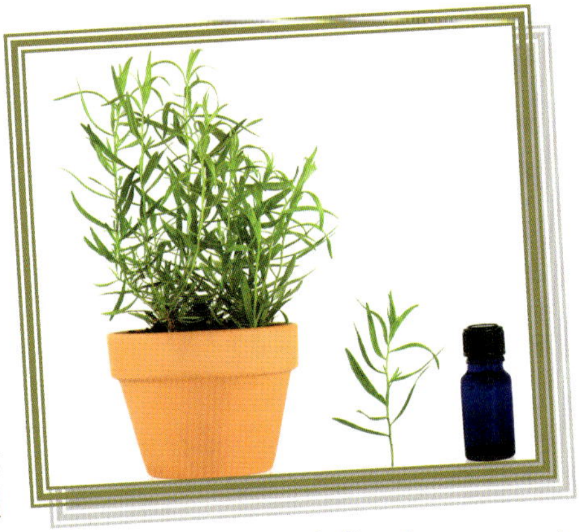

There is no doubt some herbal remedies could potentially have enormous benefits but many of the studies lack sufficient numbers or quality control to form solid conclusions. In this section herbal remedies which may cause harm are highlighted:

Caution should be taken with excessive herbal intake, especially in supplement form during chemotherapy or biological therapies. Antioxidant polyphenols in green tea may potentially decrease the efficacy of the cancer drug bortezomib (Velcade) and other boronic-acid proteasome inhibitors. Among the most widely used herbal supplements is St John's Wort (Hypericum perforatum), believed to have anti-depressant properties. This interacts with the liver enzyme (CYP3A4) decreasing the concentration of the chemotherapy drugs irinotecan, docetaxol and the biological agent imatinib. Although the evidence for a number of other supplements is less positive, potential interactions have been reported with echinacea, grape seed and gingko. Ephedra can increase blood pressure during cancer therapies and can compromise biological agents such as sutent and nexavar, and kava-kava can increase the risk of liver damage.

Yerba mate tea: Lifelong drinkers have been shown to be at increased risk of developing some cancers. Two studies finding that regular consumption of yerba mate – a tea native to South America that is gaining popularity for its high caffeine and antioxidant content – increased the risk of lung, respiratory or digestive cancers by as much as 60 percent. This study was complicated by the high smoking rates among these tea drinkers, but certainly excess intake should be avoided.

Aristolochic acid found in some Chinese herbal products such as Mu Tong and Fangchi, has been shown to significantly increase the risk for urinary tract cancer, according to a study published in the Journal of the National Cancer Institute. Investigators found that the prescription of more than 60 grams of Mu Tong and consumption of more than 150 mg aristolochic acid were independently associated with an increased risk for urinary tract cancer. This Chinese herbal preparation, taken for weight loss or urinary tract infections, has been banned in several countries, including in Taiwan and in the US.

Acupuncture

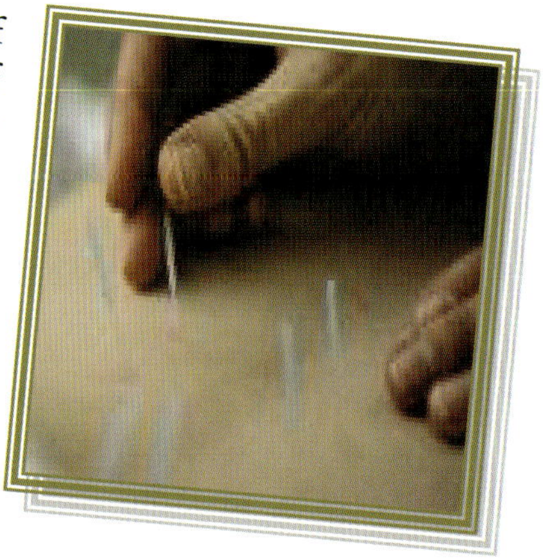

The term "acupuncture" describes a family of procedures involving the stimulation of anatomical points on the body using a variety of techniques. The acupuncture technique that has been most often studied scientifically involves penetrating the skin with thin, solid, metallic needles that are manipulated by the hands or by electrical stimulation. Practiced in China and other Asian countries for thousands of years, acupuncture is one of the key components of traditional Chinese medicine (TCM). In TCM, the body is seen as a delicate balance of two opposing and inseparable forces the *yin* and the *yang* The yin represents the cold, slow, or passive principle, while yang represents the hot, excited, or active principle. According to TCM, health is achieved by maintaining the body in a "balanced state", while disease is due to an internal imbalance of yin and yang. This imbalance leads to blockage in the flow of vital energy along pathways known as meridians. These can apparently be unblocked by using acupuncture at certain points on the body that connect with these meridians. There is some evidence that after cancer acupuncture may help some situations.

Hot flushes:

More recently there was a study published in the well respected Journal of Oncology which demonstrated a benefit for women with hot flushes. The study involved 50 women and compared a standard treatment for hot flushes called venlafexane, an antidepressant, with acupuncture. In the acupuncture group women received treatment twice a week for 12 weeks. They were analysed for a year. Although at two months there was no difference in the number or severity of hot flushes and night sweats, by three months there was a significant reduction from baseline. There was no variance between the two group,s showing that acupuncture was at least as good as the antidepressant. There was however a significant difference in other symptoms between the two groups. Sex drive, fatigue, energy levels, clarity of thought and a sense of well being were all better in the acupuncture group. What's more, acupuncture was safe and had no side effects in this group of women. Results of the study suggest that as well as the measures suggested in the "Tips for hot flushes" section of this book, before considering antidepressants it may be worth considering a course of acupuncture.

Chemotherapy induced nausea:
There have previously been some small studies which have shown that acupuncture can help nausea associated with chemotherapy but these were not particularly convincing. More recently, a study from the University of Rochester USA involving 586 patients receiving chemotherapy randomly evaluated the effect of acupupressure wrist bands which stimulate the P6 acupuncture point. Overall there was a moderate benefit. For women with breast cancer receiving chemotherapy agents which have a high chance of causing nausea, the benefit was greater. No adverse effects were found.

Dry mouth (xerostomia):
A study from Ontorio Canada, evaluated 46 patients who had had radiotherapy to the head and neck area and were suffering from a severe dry mouth. A common side effect if the salivary glands were including the radiotherapy fields. They used an acupuncture point stimulation device twice a week for six weeks and found that dry mouth symptoms significantly improved over the 3-6 month trial. No adverse effects were reported.

Advice when considering acupuncture

Check a practitioner's credentials. Most countries require a licence to practice acupuncture; however education and training standards and requirements for obtaining a licence to practice vary. Although a license does not ensure quality of care, it does indicate that the practitioner meets certain standards regarding the knowledge and use of acupuncture.

Do not rely on a diagnosis of disease by an acupuncture practitioner who does not have substantial conventional medical training. If you have received a diagnosis from a doctor, you may wish to ask your doctor whether acupuncture might help.

Use a reputable source; shop around and ask your GP, as some have trained and qualified in acupuncture, although this usually requires payment from yourself. Alternatively, ask your GP if they have a funding link to the Royal Homeopathic Hospital where it may then be available on the NHS.

Chapter Twenty one

Conclusions

Final comments

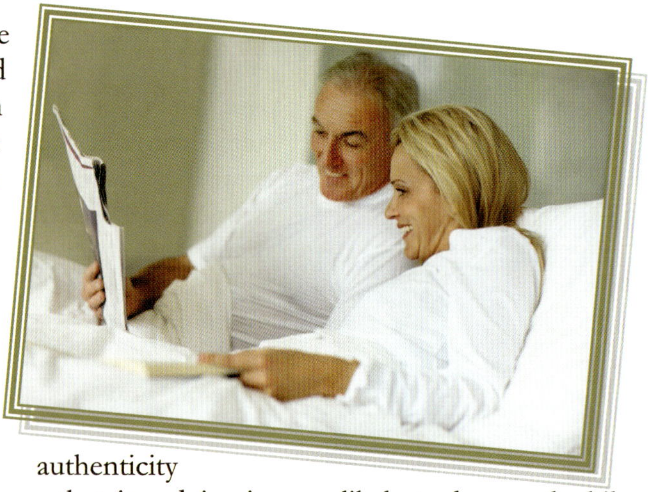

It is hoped that the information, background explanation and guidance in the chapters you have just read have provided you with the motivation and incentive to take up the challenge of a change in lifestyle. As emphasised in several chapters, the source information for this book is based solely on bona fide published evidence; its authenticity hopefully bestows a reassurance that its advice is very likely to be worthwhile despite the hard work and determination which would be required to achieve this. There is no doubt that many people will benefit in one way or another, whether to reduce the risks or side effects of treatments, to slow the cancer growth, or help prevent it relapsing after the initial intensive treatments have subsided. Despite these reassurances, it must be emphasised that not everyone will benefit from these lifestyle changes and, likewise, not everyone will have the physical capacity or resources to do so. Furthermore, not everyone will want to embark on a major change in the way they live, even if they understand the risks. This, of course, is entirely up to them – it is their choice and they should not be made to feel guilty. There may be many good reasons why a citizen of our society, with cancer or otherwise, chooses to live as they do. As long as they do not harm other people, then the choice is entirely their own. If a person chooses a greater or lesser level of intensity of treatment, or one treatment over another, then, provided they are fully informed, the decision is correct for them and should be respected. Likewise, a patient's choice for the intensity of lifestyle they wish to lead is also entirely their own.

In the meantime, although it has been said many times before, the premise to a healthy diet lies in diversity and balance. The body's cancer defence mechanisms do not work efficiently either when deprived of essential nutrients or when poisoned by excess unwanted chemicals. A balanced diet is likely to avoid these extremes. The definition of balance, however, needs clarifying further as there is a popular misconception that it refers to the balance between healthy and unhealthy lifestyle factors. A classic example is the popular excuse amongst smokers, "Well, I don't drink, so I can smoke".

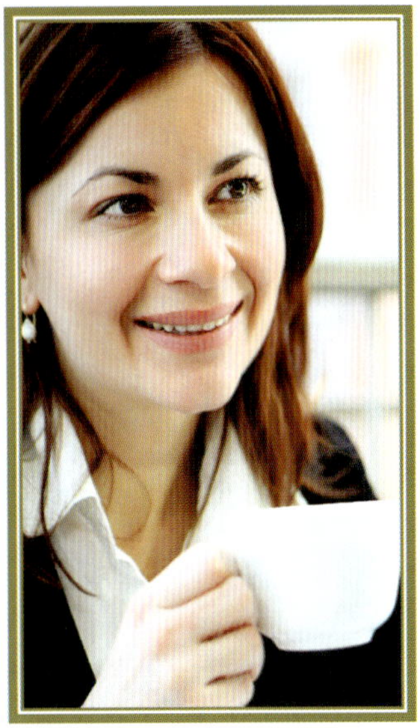

Balance, in anti-cancer dietary terms, refers to the interaction of different types of healthy foods. Bad or carcinogenic foods should simply be avoided as much as is feasible, within the parameters of our lifestyles, societies and the cultures in which we live. If, for example, you are invited to a barbeque, instead of being a martyr and refusing all food, making your host uncomfortable, simply make sure you consume foods or drinks with plenty of antioxidants at the same time to counterbalance the acrylamides present on the burnt meat. The remaining part of this book gives a guide to how best to achieve a healthy balanced cancer diet. For ease of explanation, this section has been divided into two sections: *What to do* in order to avoid substances that can promote cancer growth and progression, and *what not to do.*

When is the best time to start acting?

Shortly after a diagnosis of cancer you and your relatives would have been confronted by a sudden deluge of activity, often travelling back and forth to the hospital for blood tests, x-rays, scans, biopsies, operations, chemotherapy, radiotherapy, hormones and, more recently, biological therapies such as herceptin. This causes enormous upheaval to the daily routine – both socially and at the work place. Most of the available time is taken up adjusting to the new diagnosis, coping with the side effects of therapy and the difficulties of remembering where and when they have to be and what to do when they get there! Forcing yourself, or a patient you may be close to, into a lifestyle strategy which cannot be adhered to for practical or physical reasons would be inappropriate, and may project an unnecessary feeling of guilt. The timing is paramount; too early and the anxieties of the circumstances will be confounded, too late and the benefits of lifestyle will be overlooked. In practical terms a sensible approach, depending on your circumstances, would be to gradually introduce the concept of a life change agenda at an early point in the treatment pathway, and build up to it gradually, aiming for a long-term change.

Getting started is nearly always a daunting task for those recovering from the battering of cancer and its therapies. Even those who ate well and exercised regularly before their diagnosis may not have the same motivation or abilities afterwards. The cancer itself, surgery or the anti-cancer treatments may have caused physical disability, fatigue, weight gain, reduced esteem and created body image worries. Many, when contemplating exercise, see it as an insurmountable hurdle and regress into the immediate comfort of ignorance. Before this happens it is important that patients and their carers recognise the barriers to their expectations and ask for help, especially as following cancer therapies a more flexible and innovative approach to lifestyle is usually required. With help, patients can relearn their exercise and dietary patterns, often with a broader range of activities they may not have previously contemplated. Hopefully this book has provided some of these new ideas, but you should not be afraid to approach other sensible sources available, such as hospital specialist nurses, your family doctor, physiotherapists and exercise professionals in your local gym. You should not be shy to recruit as many friends and relatives onto the cause as possible because exercising, giving up smoking or dietary change is usually easier with someone else, and can ensure a higher level of motivation, activity and longevity. Furthermore, most people are keen to help, so what better way to make them feel more involved!

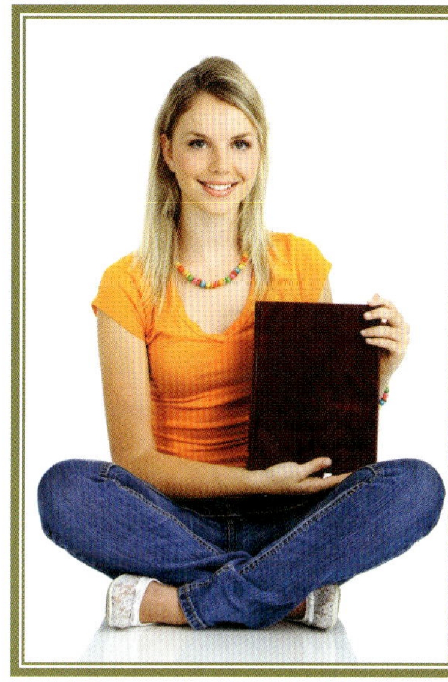

Ignore the 'burger and chips' aficionados:

Despite the overwhelming evidence available from the clinical studies presented in this book, there will remain many clinicians and patients who are not convinced. If an individual does not want to change their own lifestyle for the better this is, of course, entirely their own prerogative. The problem is that these individuals, probably to conceal their own guilt, tend to be quite vocal in the criticism of lifestyle change, often persuading everyone around them that it is not worthwhile. Please smile politely but ignore them.

I always remember one of my first ward rounds as a junior doctor. We were stunned into silence following the comments of one pleasant, but disillusioned, elderly patient when the consultant, rather optimistically, advised him to give up smoking. He had been an in-patient for nine weeks, recovering from bilateral, above-knee amputations of both legs. The years of smoking had hardened his leg arteries so much that he had developed gangrene. He was also a walking, or rather sitting, 'textbook' of smoking-related diseases, keeping medical students entertained for hours. His bladder had been removed due to cancer, so his urine drained into a bag, which had to be changed by nurses. The stroke he had suffered two years previously impaired the use of his left arm. His vision was poor, caused by smoking induced retinal degeneration. He had chronic indigestion and a barrel chest from emphysema. To top it all, a routine chest x-ray that day had picked up a shadow on his lung, which turned out to be cancer. After the consultant asked his pertinent question the guy turned to us, smiling triumphantly and holding a fag in his only good limb (yes, in those days you could smoke in hospital), and with complete sincerity answered; ***'I've been smoking for 25 years and it hasn't done me any harm!'***

This is, of course, an extreme example, but the underlying philosophy of denial adopted by this gentleman is commonplace. We have probably all had brief spells in our past when we have argued to ourselves "Well, I know it's harmful, but it's not going to happen to me". A healthy degree of nihilism from time to time is inevitable. Lets face it, we are human after all! The problem starts arising when this approach to lifestyle becomes the norm. This is often perpetuated by our society. Eating berries, nuts and fruit is often portrayed as 'geeky'. In the movies, healthy eaters are often a source of ridicule, cast as thin, spotty, cycling misfits who never 'get the girl'. You wouldn't see James Bond tucking into a rocket salad or Bruce Willis snacking on Brazil nuts and goji berries. The Marlborough cowboy always looked cool and tough, lassoing a steer whilst smoking. Well, he wasn't asked to model in the adverts after his laryngectomy! On a positive note, society is changing, particularly with attitudes to smoking, and hopefully diet and exercise will follow. In the meantime, it remains a considerable challenge to get the whole cancer patient community to embrace the virtues of a healthy lifestyle.

Other benefits of a lifestyle change:

What has not been described so far are the other, less obvious advantages of taking control of your own activities of daily living. So before you put the book down to rush out to buy a leotard and some organic goji berries, these are worth a mention, as for some of you they may be the most important aspects. They include empowerment, peace of mind and an overall sense of well-being.

Empowerment: Probably the question most frequently asked by patients, their friends or relatives after a diagnosis of cancer is: ***"What can we do to help ourselves?"*** The act of changing your lifestyle will empower you with a feeling of control. Several studies have demonstrated that patients who consider that they have been involved in their own treatment management, and share involvement with their clinicians, have a significantly better sense of well-being compared with those who feel their treatments have been dictated to them by paternalistic carers. Furthermore, patients who embarked on a self-help lifestyle change were better able to distract their minds from more sombre thoughts – and to feel more positive about their own destiny.

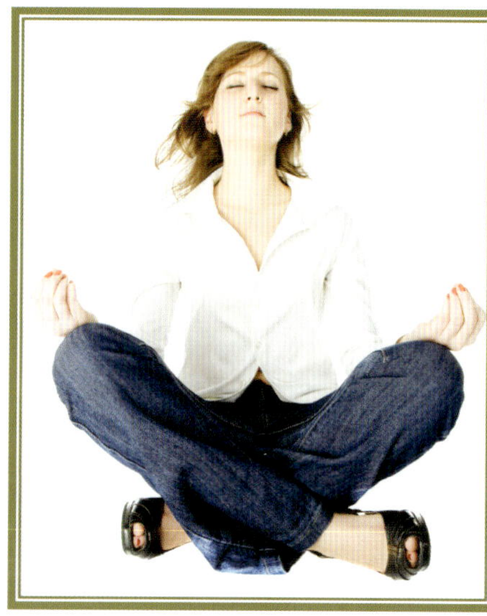

Peace of mind: There is usually an ominous feeling of foreboding among patients after their initial treatment, even if the prognosis is good. What seems to help to alleviate some of these anxieties is the understanding that everything possible has been done to reduce the risk of relapse. It is usually comforting to point out that patients have received good surgery, radiotherapy and well delivered chemotherapy or biological therapies. If patients then undertake a healthy lifestyle programme, there is really nothing else they could do to prevent their cancer coming back. In my experience as a cancer specialist, and having the privilege of meeting over 3,000 patients in the last ten years, the peace of mind that everything possible has been done is a major reassurance as time goes by. If cancer does return or progress, although of course devastating, patients don't have to contend with the nagging doubt that it could have been prevented.

General health and well-being: There are numerous other benefits to an improved lifestyle. Exercise, particularly group classes, gets you out of the house, meeting people and making friends. Diets with reduced saturated fats, more fruit and vegetables and less meat, reduce cholesterol and blood pressure, preventing the need for expensive statins and blood pressure lowering medication. A healthy lifestyle has a positive influence on your digestive system, reducing the need for anti-indigestion medication and laxatives, both of which cost the health service in the UK millions of pounds each year.

The personal cost of unhealthy living is a lot higher. Keeping fit and healthy means more energy and stamina to play and interact with your children and grandchildren, as well as participating in sport and social interaction with friends and relatives. It keeps your mind clear to enjoy intellectual conversations and can improve your ability to enjoy a loving and sensual relationship.

Very often patients with an early cancer who have changed to a healthy lifestyle start feeling the benefits, and have even been heard to comment: "This is the best I've felt for years!"

No blame – just encouragement

This book is designed to encourage individuals to optimise their lifestyle and those who do so should be rewarded and congratulated for their efforts. This book, however, does not aim to blame any patients for their cancer diagnosis, or even suggest that a previous way of life has contributed to their current situation. If that message has emerged, then this book has failed in its endeavours. In any case, even if a previous lifestyle has been a factor in the diagnosis, there is no use worrying about it now. Instead, the book aims to encourage and reassure individuals that an improvement in lifestyle is worthwhile at any stage – from now or in the future. Likewise, although it guides individuals to sensible and useful strategies relevant to a post-cancer diagnosis, it does not aim to exert blame if you cannot, or do not, wish to participate. Furthermore, although the evidence described shows that a healthy lifestyle after cancer improves the chances of a better outcome, it does not guarantee these benefits. Even the most motivated of individuals may well suffer a relapse of their disease or see their cancers growing, despite the best will in the world.

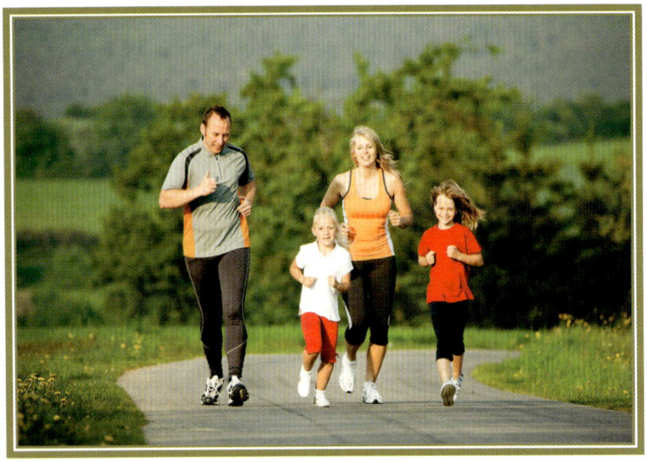

Keep focused and aim for the long-term.

Having bought the kitchen gadgets, stocked your pantry with healthy food, joined the gym and squeezed into a leotard, these would be hollow gestures unless they are kept up for the long-term. Although getting started is difficult, keeping going for the long term requires focus and determination, especially if no immediate benefits are seen. Losing weight can appear particularly unrewarding. Despite pounding the streets, living off lettuce leaves and standing on the scales, at least initially seeing no change can be especially discouraging. It is only those who are able to keep motivated, when the novelty has worn off, that see the favourable results start to appear. The path to a healthy lifestyle may also not be easy and not everyone around you will be supportive. Some people, even if their intention is humorous, can make you feel self-conscious when taking part in healthy activities, implying they are the domain of the rich and beautiful! Likewise, if anyone makes comments like "It's a bit late now", smile and give them a copy of this book.

Some years ago now a very overweight man was jogging around a running track at the same time that our athletics team was training. He was sweating profusely, despite running painfully slowly, and clearly not enjoying himself; nevertheless every member of the athletics team had complete respect for his efforts. But shortly after he started two youths walking past shouted: ***" Come on fatty, get your knees up"*** . The coach, normally a mild tempered man, approached the two boys with a pair of running spikes and asked them, with polite sarcasm, if they would like to join in? They looked embarrassed and we laughed – at them. We all went for a drink afterwards with the man, who, it turned out, had an older brother who had died recently of bowel cancer. He had decided to change his life. He became known as the 'big guy', not because he was overweight, but because of his courage to get out there and exercise despite the taunts. That was ten years ago and he has now lost five stone and regularly runs ten kilometre 'fun runs' in less than 55 minutes.

It is most important to ensure that all patients and their carers are sufficiently empowered with the correct lifestyle knowledge, so that whatever choices are made are based on accurate, relevant and proven facts. Unfortunately, formal and anecdotal reports from patients have repeatedly shown that this was not always possible, as lifestyle advice was often less than forthcoming. For this reason, I have been prompted to write this book, with the enormous support and input from colleagues and, above all, patients and relatives who have been affected by cancer. Hopefully the guidance in these chapters will fill the gaps in the advice given to you by mainstream oncology centres, and will help you and others with the fundamental lifestyle choices which are inevitable in the ups and downs of the cancer treatment pathway ahead.

Good luck!

APPENDIX

Professor Robert J Thomas Mb ChB MRCP MD FRCR

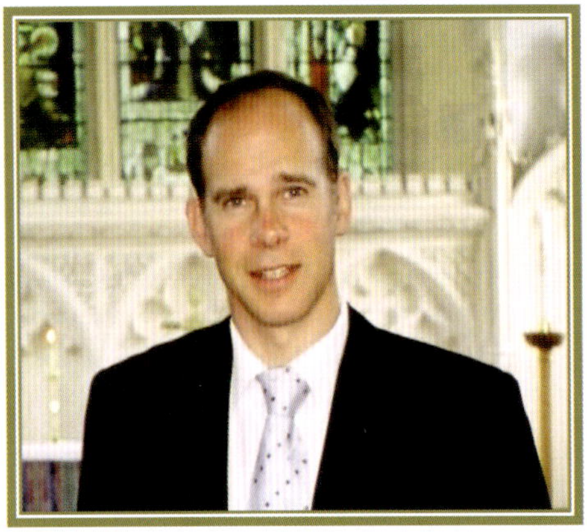

Trained in cancer medicine (Oncology) and research at a number London Hospitals including The Royal Free, Mount Vernon, Middlesex and Royal Marsden Hospitals. Current posts include: Visiting Professor of Postgraduate Medicine at Cranfield University; Director of the Primrose Oncology Research Unit, Bedford; Consultant Oncologist at Addenbrooke's Hospital Cambridge; Clinical teacher of medical students at Cambridge University.

Medical interests include the treatment of breast, colon and prostate cancers with chemotherapy, hormone therapy, biological therapies, radiotherapy and brachytherapy (radioactive seed insertion into tumours).

Research interests include designing and conducting studies to find out how lifestyle affects the development and progression of cancer. This includes the world's largest prospective lifestyle trial involving men with progressive prostate cancer. These works have been recognised by the UK Hospital Doctor Magazine "Hospital Doctor of the Year" and the Pfizer / British Oncology Association "Oncologist of the Year" and the UK NHS Communication Prize. The results of these studies have been published and presented in talks and conferences in throughout Europe as well as the USA, Australia and Mexico.

Since the first edition of this book, he was commissioned by Macmillan Cancer Relief to summarise the world evidence for their National Survivorship Programme and now leads their National Exercise Advisory committee. He has written the UK National Standards (for Skills Active) for the first Cancer Rehabilitation training course for level 4 registered Exercise Professionals. He has been appointed a member of the National Cancer Research Network committee on Complementary Medicine.

Where to find extra resources?

Cancernet-UK (www.cancernet.co.uk) has over 500 pages of information related to cancer management and therapies, ranging from chemotherapy, active surveillance, hormones, radiotherapy, cryotherapy and biological therapies. It includes information on the side effects and advice to help cope with them. It has links to services which are often required by individuals with cancer such as travel insurance, support groups and clinical trials. It has links to web sites which can search for exercise facilities in your area based on your local post code. Through cancernet.co.uk you can order a number of products which have been referred to in this book, which may be useful during cancer therapies and afterwards:

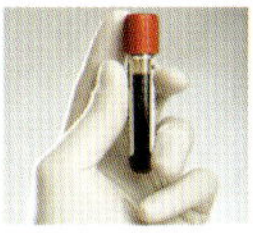

Micro-nutritional blood analysis and advisory report – a blood test which measures over 50 essential nutrients which are important for the body to help fight cancer and other diseases.

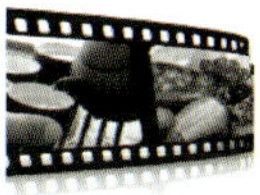

A preparatory information video "Chemotherapy & Radiotherapy" which as been evaluated in a randomised trial and shown to reduce anxiety and depression.

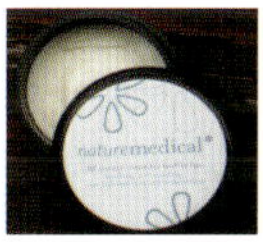

Natural essential oil based organic skin products from "*natureMedical*"

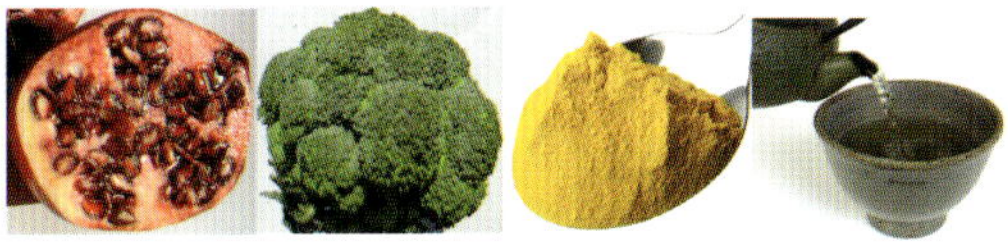

Super-food anti-oxidant boost: A combination of four whole foods simply dried and put into a dietary capsule.

Other useful websites:

- Cancer relief Macmillan; Macmillan.org.uk
- Breast cancer information and support; Breakthrough.org.uk
- Independent breast research; Breastcancercampaign.org
- Prostate cancer Information; Prostate-cancer.co.uk
- Keep health website; Keep-healthy.com
- Lung cancer information and support; Roycastle.org
- UK cancer research; Cancerresearchuk.org

Other relevant publications by the author

'Patient Information materials in Oncology: Are they needed and do they work?' Thomas R, and H Thorton. *Clinical Oncology,* 1999; 11; 225-231.

'The changing face of informed consent'. R Thomas. *British Journal of Cancer Management*, 2004, vol. 1 No. 1. pp 11-15.

'NICE guidance on supportive and palliative care – Implications for Oncology Teams'. R Thomas and Alison Richardson. *Clinical Oncology,* 2004, 16: 420-424.

'How to deal with the complexities of patient consent?' R Thomas. *Pulse Clinical*, 2003; 1,42-43.

'Complementary and alternative medicine evidence for cancer'. J Richardson, K Pilkington, R Thomas. *British Journal of Cancer Management*, 2005, vol.2, 2:10-12.

'Diet, salicylates and their effect on prostate cancer'. Robert Thomas, Cathryn Woodward, Peter Williams. *British Journal of Cancer Management*, 2006, vol. 3, 1:5-9.

'Adjuvant breast cancer drugs- blockbusters or bankrupters?' Thomas R, Glen J and Callam M. *British Journal of Cancer Management*, 2006, vol. 24, 3: 5-9

'Can dietary intervention alter prostate cancer progression'. R Thomas, Mabel Blades and Madeleine Williams. *Nutrition & Food Science*, 2007, vol. 37, 1: 24-36.

'Cancer – the roles of exercise in prevention and progression'. Robert Thomas and Nichola Davies. *Nutrition & Food Science*, 2007, vol. 37, 5: 3-10.

'Lifestyle During & after cancer treatments'. Thomas R, Davies N. *Clinical Oncology*, 2007, 19: 616-627

'Modifying the Barthel index score for use with patients with brain tumours'. R.Thomas, F Hines, M Brada. *European Journal of Cancer Care,* 1995, vol.4,. 63-68.

'Modifying the Quality of Life Barthel index for use in patients with brain tumours – an update'. R Thomas. *European Journal of Cancer Care*, 1997, 6:2-6.

'Patient preferences for video cassette recorded information. Effect of age, sex and ethnic group'. Thomas R, Deary A and Kaminski E. *European Journal of Cancer Care*, 1999, 8, 1999

'Forewarned is forearmed – benefits of information on video for patients receiving chemotherapy and radiotherapy- a randomised trial'. Thomas R. *European Journal of Cancer,* 2000, 36: 1536-1543.

'Examining quality of life issues in relation to endocrine therapy for breast cancer'. Robert Thomas. *American Journal of Clinical Oncology*, 2003, 26, 4: 40-44

'Measuring information strategies in oncology – developing an information satisfaction questionnaire'. Thomas R et al. *Euro J Cancer Care*, 2004, 13, 65-70.

'Black Cohosh for menopausal symptoms in women with breast cancer'. J Smith, J Richardson, R Thomas and K Pilkington. 2003.

'Patient Information – patients in clinical trials are more satisfied'. R. Thomas and M Williams. *European Journal of Cancer*, 2005, vol. 3, 2: 384.

'Can we move to a paperless information system?' A Deary and R Thomas. *European Journal of Cancer*, 2005, vol. 3, 2: 460.

'Giving patients a choice improves quality of life: A multi-centre, investigator-blind, randomised, crossover study comparing letrozole with anastrozole'. R. Thomas, S.et al *Clinical Oncology*, 2004, 16: 485-491.

'Dietary advice combined with a salicylate, mineral and vitamin supplement has some tumour static properties'. R Thomas, M Blades and M Williams. *Nutrition & Food Science,* 2005, vol. 35, 6: 436- 451

'Aloe Vera for preventing radiation-induced skin reaction: A literature review'. J Richardson, R Thomas and K Pilkington. *Clinical Oncology*, 2005, 17:478-484.

'Empowering patients to make informed decisions by measuring their needs and satisfaction'. N Davies, R Thomas. *Clinical Focus Cancer Medicine*, 2007, vol. 1, 1:3-8

'Is there a need for lifestyle clinics in Oncology?' R Thomas and M Williams. *Clinical Focus Cancer Medicine*, 2008, vol. 2, 1: 10-12.

Other reference sources for this book

Ades PA et al (1992) Cardiac rehabilitation participation predicts lower rehospitalization costs. Am Heart J. 1992 Apr; 123(4 Pt 1):916-21.

Adlercreutz H et al (1986) Urinary estrogen profile determination in young Finnish vegetarian and omnivorous women. J Steroid Biochem. 24: p. 289-95.

Allen N et al. (2009). "Moderate Alcohol Intake and Cancer Incidence in Women." J. Natl. Cancer Inst. 101(5): 296-305.

Amling C, et al (2004) Pathologic variables and recurrence rates as related to obesity and race in men with prostate cancer undergoing radical prostatectomy. J Clin Oncol., 22: 439-445.

Augustsson K, et al. (2003) A prospective study of intake of fish and marine fatty acids and prostate cancer. Cancer Epidemiol Biomarkers Prevent, 12: 64-67.

Baron JA, et al (2003) A randomised trial of aspirin to prevent colorectal adenomas. The New England Journal of Medicine, 348(10): p. 891-899.

Baxter RC and Turtle JR (1978) Regulation of hepatic growth hormone receptors by insulin. Biochem Biophys Res Commun, 84: p. 350-7.

Berwick M, et al (2005)Sun exposure and mortality from melanoma. J Natl Cancer Inst ;97:195–9.

Blacklock CJ, et al (2001) Salicylic acid in the serum of subjects not taking aspirin. Comparison of salicylic acid concentrations in the serum of vegetarians, non-vegetarians, and patients taking low dose aspirin. J Clin Pathology, 54: p. 553-5.

Blot W et al (1993) Nutrition intervention in Linxian, China: supplementation with specific vitamin/mineral combinations, cancer incidence, and disease-specific mortality in the general population. J. Natl. Cancer Inst, 85: 1483-1492.

Blutt SE, et al (2000) Calcitriol-induced apoptosis in LNCaP cells is blocked by overexpression of bcl-2. Endocrinology, 141: p. 10-17.

Campell MJ, Koeffler HP (1997) Toward therapeutic intervention of cancer by vitamin D compounds. J Natl Cancer Inst, 89: p. 182-185.

Chan JM, Gann PH, and Giovannucci EL (2005) Role of diet in prostate cancer development and progression. Journal of Clinical Oncology, 23(32): p. 8152-60.

Chaudry AA, et al (1994) Arachidonic acid metabolism in benign and malignant prostatic tissue in vitro: Effects of fatty acids and cyclooxygenase inhibitors. Int J Cancer, 57: p. 176-180.

Chen L, et al. (2001) Oxidative DNA damage in prostate cancer patients consuming tomato sauce-based entrees as a whole-food intervention. J Natl Cancer Inst, 93: p. 1872-1879.

Cheng, M (2009) Tanning beds are as deadly as arsenic, cancer study says. http://www.boston.com/news/nation/articles/2009/07/29/cancer_study_shows_tanning_beds_as_deadly_as_arsenic/.

Chlebowski R, Aiello E, and McTiernan A. (2002) Weight loss in breast cancer patient management. J Clin Oncol., 20: p. 1128-1143.

Chlebowski RT, et al The WINS Investigators (2005) Dietary fat reduction in post menopausal women with primary breast cancer. Journal of Clinical Oncology, (10): p. 3s.

Clark LC, et al. (1998) Decreased incidence of prostate cancer with selenium supplementation: results of a double-blind cancer prevention trial. British Journal of Urology, 81: p. 730-734.

Coombs GF (2004) Status of selenium in prostate cancer prevention. British Journal of Cancer, 91: p. 195-199.

Demark-Wahnefried W, et al (2005) Riding the Crest of the Teachable Moment: Promoting Long-Term Health After the Diagnosis of Cancer Journal of Clinical Oncology, Vol 23, No 24 , pp. 5814-5830.

Dieppe P, Ebrahim S, and Juni P (2004) Lessons from the withdrawl from rofecoxib. BMJ, 329: p. 867-868.

Dignam JJ, et al (2006) Effect of body mass index on outcome in patients with dukes B and C colon cancer: An analysis of NSABP trials. Journal of Clinical Oncology, 3533: p. 254s.

Dignam, J. J., B. N. Polite, et al. (2006). "Body Mass Index and Outcomes in Patients Who Receive Adjuvant Chemotherapy for Colon Cancer." J. Natl. Cancer Inst. 98(22): 1647-1654.

Ebbing M, et al (2009) Cancer Incidence and Mortality After Treatment With Folic Acid and Vitamin B12 JAMA. 2009;302(19):2119-2126.

Egan KM, (1996) Prospective study of regular aspirin use and the risk of breast cancer. Journal of the National Cancer Institute, 88: p. 988-993.

Evans BA, (1995) Inhibition of 5 alpha-reductase in genital skin fibroblasts and prostate tissue by dietary lignans and isoflavonoids. Journal of Endocrinology, 147: p. 295-302.

Figueiredo, J., et al. (2009). "Folic Acid and Risk of Prostate Cancer: Results From a Randomized Clinical Trial." J. Natl. Cancer Inst. 101(6): 432-435.

Flowers, M. (2009). Conjugated Linoleic Acid Suppresses HER2 Protein and Enhances Apoptosis in SKBr3 Breast Cancer Cells: Possible Role of COX2." PLoS ONE 4(4): e5342.

Food and Drug Administration (FDA) (2006) Carcinogens and antioxidants.

Fraga CU (1991) Ascorbic acid protects against endogenous oxidative DNA damage in human sperm. Proc Nati Acad Sci USA, 8(8(24)): p. 11003.

Freier S,. (1999) Expression of the insulin-like growth factors and their receptors in adenocarcinoma of the colon. Gut, 44: p. 704-8.

Fuchs C, Mayer RJ (2005) Influence of regular aspirin use on survival for patients with stage III colon cancer: Findings from intergroup trial CALGB 89803. American Society of Clinical Oncology Abstract Book, 2005.

Giles GG and English DR (2002) The Melbourne Collaborative Cohort Study. IARC Sci Publ, 156: p. 69-70.

Giovannucci E, (2002) A prospective study of tomato products, lycopene, and prostate cancer risk. Journal of the National Cancer Institute, 94: p. 391-398.

Gold EB,. (2009) Dietary Pattern Influences Breast Cancer Prognosis in Women Without Hot Flashes: JCO vol 27, no.3; 352-359.

Golden, E., et al. (2009). "Green tea polyphenols block the anticancer effects of bortezomib and other boronic acid-based proteasome inhibitors." Blood 113(23): 5927-5937.

Gong, Z., et al. (2009). "Alcohol consumption, finasteride, and prostate cancer risk." Cancer 115(16): 3661-3669.

Goodwin PJ, (2009) Prognostic Effects of 25-Hydroxyvitamin D Levels in Early Breast Cancer. Journal of Clinical Oncology, Vol 27, No 23: pp. 3757-3763.

Gritz ER (1993) Cancer Smoking Epidemiology Biomarkers & Prevention, 2;(3); 261-270.

Gross M, (2006) Obesity, ethnicity and surgical outcome for clinically localized prostate cancer. Journal of Clinical Oncology, 5(9615 supplement): p. 865.

Hamilton M, (2006) Effects of Smoking on the Pharmacokinetics of Erlotinib. Clinical Cancer Research doi: 10.1158/1078-0432.CCR-05-2235 Clinical Cancer Research April 1, 12, 2166.

Harris RE,. (1996) Nonsteroidal antiinflammatory drugs and breast cancer. Epidemiology, 7: p. 203-205.

Harvei S (1997) Prediagnostic level of fatty acids in serum phospholipids: Omega-3 and omega-6 fatty acids and the risk of prostate cancer. Int J Cancer, 71;545-551.

Hayes SC (2009) Australian Association for Exercise and Sport Science position stand: Optimising cancer outcomes through exercise. J.Sci.Med.Sport. 2009;12:428-434.

Haydon A (2006) The effect of physical activity and body size on survival after diagnosis with colorectal cancer. Gut, 55: p. 62-67.

Heinonen OP. (1998) Prostate cancer and supplementation with alpha-tocopherol and beta carotene: Incidence and mortality in a controlled trial. J Natl Cancer Inst, 90: p. 440-446.

Hippisley-Cox J (2005) Risk of myocardial infarction in patients taking cyclo-oxygenase-2 inhibitors or conventional non-steroidal anti-inflammatory drugs: population based nested case-control analysis. BMJ 330: p. 1366-1369.

Holick CN, (2008)Physical Activity and Survival after Diagnosis of Invasive Breast Cancer. Cancer Epidemiological Biomarkers Prev., PP. 379-386.

Holmes MD, (1999) Dietary factors and the survival of women with breast cancer. Cancer, 85(5): p. 826-35.

Holmes MD, (2005) Physical activity and survival after breast cancer diagnosis. JAMA, 293: p. 2479-86.

Hsieh T and Wu JM, (1997) Induction of apoptosis and altered nuclear - cytoplasmic distribution of the androgen receptor and prostate-specific antigen Biochemical and biophysical research communications, 235: p. 539-544.

Hsu AL, CS (2000) The cyclooxygenases-2 inhibitor celecoxib induces apoptosis by blocking Akt activation in human prostate cancer cells independently of Bcl-2. Journal of Biological Chemistry, 275: p. 11397-11403.

Jackson MJ, (2004) Are there functional consequences of a reduction in selenium intake in UK subjects? Proceedings of the Nutrition Society, 63: p. 513-517.

Jolliffe JA, (2000) Exercise-based rehabilitation for coronary heart disease Jolliffe JA, Rees K,Cochrane Database Syst Rev.;(4):CD001800.

Joseph A, (2007) Cruciferous Vegetables, Genetic Polymorphisms in Glutathione S-Transferases M1 and T1, and Prostate Cancer Risk Michael A. NUTRITION AND CANCER, 50(2), 206–213.

Kaaks R (2002) Effects of weight control and physical activity in cancer prevention: role of endogenous hormones. Ann N Y Acad Sci, 963:. 268-81.

Klein A (2009) SELECT STUDY. JNCI Journal of the National Cancer Institute 2009 101(5):283-285.

Knols R, (2005) Physical exercise in cancer patients during and after medical treatment: A systemic review of randomised clinical trials. JCO, 23(16): 3830-42.

Kristal AR, (2002) Associations of energy, fat, calcium and vitamin D with prostate cancer risk. Cancer Epidemiol Biomarkers Prevent, 11: p. 719-725.

Kroenke CH, et al., Dietary patterns and survival after breast cancer diagnosis. Journal of Clinical Oncology, 2005. 23(36): p. 9295-0303.

Kucuk O, . (2002) Effects of lycopene supplementation in patients with localized prostate cancer. Exp Biol Med (Maywood), 227: p. 881-885.

Lahmann PH, (2007) Cancer Epidemiol Biomarkers Prev. Jan;16(1):36-42. Epub 2006 Dec 19.

Leatham A (2006) DietComplyf: The role of diet, complementary treatment, and lifestyle in breast cancer survival. http://www.ucl.ac.uk/abc-research-group/Documentations/DietCompLyf%20Protocol%20v6,%20Jan%2006.pdf.

Lee CY (2002) Phytochemicals and apples. The Lancet. 359(12): p. 9301.

Lee M, (2003) Soy, Isoflavone Consumption & Relation to Prostate Cancer Risk in China. Cancer Epidemiology, Biomarkers & Prevention July 1, 2003 12, 665.

Land, C. E. (1995). "Studies of Cancer and Radiation Dose Among Atomic Bomb Survivors: The Example of Breast Cancer." JAMA 274(5): 402-407.

Li C, (2009). Relationship between potentially modifiable lifestyle factors and risk of secondary contralateral breast cancer Journal of Clinical Oncology vol. 27, No.32, pp4312-5302

Ma J, (2004) A prospective study of plasma C-peptide and colorectal cancer risk in men. J Natl Cancer Inst, 96: p. 546-53.

Ma J, (1999) Prospective study of colorectal cancer risk in men and plasma levels of insulin-like growth factor (IGF)-I and IGFbinding protein-3. J Natl Cancer Inst, 91: p. 620-5.

Madaan S, (2000) Cytoplasmic induction and over-expression of cyclooxygenase-2 in human prostate cancer: implications for prevention and treatment. International Journal of Urology, 86: p. 736-741.

Mahmud S, (2003) Prostate cancer and use of nonsteroidal anti-inflammatory drugs: systematic review and meta-analysis. BJC 90: p. 93-99.

Marklund SL, (1982) Copper- and zinc-containing superoxide dismutase, manganese-containing superoxide dismutase, catalase, and glutathione peroxidase in normal and neoplastic human cell lines. Cancer Research, 42(5): p. 1955-61.

Mehta RG (1991) Characterization of effective chemopreventive agents in mammary gland in vitro using an initiation-promotion protocol. Anticancer Research, 11: p. 593-596.

McLarty J (2009) Tea Polyphenols Decrease Serum Levels of Prostate-Specific Antigen, Hepatocyte Growth Factor, and Vascular Endothelial Growth Factor in Prostate Cancer Patients. Cancer Prev Res: 1940-6207.CAPR-08-0167.

McTiernan A, (1998) Physical activity and cancer etiology: associations and mechanisms. Cancer Causes Control, 9: p. 487-509.

Meyerhardt JA, (2005) The impact of physical activity on patients with stage III colon cancer: Findings from Intergroup trial CALGB 89803. Proc Am Soc Clin Oncol, 24: p. 3534.

Nomura A, et al. (2003) Serum insulin-like growth factor I and subsequent risk of colorectal cancer among Japanese-American men. Am J Epidemiol, 158:424-31.

Ng, K.(2008). "Circulating 25-Hydroxyvitamin D Levels and Survival in Patients With Colorectal Cancer." J Clin Oncol 26(18): 2984-2991.

Nguyen, T (2002). "Nonmelanoma skin cancer." Current Treatment Options in Oncology 3(3): 193-203.

Oldridge NB, (1988) Cardiac rehabilitation after myocardial infarction. Combined experience of randomized clinical trials. JAMA vol.2 60, 7.

Omenn GS, et al., (1996) Risk factors for lung cancer and for intervention effects in CARET, the beta-carotene in retinol efficacy trial. Journal of the National Cancer Institute, 88: p. 1550-1559.

Onland-Moret, N. C. (2005). "Alcohol and Endogenous Sex Steroid Levels in Postmenopausal Women: A Cross-Sectional Study." J Clin Endocrinol Metab 90(3): 1414-1419.

Ornish D, et al. (2005) Intensive lifestyle changes may affect the progression of prostate cancer. The Journal of Urology, 174: p. 1065-1070.

Ostroff JS, (1995) Prevalence and predictors of continued tobacco use after treatment of patients with head and neck cancer. Cancer; Jan 15;75(2):569-76.

Palmqvist R, et al., (2002) Plasma insulin-like growth factor 1, insulin-like growth factor binding protein 3, and risk of colorectal cancer: a prospective study in northern Sweden. Gut, 50: p. 642-6.

Pantuck AJ, et al. (2006) Phase 11 study of pomegranate juice for men with rising PSA following surgery or RXT for prostate cancer. Clin Cancer Res, 12(13): p. 4018-4026.

Payne JK, (2008) Effect of exercise on biomarkers, fatigue, sleep disturbances, and depressive symptoms in older women with breast cancer receiving hormonal therapy. Oncol.Nurs.Forum; 35:635-642.

Peehl DM, et al. (1994) Antiproliferative effects of 1, 25-dihydroxyvitamin D3 on primary cultures of human prostatic cells. Cancer Research, 54: p. 805-810.

Pierce, J. P, (2007). "Influence of a Diet Very High in Vegetables, Fruit, and Fiber and Low in Fat on Prognosis Following Treatment for Breast Cancer: The Women's Healthy Eating and Living (WHEL) Randomized Trial." JAMA 298(3): 289-298.

Quadrilatero J, (2003) Physical activity and colon cancer. Asystematic review of potential mechanisms. J Sports Med Phys Fitness, 43: p. 121-138.

Reeves G, (2007) Cancer incidence andmortality in relation to BMI in the Million Women Study. BMJ, 335, 1134.

Richardson, G. E. (1993). "Smoking Cessation after Successful Treatment of Small-Cell Lung Cancer Is Associated with Fewer Smoking-related Second Primary Cancers." Annals of Internal Medicine 119(5): 383-390.

Rodriguez C et al, (2004) Vitamin E supplements and the risk of prostate cancer. Cancer Epidemiol Biomarkers Prevent, 13: p. 378-382.

Rogers L, et al. (2009) Physical Activity and Health Outcomes Three Months After Completing a Physical Activity Behavior Change Intervention: Persistent and Delayed Effects. Cancer Epidemiol Biomarkers Prev, 18(5):1410–8.

Rohan TE, Hiller JE, and McMichael AJ. (1993) Dietary factors and survival from breast cancer. Nutr Cancer, 1993. 20: p. 167-77.

Rose DP (1992) Dietary fibre, phytoestrogens and breast cancer. Nutrition, 8: p. 47-51.

Sandler RS, et al. (2003) A randomised trial of aspirin to prevent colorectal adenomas in patients with previous colorectal cancer. The New England Joural of Medicine, 348(10): p. 883-890.

Schoonen WM, et al. (2005) Alcohol cosumption and the risk of prostate cancer in middle-aged men. Int J Cancer, 113: p. 133-140.

Schreinemachers DM and Everson RB. (1994) Aspirin use and lung, colon and breast cancer incidence in a prospective study. Epidemiology, 5: p. 138-146.

Schwartz GG et al. (1994) Human prostate cancer cells: Inhibition of proliferation by vitamin D analogs. Anticancer Research, 1994. 14: p. 1077-1081.

Schwartz, L. H., M. Ozsahin, et al. (1994). "Synchronous and metachronous head and neck carcinomas." Cancer 74(7): 1933-1938.

Schwarz S, Obermu UC, ller-Jevic, Hellmis E, Koch W, Jacobi G, and Biesalski HK (2008) Lycopene Inhibits Disease Progression in Patients with Benign Prostate Hyperplasia. Journal of nutrition and disease J. Nutr. 138: 49–53, 2008.

Segar M, et al. (1998) Affect of aerobic exercise on self-esteem, depressive and anxiety symptoms in breast cancer survivors. Oncol Nurs Forum, 25:107-113.

Smedby KE, (2005) Ultraviolet radiation exposure and risk of malignant lymphomas. J Natl Cancer Inst;97:199–209.

Soliman, S. (2009). "Analyzing Serum-Stimulated Prostate Cancer Cell Lines After Low-Fat, High-Fiber Diet and Exercise Intervention." eCAM: nep031.

Sonn GA, Aronson W, and Litwin MS (2005) Impact of diet on prostate cancer: A review. Prostate cancer and prostate disease, 8: p. 304-310.

Spentzos D, Mantzoros C, Regan MM, Morrissey ME (2003) Clinical Cancer Research August 2003 9, 3282.

Sprod LK (2009) Considerations for Training Cancer Survivors Strength and conditioning journal volume 31, number 1. Rocky Mountain Cancer Rehabilitation Institute, University of Northern Colorado, Greeley, Colorado.

Stivala LA, et al. (2000) The antiproliferative effect of beta-carotene requires p21waf1/cip1 in normal human fibroblasts. J.Biochemistry, 267: p. 2290-2296.

Suikkari AM, et al. (1988) Insulin regulates the serum levels of low molecular weight insulin-like growth factor-binding protein. J Clin Endol Metab, 66: 266-72.

Svilaas A, et al. (2004) Intake of antioxidants in coffee, wine and vegetables are correlated with human plasma carotenoids. Journal of Nutrition, 134: 562-567.

Terry P, et al. (2001) Fatty fish consumption and risk of prostate cancer. Lancet, 357: p. 1764-1766.

Terry PD, (2003) Intakes of fish and marine fatty acids and the risks of cancers of the breast and prostate and of other hormone-related cancers: A review of the epidemiologic evidence. American Journal of Clinical Nutrition, 77: p. 532-543.

Thomas R, (2000) Forewarned is forearmed - Randomised evaluation of a preparatory information film for cancer patients. Eur J Cancer, 36(2): p. 52-53.

Thomas R, et al. (2005) Dietary advice combined with a salicylate, mineral and vitamin supplement (CV247) has some tumour static properties - a phase II study. Nutrition and science, 2005. 35(6): p. 436-451.

Thomas R et al. (2006) Diet, salicylates and Prostate cancer. British Journal of Cancer Management,.

Thomas R et al, (2009) Development of a lifestyle exit tool box abstract and poster ECCO 2009 EJC vol 7, no.2 page210 sup3608.

Thun, M. J., R. Peto, et al. (1997). "Alcohol Consumption and Mortality among Middle-Aged and Elderly U.S. Adults." N Engl J Med 337(24): 1705-1714.

van der Bol JM, (2007) Cigarette Smoking and Irinotecan Treatment: Pharmacokinetic Interaction and Effects on Neutropenia. Journal of Clinical Oncology, Vol 25, No 19 (July 1), pp. 2719-2726.

Warren RS, et al. (1996) Induction of vascular endothelial growth factor by insulin-like growth factor 1 in colorectal carcinoma. J Biol Chem, 271: p. 29483-8.

Westerlind KC (2003) Physical activity and cancer prevention-mechanisms. Med Sci Sports Exerc., 2003. 35: p. 1834-40.

Wilkinson S (2003) Critical review of complementary therapies for prostate cancer. Journal of Clinical Oncology, 21(11): p. 2199-2210.

Wu A, Pike M, and Stram D (1999) Dietary fat intake, serum estrogen levels, and the risk of breast cancer. J Natl Cancer Inst, 91: p. 529-534.

Yu GP et al. (1997) The effect of smoking after treatment for Cancer. Cancer Detect Prev 21:487-509.

Yu H and Rohan T (2000) Role of the insulin-like growth factor family in cancer development and progression. J Natl Cancer Inst; 92: p. 1472-89.

Zhao XY, et al. (1999) Induction of androgen receptor by 1 alpha, 25-dihydroxyvitaminD3 and 9-cis retinoic acid in LNCaP human prostate cancer cells. Endocrinology, 140: p. 1205-1212.

Other books by the author

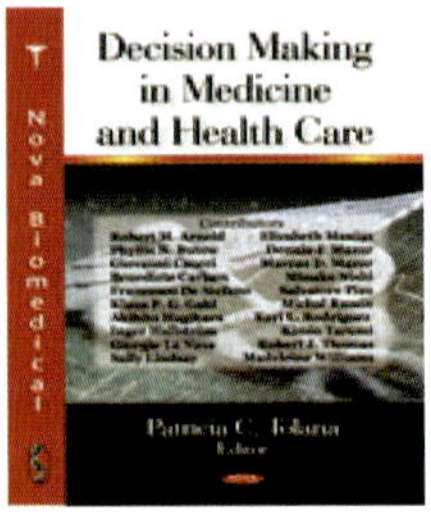

Decision making in medicine and health by Novo publications 2008.
Available from www.novopublications.com

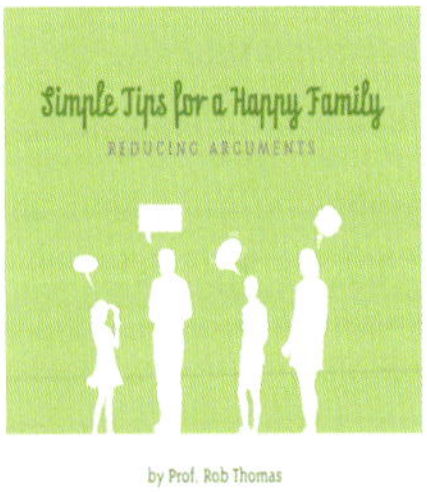

Simple tips for a Happy Family – reducing arguments after a diagnosis of cancer. Published by Health Education Publications, 2008.
Available from www.lulu.com

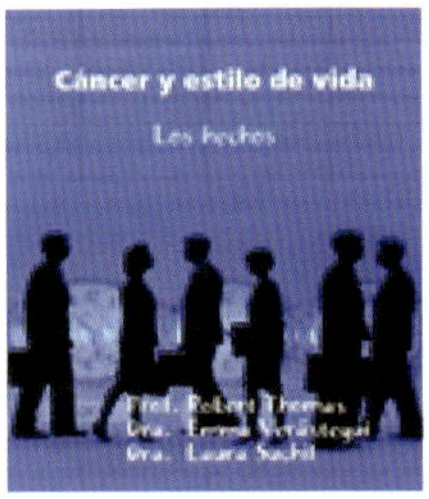

Cancer y estilo de vida. (Spanish version). Published by Health Education Publications, 2009.
Available from www.lulu.com

GLOSSARY

A

Acrylamides – a common carcinogen formed by heating carbohydrates.

Adjuvant – treatments given in addition to the main treatment.

Angiogenesis – development of new blood vessel formation, needed to feed cancer cells.

Antioxidants – chemicals known to reduce the risk of cancers and other disease.

Anthocyanin – a blue, violet or red flavanoid pigment found in plants.

Arachidonic acid – a polyunsaturated fatty acid present in animal fats.

Arimidex (anastrozole) – a hormonal drug which reduces oestrogen levels.

Aromasin (exemestane) – a hormonal drug which reduces oestrogen levels.

Apoptosis – programmed cell death (cells die when they should).

B

Baseline oxidative state (BOS) – measure of carcinogenic attack.

Benzoic acid – a cancer-forming chemical.

Biological agents – anti-cancer drugs targeting biological or genetic pathways.

Blinded trial – participants do not known which test treatments they are taking.

BMI – body mass index.

C

Caffeic acid – antioxidant found in fruit, vegetables, herbs and coffee

Catechins – a polyphenolic antioxidant found in tea.

Cancer – a malignant growth.

Carcinogen – a chemical that can cause cancer.

Carotenoids – antioxidants in the vitamin A family.

Cinnamic acid – a chemical widely used in manufacturing, can irritate the skin.

Chemotherapy – chemicals that poison and kill cancer cells.

Cholesterol – fats in the body, which if in excess, are harmful.

C peptide – a component of insulin, which regulates blood sugar levels.

Cyclooxidase – an enzyme needed to help regulate the hormone levels.

Cyclooxidase I (COX-1) inhibitor – reduces development of some cancers.

Cyclooxidase II (COX-II) inhibitor – enzyme found at sites of inflammation.

D

DNA – Deoxyribonucleic acid, the template for the body's genetic code.

E

Exemestane (aromasin) and aromatase inhibitor

F

Flavonoids – pigments found in a large number of plants, with antioxidant properties.

Femara (letrozole) – a hormonal drug which stops oestrogen feeding breast cancer cells.

Free radicals – short lived particles, generated by carcinogens which damage DNA.

Free radical scavengers – chemicals that stop free radicals damaging DNA.

G

Gallic acid – an acid extracted from oak galls and other vegetable products.

Genes – packets of nuclear codes found on DNA.

Grade – how aggressive cancer cells look like down the microscope.

H

Hormone therapy – treatments that attack cancer, via a hormone route.

Hydroxybenzoic acid – used to make pesticides and can accumulate in fish.

I

Incidence – number of cases at that time.

IGFR – Insulin-like growth factor.

IGFRBP-3 – insulin-like Growth Factor Binding Protein.

Invasion – cancer cells ability to invade into adjacent organs.

J

Juices – squeezed fruits

K

Kaempferol – a non-oestrogenic flavanol found in teas and broccoli.

L

Lignans – an antioxidant and phytoestrogen found in plants, especially flax seeds.

Lipids – fatty acids which are insoluble in water.

Legumes – pulses such as beans, peas and lentils

M

Malignancy – cancer.

Metastasis – cancer's ability to spread to, and grow in, another part of the body.

Monoclonal antibodies – identical antibody molecules produced by a single clone of cells.

Mutation – cells changing their genetic makeup.

N

Non-oestrogenic flavanoids – antioxidant found pigment in plants; not oestrogenic.

N-nitrosification – cancer-forming chemical produced by meat

Nitroso compounds – compound of iron found in meat, which can become a carcinogen.

O

Obesity – clinical definition of being overweight.

Oestrogen – the female sex hormone, which can feed oestrogen sensitive breast cancer.

Oestrogenic polyphenols – antioxidant found in plants, having oestrogen-like properties.

ORAC – The Oxygen Radical Absorbance Capacity; grades antioxidant activity.

P

Phytochemicals – Plant based chemicals.

Phytoestrogens – substances found in plants; having oestrogen-like properties

Polyphenols – antioxidant found in plants and reduces risk of cancer and heart disease.

Phenolic acids – antioxidants found in plants.

Placebo – a non-active substance used in clinical trials to compare with the active drug.

Polyphenol epigallocatechin gallate – the antioxidant found in green tea.

Primary endpoint – the main factor being investigated within a clinical trial.

Proanthocyanidins – a non-oestrogenic flavanoid.

Proliferation – growth and spread of cells.

Prostaglandin – compounds with varying hormone-like effects.

PSA – prostate specific antigen, a tumour marker for prostate cancer and disease.

PSAdt – PSA doubling time i.e. the time it takes for a prostate cancer to double in size.

PSA kinetics – another way of describing PSAdt.

Q

Quinic acid – a sugar compound found in many plants, with anti-bacterial properties.

R

Radiation – rays or particles of energy that can cause DNA damage.

Radiotherapy – the therapeutic use of radiation to kill cancer cells.

Randomized controlled trial – clinical trial which randomly allocates treatment groups.

S

Selenium – powerful antioxidant essential for all cell functions, mainly found in Brazil nuts.

Sodium salicylate – a chemical found in painkiller and anti-inflammatory drugs.

Stage – clinical definition of how far a tumour has spread.

Stilbens – A non-oestrogenic flavoncl.

Superfoods – foods with a high ORAC concentration.

T

Thalidomide – a sedative drug causing malformation of limbs of a developing embryo.

Tumour – an abnormal mass of any kind.

U

Uracil – one of the DNA chemical bases

V

Vitamins – chemicals found in foods essential for the body's healthy function.

Vioxx – an anti-inflammatory painkiller, now withdrawn due to safety concerns.

W

Watercress – high in iron, vitamins, fibre and antioxidants

X

Xenoestrogens – harmful environmental oestrogenic chemicals.

Disclaimer

This book is for educational interest. The lifestyle advice is aimed to complement the established management of malignant disease. It should not be considered as offering alternative medical advice. Never disregard medical advice or delay in seeking it because of something you have read or that may be misinterpreted in this book. The issues provided in this book are for informational purposes and are not intended for use as diagnosis or treatment of a health problem or as a substitute for consulting a licensed medical professional. ThrCheck with a family doctor or specialist physician if you suspect you are ill, or believe you may have one of the problems discussed in this book, as many problems and disease states may be serious and even life threatening.

Also note that while the information was up to date at the time of initial publication, medical information changes rapidly, so it is possible that some information may be out of date or even possibly inaccurate and erroneous at the time of reading. If you find information on our site that you believe is in error, please let us know by emailing health-education@clara.co.uk. The author makes no representations or warranties with respect to any information offered or provided through this book regarding treatment, action, or application of medication. The author or his affiliates will not be liable for any direct, indirect, consequential, special, exemplary, or other damages.